ADVANCES IN MEDICINE AND BIOLOGY

VOLUME 77

ADVANCES IN MEDICINE AND BIOLOGY

Additional books in this series can be found on Nova's website
under the Series tab.

Additional e-books in this series can be found on Nova's website
under the e-book tab.

ADVANCES IN MEDICINE AND BIOLOGY

VOLUME 77

LEON V. BERHARDT
EDITOR

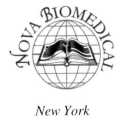

New York

Library of Congress Cataloging-in-Publication Data

ISSN: 2157-5398

ISBN: 978-1-63117-444-5

Published by Nova Science Publishers, Inc. † New York

Contents

Preface

This continuing series gathers and presents original research results on the leading edge of medicine and biology. Each article has been carefully selected in an attempt to present substantial topical data across a broad spectrum. Topics discussed in this book include microbiological hazards associated with infant formula; spontaneous bacterial peritonitis; rheumatoid arthritis; chronic subdural hematomas; metabolic acidosis; ankle joints; hemorrhagic shock; hematoma enlargement; thoracic hematoma; peritoneal dialysis; renal tubular acidosis; metabolic diseases; and lactic acidosis in HIV-infected patients.

Chapter 1 – Powdered infant formula constitutes the majority of infant formula fed to infants worldwide. This product is formulated to mimic the nutritional profile of human breast milk. Powdered infant formula is not a sterile product, and can act as a potential source of harmful pathogens. Being a nutrient-rich medium, reconstituted powdered infant formula can support bacterial growth when favorable conditions of water availability, time and temperature are provided. Therefore once rehydrated the only limiting conditions for bacterial growth are storage time and temperature. In addition, infants and young children do not have a well-developed immune system, and hence are more vulnerable to food-borne infections. Therefore the microbiological safety of the infant formula and follow-up formula is critical.

During the last 20 years, there have been multiple reports associating infant formula pathogens with infection among infants who have been fed with these products. Contaminated infant formula has been implicated in the etiology of nosocomial infections, especially when administered to infants and neonates. To assure the microbiological safety of infant formula, several microbiological tests are recommended and compared with the microbiological criteria set by the Codex Alimentarius Commission. The specific microbes commonly tested include *Staphylococcus aureus*, *Bacillus cereus*, *Cronobacter sakazakii* and other Enterbacteriaceae and *Salmonella*. Among the specific microbes tested for presence in powdered infant formula, *C. sakazakii* is placed under category A by FAO-WHO, and is considered a potential agent for causing neonatal infections.

There are four routes by which pathogens can enter prepared formula. These include the ingredients added in dry mixing operations during the manufacturing of prepared formula, through contamination of the formula from the processing environment in the steps during or following the drying, through contamination of the prepared formula after the package is opened, and through contamination during or after reconstitution by the caregiver prior to feeding. Since most of the formula associated pathogens may be found in many environments such as food factories, hospitals, institutions, day-care facilities and homes, they can have potential access for entry in to the infant formula. Therefore, ensuring infant formula safety requires a multipronged approach in which manufacturers, regulators, and caregivers to infants can all play a role.

This chapter will discuss the predominant microbiological hazards in infant formula. It will focus specifically on i) bacterial hazards in infant formula, ii) sources and routes of entry for pathogens into the formula, iii) outbreaks associated with infant formula and iv) microbiological standards for infant formula,.

Chapter 2 – Spontaneous bacterial peritonitis (SBP) is defined as the primary infection of peritoneum not directly related to an intraabdominal process. It is a frequent and severe complication seen in patients with cirrhosis and ascites. The basic pathophysiology is the translocation of bacterial flora into the peritoneal fluid. Most patients who develop SBP are in Child Pugh C class of liver disease severity. Renal failure following SBP is the most predictive factor for mortality. The most common symptoms and signs of SBP are abdominal pain and fever followed by vomiting, hepatic encephalopathy, gastrointestinal bleeding and renal impairment. The diagnosis is confirmed by cell counts, protein, glucose and microbiological evaluation of ascitic fluid. The pathogens are of enteric origin in more than two-thirds of cases. Antibiotic resistant bacteria including Pseudomonas aeruginosa, methicillin resistant Staphylococcus aureus and extended spectrum betalactamase producing E.coli are seen in hospitalized patients and those with prior antibiotic therapy. Initial presumptive antimicrobial therapy should have a broad spectrum of coverage and includes third generation cephlosporins like cefotaxime and ceftriaxone, extended spectrum penicillin like piperacillin-tazibactam, carbapenems like meropenem and newer fluoroquinolones like moxifloxacin. Patients with risk factors for multiple drug resistant bacteria should receive appropriate therapy based on local microbiology. For long term antibiotic prophylaxis following an episode of SBP fluoroquinolones like norfloxacin and trimethprim/ sulfamethoxazole have been used resulting in resistance to these agents. Recently, Rifaximin a non-absorbable antibiotic has been shown to cause a significant reduction in the rate of SBP and a transplant-free survival benefit.

Chapter 3 – Rheumatoid arthritis (RA) is a chronic disease primarily affecting the joints and producing marked inflammatory changes in the synovial membrane and adjacent structures. Although any joint can be affected the disease normally affects the hands, feet, knees and wrists. Disease activity and the rate of progression to involve new joints are variable. The pain and disability associated represent a real burden both for the patients and society and the disease is also associated with premature mortality [1, 2].

There is currently no cure for RA. Historically, treatments which deplete T-cells led to reduction of symptoms supporting the notion of a T cell mediated disease. Today, the pathology is thought to be the product of a series of complex cellular interactions where synovial T-cells orchestrate disease through their interaction with fibroblasts, B-cells, dendritic cells, and macrophages. Modern treatment options include the use of "biological" drugs, which block cytokines such as TNF alpha, IL-1, IL-6, limit co-stimulation between B and T-cells or deplete B-cells. Although their use bring great benefit, a wide range of adverse events have been reported (including infections, cancer, vasculitis, lupus-like and multiple sclerosis, liver disease, hematologic abnormalities (such as aplastic anemia, lymphoma) and aseptic meningitis). In addition resistance to these agents or loss of response, relapse on cessation of treatment, side effects occurs in more than 40% of patients. The cost of these therapies is also major pitfall.

The complex cellular interactions in the synovium between stromal cells, T-cells and their subsequent effect on B-cells, macrophages and endothelial cells provide a large panel of alternative targets, both cellular and molecular, for therapeutic intervention in RA. Inhibiting cytokines signalling has proven successful and the authors (and others) hypothesise that IL-7 may be an appropriate therapeutic target in RA as well as in several other autoimmune diseases. The main rational for targeting IL-7 is that it is (i) over expressed specifically at the disease site, however only in active disease, (ii) not capable of exiting the joint (due to its retention and presentation by extra-cellular matrix) (iii) produced by local resident cells with no mobility (i.e. fibroblasts). In addition, low levels of circulating IL-7 in RA patients suggest that efficient inhibition of IL-7 signalling may only take place in the joint. The role of IL-7 in the disease itself is slowly being dissected and will be reviewed to support this statement.

Chapter 4 – Peritonitis is a pathologic inflammation of the serosal membrane that lines the abdominal cavity and can be classified as primary, secondary or tertiary. Primary peritonitis, most often spontaneous bacterial peritonitis (SBP), is a common and severe complication in patients with advanced cirrhosis. Additional risk factors have been identified, as an ascitic fluid total protein <1.5 g/dL with Child-Pugh score ≥9 points and serum bilirubin ≥3 mg/dL or serum creatinine ≥1.2 mg/dL, blood urea nitrogen ≥25 mg/dL or plasma sodium ≤130 mEq/L. SBP is defined as an ascitic fluid infection without an evident intra-abdominal surgically treatable source.

The clinical presentation is non-specific and may range from abdominal pain to subtle changes of mental status, or even, no symptoms. Diagnosis is established with a diagnostic paracentesis, when the number of polymorphonuclear leucocytes in the ascitic fluid exceeds 250 cells/mm3. Antibiotics should be started at diagnosis and adjusted, if necessary, according with the ascitic fluid cultural results. Considering Gram-negative bacteria are the most frequent pathogens involved, the first-line antibiotic treatment is often a third-generation cephalosporin, however, the reports of resistance cases to first-line antibiotics are increasing. Intravenous albumin should be given together at day 1 and day 3. Patients with prior SBP, acute gastrointestinal haemorrhage and patients with low total protein concentration in ascitic fluid should be on a prophylaxis antibiotherapy due to a higher risk of SBP. Approximately half of all deaths in patients with SBP occur after the resolution of the infection, usually as a result of gastrointestinal hemorrhage, liver or renal failure. Given the complex nature of SBP, it is not surprising that it heralds increased morbidity and mortality in cirrhotic patients and increased cost-utilization upon the health-care system. This review will detail the risk factors, diagnosis and preventive care of cirrhotic patients with SBP.

Chapter 5 – Chronic subdural hematoma (CSDH) is frequently seen in daily neurosurgical practice. It is becoming more and more a disease of the elderly, often following a trivial head trauma. Even if diagnosis and treatment are well established, there are still debated questions about recurrences, complications and outcome, especially in elderly patients. In this study the authors evaluated clinical characteristics, surgical results and long term follow-up in 142 consecutive patients (109 males and 33 females) surgically treated at the authors' Department between 1th January 2009 and 31th December 2010, extracted by a total population of 257 patients (172 males and 84 females) harboring CSDH. Patients were followed up by neurological examinations and CT scan, one, three and twelve months after surgery. The authors obtained good results in 105 cases (73,9%) after one month, 103 cases (72,5%) after three months and 99 cases (69,7) after one year, with a recurrence rate of 9,1% and a mortality rate of 6,3%. Burr hole craniostomy is a good therapy for management of

CSDHs, leading to a good outcome in a significant percentage, even in elderly people. The distinctive feature of this study is the remarkably large series of patients treated through the same surgical technique at the same Department and followed up for at least one year. At the authors' knowledge, no previous study has examined the outcome of CSDHs such a long time after surgery in a relatively homogeneous population of elderly patients, who all underwent the same surgical technique, with a steady cure rate of almost 70% one year after surgery.

Chapter 6 – Metabolic acidosis is a disorder of the acid-base balance due to excessive acid production, kidney maladjustment to such production or excessive loss of base. The consequence is the reduction of serum bicarbonate (when combined with excess acid or lost by the kidney or gastrointestinal tract), the secondary decrease in partial carbon dioxide blood pressure and the reduction in blood pH.

It is a symptom of various diseases and its severity can range from mild discomfort to the possibility of imminent death.

Depending on the anion gap [$Na+ - (Cl - + HCO3-)$], metabolic acidosis are classified into two types: hyperchloremic (normal anion gap), which are caused by bicarbonate losses through the digestive or urinary tract and normocloremic (anion gap increased), caused by acid gain, which can be endogenous or exogenous. The latter group includes lactic acidosis, ketoacidosis, renal failure acidosis, and intoxication by ethanol, methanol, ethylene glycol, aldehydes and acetyl salicylic acid.

Any type of metabolic acidosis significantly alters both hydroelectrolytic balance and extracellular volume. Thus, in acute stages hyperkalemia, distal reuptake inhibition of sodium, volume depletion and hypercalcemia (protein bound calcium displacement) occur. At this stage the cardiovascular system is affected in a very obvious way, as both contractility and cardiac output are reduced and arterial vasodilation occurs, which contributes to the development of hypotension. Other signs include tachypnea, diaphoresis, gastrointestinal discomfort and depression of the central nervous system.

In chronic stages hypokalemia, increased natriuresis (as sodium gets out of the bone, this acting as acid buffer) and increased renal loss of calcium, phosphorus and magnesium occur. At this stage the musculoskeletal system is most affected, since metabolic acidosis can cause or exacerbate pre-existing bone disease, accelerate muscle breakdown to produce muscle loss and cause growth deficiency in children.

The diagnosis of metabolic acidosis is based on four points: confirmation of the state of acidosis, respiratory compensation assessment, quantification of the anion gap and comparison of the anion gap increase with decreasing plasma bicarbonate. This requires having a blood gas test, which can be venous, arterial or capillary and quantifying the plasma sodium, potassium and chlorine.

Regarding the treatment it is essential to assess the magnitude and speed of the onset of acidosis, determine the cause, apply a specific treatment and ensure advanced life support for severe cases. The general treatment is to stop the production of acid, increase endogenous bicarbonate production, apply exogenous bicarbonate and maintain homeostasis of the internal environment.

Chapter 7 – Ankle joint is one of the most complex joints in the human body. Anatomists, biomechanical engineers, and clinicians have studied the foot and ankle complex for centuries.

Each discipline has provided its unique insight into the structure and function of this unit. The differences of approaches have also led to varying interpretations, resulting in considerable confusion regarding the operation of this complex.

The purpose of this article is to discuss the basic biomechanical characteristics and forces acting on the ankle under static conditions and their influences on artificial total ankle replacement designs.

Chapter 8 – Severe or irreversible shock is the late stage of shock with persistent or refractory hypotension and often is a life-threatening situation, in which the therapeutic anti-shock measures including infusion, transfusion, and vasoactive agent are generally ineffective, indicating that besides microcirculatory disturbance, other events may be involved in the genesis. It was shown by us and others that the depletion of ATP in arteriolar smooth muscle cells (ASMCs) in severe shock led to activate ATP-sensitive potassium channels (K_{ATP}) with hyperpolarization of ASMCs, which inhibited L-type calcium channels in norepinephrine-stimulated ASMCs. The consequently reduced influx Ca^{2+} resulted in depression of contractile vasoresponsiveness and persistent hypotension. The depressed ASMCs ATP levels, with ensuing activation of K_{ATP} channels, existed even after improvement of microcirculation, which indicated that lower ATP level might not only result from insufficient delivery of nutrient and oxygen, but also from damage of ATP factory. Mitochondrion is the power plant with 90% ATP production in cell. Mitochondrial injury may lead to energy exhaustion with ROS production, release of apoptosis enzymes, and calcium overload, which finally results in cell damage or death. Therefore, an acute severe hemorrhagic shock rat model (the duration of 4 h in the experiment including 2 h for hemorrhage and 2 h after reinfusion of shed blood) was reproduced in the authors' lab, then the arteriolar smooth muscle cells were isolated and the mitochondrial function including 5 indices was measured. In the shock group, the mitochondria appeared apparently swollen with poor defined cristae under electron microscope; the mitochondrial permeability transition pore often opened with the calcein-Co^{2+} technique; the inner mitochondrial membrane potential (ψm) was reduced with JC_1 method; the lysosomal stability was decreased with acridine orange base method and LPO content was increased using LPO assay kit, which led to injury mitochondria through the lysosomal-mitochondria axis; and the intracellular ATP level apparently decreased to 17.6 ± 7.9% of normal condition, although treatment of reinfusion was taken. The above change of morphology (ultrastructure), metabolic (ψm, mPTP), and function (ATP content) indicated the presence of ASMCs mitochondrial damage or mitochondrial dysfunction. Administration of mitochondrial protector (cyclosporine A, resveratrol, and polydatin) could partially recover the variables mentioned above. Among them the best one was polydatin, which could return intracellular ATP level to 90.7±7.5% with prolonged survival time. With ATP level recovery in ASMCs, PD also suppressed the activation of K_{ATP} channels, ASMCs hyperpolarization, and reduced vasoresponsiveness, which led recover the MAP and significantly prolong the survival time. Besides ASMCs and brain neurons, hepatocytes and platelets were also studied in rat with severe shock, which showed similar alterations of mitochondrial dysfunction including ultrastructure alterations, ψm, mPTP, activation of lysosomal-mitochondrial axis, and ATP content. The study demonstrated that mitochondrial dysfunction was a common phenomenon among diverse organs, which involved in the genesis of severe shock, and administration of mitochondrial protector might be a new approach to treatment of severe shock.

Chapter 9 – Hematoma enlargement is reported in a significant proportion of patients with intracerebral hemorrhage (ICH). Early hematoma enlargement is associated with poor clinical outcome after ICH. Imaging studies play an important role in prompt identification of high risk patients for hematoma enlargement. Selection of patients at high risk for hematoma enlargement is crucial for treatment. Current knowledge of the clinical and imaging predictors for hematoma enlargement is discussed in detail. The contrast extravasation on CT angiography (CTA) is a well-established imaging predictor for subsequent hematoma expansion. The presence of contrast extravasation may be used as a useful imaging marker to guide therapies. The CTA spot sign is also associated with early hematoma enlargement. Hemostatic treatment may limit hematoma expansion, but fail to change clinical outcome. Rapid intensive lowering of blood pressure reduces hematoma growth, but fails to result in a significant reduction in death or major disability. However, intensive lowering of blood pressure may improve functional outcomes in selected patients. The safety and possible benefit of intensive blood pressure lowering in treatment of patients with intracerebral hemorrhage needs further validation.

Chapter 10 – Many are the causes of hematomas within the boundaries of the chest, these span from a natural origin such as vascular malformations or tumors; traumatic such as rib fractures, intra-parenchymal bleeding or vascular rupture; infectious such as chronic tuberculous lesions; post-operative complications, anticoagulation and idiopathic are also other type of associated etiologies. In this chapter a thorough review is made of each, emphasizing the mechanisms that led to a thoracic hematoma, weather it occurred in the chest wall, the mediastinum, cardiac tissue, lung parenchyma, diaphragm or pericardium, a conscious analysis is made with each case towards what produced it and how it is approached and managed with the best evidence based treatment available. This rare entity which usually transcends with a benign course, left unattended or undermined could lead to fatal consequences, hence the importance of understanding and applying today's technological tools and knowledge for the accurate diagnosis and treatment of these patients.

Chapter 11 – The worldwide increases of programs to treat chronic uremia with peritoneal dialysis does not ignore that the main complication still is peritonitis and has taken special interest in the field. This type of peritonitis is different to other processes, it involves the peritoneum, as happens in abdominal trauma, perforations and surgical process.

At the earliness time (1960, the PD procedure was done with rigid catheter, fluid in glass container, added with heparin, xylocaine, and tetracycline for treating acute kidney failure, drugs intoxication and severe complications of chronic renal failure.

In June 1978, the initial group of continuous ambulatory peritoneal dialysis, results of 27 patients were shown during the First International Symposium of PD held in Chapala, Jalisco, México the incidence of episode of PD/P peritonitis was around 6 to 8 months, later the benefits of use plastic bags and soft catheter make an enormous difference. It was considered that adequate training, and treatment with new contactology and prophylaxis was the way to diminish those figures and it happens, the use of titanium connector and double bag system as the use of cyclers or automated machines the incidence of PD/P episode diminish to one episode every 18-24 months even less in the best centers. But PD/ still is the "Achilles' heel" that cause technical and patients failure, relapse episodes of peritonitis most of them severe or chronically that require prolonged hospitalizations, expenses antibiotics and surgical reinsertion of catheters. All of these troubles have dropped the figures of patients in selected countries (Canada, UK, Mexico) in chronic PD from 50% to 12% or 15% or less, except Colombia, Taiwan and Hong Kong that maintain figures 40 to 70 %.

In fact there are different types of PD-peritonitis depending of the cause, bacterial, fungi, aseptic, relapse and the worse form is sclerosing peritonitis.

But it has been demonstrated that PD fluids with glucose damage the peritoneum membrane physiological and morphology so in the last decade had been developed new more physiology PD solutions changing the osmolality substance, pH, and added some other compounds. So there are some lines of investigation inhibitors of rennin angiotensin aldosterone system, the endothelial factor, peritoneal resting, application of statins, acetylcysteine and gene therapy on stem cells. So the authors need to look to the future to expect a better results of PD and to avoid or disappears all the complications including severe peritonitis that even could be fatal. Keeping in mind that PD is a very good treatment for selected patients a lower cost the hemodialysis.

Chapter 12 – Acid/base balance is tightly regulated by kidney and lung. In kidney, proximal tubules and collecting ducts are the main sites of acid/base regulation. Proximal tubules reabsorb most of the bicarbonate filtered from glomeruli. On the other hand, α intercalated cells in collecting ducts secrete proton and reabsorb the regenerated bicarbonate. Carbonic anhydrase II (CAII) is located in the cytoplasm of both tubular cells, catalyzing the transformation between CO_2 and HCO_3^-. The main acid/base transporters in proximal tubules are the sodium-bicarbonate cotransporter (NBCe1) in the basolateral side and sodium-proton exchanger type 3 (NHE3) in the luminal side. Mutations in NBCe1 cause proximal renal tubular acidosis (pRTA) with ocular abnormalities and other extrarenal manifestations. In α intercalated cells, anion exchanger 1 (AE1) in the basolateral side and vacuolar type proton ATPase (V-ATPase) in the luminal side are the main transporters. Mutations in AE1 cause autosomal recessive distal renal tubular acidosis (dRTA) and/or autosomal dominant red blood cell dysmorphologies. Among multiple subunits of V-ATPase, mutations in a4 and B1 subunits cause autosomal recessive dRTA with or without impaired hearing. Mutations in CAII cause a mixed type RTA with osteopetrosis. Recent studies using genetically modified mice have significantly clarified the pathogenesis of RTA and associated extrarenal manifestations. Clinically, cases of secondary RTA due to systemic diseases such as multiple myeloma and Sjögren syndrome, or side effects of drugs are much more common than cases of hereditary RTA. In this chapter the authors will focus on the molecular mechanisms of RTA.

Chapter 13 – The pH of body fluids is maintained constant by various internal buffering systems and acid excretion. However, in pathological metabolic conditions such as diabetes, the body fluid pH becomes acidic, mainly due to the elevated levels of production of organic acids, which further advances the disease severity. In addition, drastic changes in the interstitial fluid of the local metabolic tissues are observed even before the clinical onset of disease. It has been suggested that a reduction in the interstitial fluid pH during the early developmental stage of insulin resistance mediates the onset of insulin resistance. On the other hand, intake of several nutrients and exercise therapy can improve lipid metabolism, buffering capacity, and proton clearance in muscle, which may partly explain their preventive and therapeutic effects in metabolic diseases.

Chapter 14 – Lactic acidosis is the most serious, sometimes life-threatening, adverse effect of nucleoside reverse transcriptase inhibitor (NRTI) usage in HIV infected patients. The reported incidence rate of lactic acidosis due to an NRTI based regimen is low, but the fatality rate is estimated at around 60 - 80% in those HIV-infected patients who develop lactic acidosis during NRTI usage. The mechanism of NRTI induced lactic acidosis is based on inhibition of mitochondrial DNA polymerase - γ and consequent mitochondrial depletion and deficit in the respiratory chain function.

All NRTIs may interact with polymerase – γ, but dideoxynucleosides, such as stavudine (d4T), zalcitabine (ddC) and didanosine (ddI), also known as d-drugs, are the most potent. In resource limited settings, where d-drugs still remain the first line treatment option, the highest incidence of NRTI-induced lactic acidosis is due to stavudine (d4T), followed by didanosine (ddI) usage. Lactic acidosis developed even more frequently when stavudine and didanosine were prescribed together.

Zidovudine (AZT) could potentially induce lactic acidosis, while significant events are not reported with other NRTI drugs, such as lamivudine, abacavir and tenofovir. Risk factors associated with lactic acidosis are female sex, advanced HIV-1 induced immunodeficiency, obesity and prolonged duration of NRTI-based antiretroviral treatment. Renal and liver abnormalities, especially hepatitis B and hepatitis C virus co-infection, are associated with a higher incidence of lactic acidosis. Lactic acidosis induced with NRTI usage is treated by NRTI withdrawal, especially in life-threatening clinical conditions with serum lactate level of 5 mmol/L and higher. Within several days the outcome is favourable in most cases. Recovery is complete, especially when no other d-drug is re-administered.

Even though current HIV/AIDS treatment guidelines discourage the usage of d-drugs, national HIV treatment guidelines from low-middle income countries are still unable to abandon these drugs. Thus, NRTI-associated lactic acidosis is still issue of concern in the resource limited settings.

In: Advances in Medicine and Biology. Volume 77   ISBN: 978-1-63117-444-5
Editor: Leon V. Berhardt   © 2014 Nova Science Publishers, Inc.

Chapter 1

Microbiological Hazards Associated with Infant Formula

*Mary Anne Roshni Amalaradjou and Kumar Venkitanarayanan**
Department of Animal Science, University of Connecticut,
Storrs, CT, US

Abstract

Powdered infant formula constitutes the majority of infant formula fed to infants worldwide. This product is formulated to mimic the nutritional profile of human breast milk. Powdered infant formula is not a sterile product, and can act as a potential source of harmful pathogens. Being a nutrient-rich medium, reconstituted powdered infant formula can support bacterial growth when favorable conditions of water availability, time and temperature are provided. Therefore once rehydrated the only limiting conditions for bacterial growth are storage time and temperature. In addition, infants and young children do not have a well-developed immune system, and hence are more vulnerable to food-borne infections. Therefore the microbiological safety of the infant formula and follow-up formula is critical.

During the last 20 years, there have been multiple reports associating infant formula pathogens with infection among infants who have been fed with these products. Contaminated infant formula has been implicated in the etiology of nosocomial infections, especially when administered to infants and neonates. To assure the microbiological safety of infant formula, several microbiological tests are recommended and compared with the microbiological criteria set by the Codex Alimentarius Commission. The specific microbes commonly tested include *Staphylococcus aureus*, *Bacillus cereus*, *Cronobacter sakazakii* and other Enterbacteriaceae and *Salmonella*. Among the specific microbes tested for presence in powdered infant formula, *C. sakazakii* is placed under category A by FAO-WHO, and is considered a potential agent for causing neonatal infections.

---

* Dr. Kumar Venkitanarayanan, Professor, Department of Animal Science, University of Connecticut, Storrs, CT, USA, Email: kumar.venkitanarayanan@uconn.edu.

There are four routes by which pathogens can enter prepared formula. These include the ingredients added in dry mixing operations during the manufacturing of prepared formula, through contamination of the formula from the processing environment in the steps during or following the drying, through contamination of the prepared formula after the package is opened, and through contamination during or after reconstitution by the caregiver prior to feeding. Since most of the formula associated pathogens may be found in many environments such as food factories, hospitals, institutions, day-care facilities and homes, they can have potential access for entry in to the infant formula. Therefore, ensuring infant formula safety requires a multipronged approach in which manufacturers, regulators, and caregivers to infants can all play a role.

This chapter will discuss the predominant microbiological hazards in infant formula. It will focus specifically on i) bacterial hazards in infant formula, ii) sources and routes of entry for pathogens into the formula, iii) outbreaks associated with infant formula and iv) microbiological standards for infant formula,.

Introduction

The World Health Organization (WHO) guidelines reiterate the global recommendation that infants be exclusively breastfed for the first six months of their life to ensure optimal growth, development and health. However, breast-milk substitutes are used worldwide for feeding infants who do not have access to breast milk. *The Federal Food, Drug, and Cosmetic Act (FFDCA) defines infant formula as "a food which purports to be or is represented for special dietary use solely as a food for infants by reason of its simulation of human milk or its suitability as a complete or partial substitute for human milk" (FFDCA 201(z)). The United States Food and Drug Administration (FDA)regulations define infants as persons not more than 12 months old (Title 21, Code of Federal Regulations 21 CFR 105.3(e)).*The breast-milk substitutes are of three types, namely infant formula for normal healthy infants under six-months of age, follow-up formula for older infants, and special medical purpose formula for sick infants. In the U.S., infant formula is regulated by the Infant Formula Act of 1980, as amended in 1986. The act stipulates lower limits on 29 nutrients to support normal growth, and requires the manufacturers to follow "good manufacturing practices" and clear labeling of the contents. However, powdered infant formula preparations for feeding infants are not sterile, and are not guaranteed or required to be free of pathogenic microorganisms (Baker, 2002).

Microbial Hazards Associated with Infant Formula

The ongoing need to provide safe feeding for all infants and the incidence of formula associated infections led to the Food and Agriculture Organization/World Health Organization joint meeting in 2004. The purpose of this meeting was to provide input for the revisions to the Code of Hygienic Practice for Foods for infants and children. The committee also reviewed published refereed literature concerning bacterial infections attributed to powdered infant formula (PIF). The meeting concluded that intrinsic contamination of powdered infant formula with *Cronobacter sakazakii* and *Salmonella* has been responsible for infections, severe disease and death in infants (WHO, 2007a). The meeting also recognized the microorganisms of concern with infant formula, and classified them as following based on causal association between their presence in infant formula and illness in infants.

Category A: Clear evidence of causality, includes organisms that have been well established causes of illness in infants and have been found in powdered infant formula. Additionally, in outbreaks associated with these pathogens, contaminated infant formula has been convincingly shown to be the vehicle and source of infection in infants, both epidemiologically and microbiologically. The two organisms under this category include *Cronobacter sakazakii* and *Salmonella enterica*.

Category B: Causality plausible, but not yet demonstrated consists of microorganisms that are well-established causes of illness in infants, and have been found in infant formula, but contaminated infant formula has not been convincingly shown to be the vehicle and source of infection in infants. This category includes members of the Enterobacteriaceae family such as *Pantoea agglomerans*, *Escherichia vulneria*, *Hafnia alvei*, *Klebsiella pneumonia*, *Citrobacter koseri*, *Citrobacter fruendii*, *Klebsiella oxytoca* and *Enterobacter cloacae*. These microorganisms are becoming increasingly important as they are known to be present in low levels in infant formula, and hence are potential candidates as PIF-borne pathogens.

Category C: Causality less plausible or not yet demonstrated includes microorganisms that despite causing illness in infants have not been identified in PIF or have been identified in PIF, but not been implicated as causing such illness in infants. These organisms include *Bacillus cereus*, *Clostridium difficile*, *C. perfringens*, *C. botulinum*, *Staphylococcus aureus* and *Listeria monocytogenes*.

Although liquid formulas are sterile, PIF is not, and since most PIF-borne infections have been attributed to *Cronobacter sakazakii*, this chapter will focus on the physiology, pathology, potential routes of dissemination and entry of *C. sakazakii* into PIF.

Cronobacter Sakazakii

Cronobacter sakazakii, formerly *Enterobacter sakazakii* is a gram-negative, peritrichous, motile, non-spore forming, facultative anaerobic bacterium belonging to the family Enterobacteriaceae. The species name was given in recognition of the contributions of the Japanese bacteriologist, Dr. Riichi Sakazaki in the field of enteric bacteriology (Farmer *et al.*, 1980). The genus *Cronobacter* consists of ten species: *C. sakazakii*, *C. malonaticus*, *C. turicensis*, *C. universalis*, *C. muytjensii*, *C. dublinensis*, *C. condiment,C. zurichensis*, *C. pulveris*, and *C. helveticus* (Masood et al., 2013). Although there are several species, *C. sakazakii* has been primarily responsible for infections in infants particularly those associated with infant formula. *C. sakazakii* is an opportunistic food-borne pathogen that contaminates powdered infant formula, causing a rare, but life-threatening form of neonatal meningitis, bacteremia, necrotizing colitis and meningoencephalitis (Kleiman et al., 1981; Lai, 2001; Nazarowec-White and Farber, 1997; Sanders and Sanders, 1997; van Acker et al., 2001), with a case fatality rate of 40-80% (Bowen and Braden, 2006). Cronobacter-associated meningitis is fatal in almost 42% of patients, whereas Cronobacter-associated sepsis and necrotizing enterocolitis are fatal in approximately 10 and 20% cases, respectively (Friedemann, 2009). In addition to the high mortality rate, *C. sakazakii* infections may result in severe neurological sequelae such as hydrocephalus, quadriplegia and retarded neural development in survivors

(Forsythe, 2005). It has been reported that the delayed neurological development and poor lifelong outcomes may occur in more than 74% of survivors (Reij et al., 2009). Urmenyi and Franklin (1961) reported the first two known cases of terminal neonatal meningitis implicating the 'yellow pigmented *Enterobacter cloacae*'. Since then, there have been at least 111 reported cases of severe infection in infants and children worldwide (Iversen and Forsythe, 2003; Drudy et al., 2006; Mullane et al., 2008). In the US, *C. sakazakii*-associated neonatal infections rates continue to be low, and are reported to be one *Cronobacter* infection per 100,000 infants and one per 10,660 very low birth-weight neonates (Stoll et al., 2004). Based on the data from the US Centers for Disease Control and Prevention (CDC), it is estimated that there are approximately six new cases of *Cronobacter* infections reported each year worldwide. However, this estimate does not take into account the number of misidentifications that may occur (Healy *et al.*, 2010). Although the incidence of *C. sakazakii* infection is low, the prognosis is poor, and the infection is associated with significant morbidity and mortality (Drudy et al., 2006).

Clinical Significance

C. sakazakii is considered as an opportunistic food-borne pathogen that contaminates PIF, causing a rare, but life-threatening form of neonatal meningitis, bacteremia, necrotizing colitis and meningoencephalitis (Bar-Oz et al., 2001; Caubilla-Barron et al., 2007; Giovannini et al., 2008). The CDC estimates that there are approximately six new cases of Cronobacter infections reported each year worldwide (Healy et al., 2010). Risk analysis performed on 46 cases of infections in infants by Bowen and Braden (2006) included thirty three cases of meningitis, 12 cases of bacteremia, and 1 urinary tract infection. The results of risk analysis revealed that infants born prematurely are more prone to the invasive central nervous system disease caused by the bacterium. Since infants do not have a well-developed immune system, they are particularly vulnerable to infections transmitted via food, highlighting that the microbiological safety of infant and follow-up formula is critical. On April 12, 2002, the FDA issued an alert to U.S. health care professionals regarding the risk associated with *C. sakazakii* infections among neonates fed milk-based, powdered infant formula (FDA, 2002). In addition, the International Commission on Microbiological Specifications for Foods (ICMSF) ranked *C. sakazakii* as a 'severe hazard for restricted populations, life-threatening or substantial chronic sequelae of long duration', thereby placing *C. sakazakii* along with other common food- and waterborne pathogens such as *Listeria monocytogenes*, *Clostridium botulinum* types A and B and *Cryptosporidium parvum* (ICMSF, 2002). Although infections with *C. sakazakii* have been primarily associated with infants, recent reports have highlighted the risk posed to immunocompromised adults, particularly the elderly.

Clinical Manifestations

C. sakazakii infections have been associated frequently with sporadic cases of life-threatening illness, in particular meningitis, necrotizing enterocolitis and septicemia in infants (Lai, 2001). The symptoms include meningitis leading to ventriculitis, brain abscess, hydrocephalus and cyst formation, as well as necrotizing enterocolitis characterized by intestinal necrosis and pnuematosis intestinalis (presence of gas in the intestinal wall), pulmonary, urinary and bloodstream infections (Nazarowec-White and Farber, 1997; Gurtler et al., 2005). Meningital *Cronobacter* infection in infants is established between the fourth and fifth days post-birth, and can be fatal within hours to several days following the onset of the first clinical symptoms (Muytjens et al., 1983). Neonatal meningitis results in ventriculitis, brain abscess, or cyst formation, and the development of hydrocephalus. The fatality rate for neonatal infections has been reported to be as high as 80%; half of the reported patients die within one week of diagnosis, and all patients that recover from central nervous system infections suffer irreversible mental and physical delays (Lai et al., 2001; Lehner and Stephan, 2004). This led the International Commission on Microbiological Specification for Foods (ICMSF, 2002) to classify *Cronobacter* as a severe hazard for restricted populations, causing life-threatening or substantial chronic sequelae or illness of long duration.

Another major clinical manifestation in *C. sakazakii* infections is the development of neonatal necrotizing enterocolitis (NEC) following the consumption of contaminated powdered infant formula. The disease is characterized by intestinal necrosis and pneumatosis intestinalis, and is the most common gastrointestinal emergency in newborns. Lucas and Cole (1990) found that confirmed NEC is 10 times more common in babies fed only formula than in those fed only breast milk. Van Acker et al. (2001) investigated an outbreak of NEC in an intensive care unit of a hospital in Belgium, where 12 neonates contracted the disease in June and July 1998. In reviewing the feeding procedures, a significant correlation was found between the development of NEC, the consumption of a specific brand of powdered infant formula, and the isolation of *C. sakazakii* in neonates. Strain similarity between the milk and patient isolates was confirmed using molecular typing methods.

Food and Environmental Sources of *C. sakazakii*

C. sakazakii has been isolated from a variety of sources, including clinical specimens, environmental sources, foods and insect vectors. The first hint of the possible environmental reservoir of *C. sakazakii* was reported by Kuzina et al. (2001), who isolated *C. sakazakii* from the gut of insects such as the Mexican fly *Anastrepha ludens*. *C. sakazakii* was also isolated from the stable fly,*Stomoxys calcitrans* by Hamilton et al (2003). Stable flies are found in the vicinity of warm-blooded animals such as cattle, pigs or horses. They feed on the blood of these animals and have a worldwide distribution. Contamination of the environment by insects can play an important role in the spread of the pathogen. Researchers have investigated the presence of *C. sakazakii* in the production environment of food factories and households (Kandhai et al., 2004a; 2004b). Dry environmental samples from factories were obtained by scraping or sweeping surfaces in the production-line environment and by sampling vacuum-cleaner bags. *C. sakazakii* was isolated from nearly all the environmental samples with varying frequencies (Jaradat et al., 2009).

The sources of *C. sakazakii* in contaminated PIF include the powder itself, the equipment and possibly the personnel preparing the formula. Studies on the transmission routes of *C. sakazakii* in a milk powder-producing plant revealed that seven different pulse-filed gel electrophoresis types were detected in the spray dry area (Jacobs et al., 2011). This indicated that the pathogen probably entered the plant through an aperture for process air and an improperly controlled roller structure. Additionally, the textile fibers for the exhaust air of the spray drying towers were identified as internal reservoirs of the organism. In most cases, the powder from the textile fibers will be reintroduced into the product flow for economic reasons, thus suggesting the potential to contaminate the final product (Jacobs et al., 2011). Another area for potential transmission was identified as the roller dryer section. It was shown that contaminated milk concentrate could pass through the process without heating, thereby leading to contamination of the final product (Jacobs et al., 2011).

Besides the processing plant environment,*C. sakazakii* has been isolated from a wide range of foods, including cheese, meat, vegetables, grains, herbs, spices and ultrahigh-temperature milk (Iversen and Forsythe, 2003; Leclercq et al., 2002; Skladal et al., 1993). Additional C. sakazakii contaminated foods and drinks include fruits, legumes, cereals, herbs, tea, spices, salad and dried fruit powder (Gurtler et al., 2005; Cruz et al., 2004; Restaino et al., 2006; Mensah et al., 2002; Lehner et al., 2005). *C. sakazakii* has also been isolated from lemon rootstocks (Gardner et al., 1982), wheat rhizosphere (Forlani *et al.*, 1995) and sugar beet seeds (Kanivets and Pishchur, 2001). It has been isolated from rice- and soy-based products since it belongs to the cultivable endophytic and epiphytic flora of rice (Yang et al., 1999) and soy bean plants (Kuklinsky-Sobral et al., 2005). Traditional cereal-, herb- and legume-based foods and beverages were also found to be contaminated with *C. sakazakii* (Mensah et al., 2002; Nassereddin and Yamani, 2005). *C. sakazakii* can also be part of starter cultures used for the fermentation of traditional vegetarian food products (Coulin et al., 2006). Others have isolated *C. sakazakii* from mixed salad vegetables and fresh and deep-frozen vegetables at the retail level (Geiges et al., 1990; Osterblad et al., 1999).

Among foods of animal origin, *C. sakazakii* has been isolated from meat and meat products from camel, pig, beef and poultry, eggs, raw milk, dairy products and fish (Leclercq et al., 2002; De Clerck et al., 2004; Liu et al., 2005; Restaino et al., 2006; Gurtler et al., 2005). *C. sakazakii* has been isolated from birds and different animals (Farmer et al., 1985; Goullet and Picard, 1986), especially lizards, rats and piglets (Gakuya et al., 2001; Montgomery et al., 2002). In vertebrate animals, *C. sakazakii* is a member of the normal oral and intestinal flora (Montgomery et al., 2002; Zogaj et al., 2003). *C. sakazakii* has been isolated from the secretions of an infected mammary gland of dairy heifers (Salmon et al., 1998). *C. sakazakii* has been found in fresh and prepared fish (Miranda et al., 2003). It has also been isolated from smoked sardines that were irradiated and stored for 12 weeks (Nketsia-Tabiri et al., 2003). In addition to all the above mentioned sources, *C. sakazakii* has been isolated from foods such as biscuits, baby foods, dumplings and sweets (Liu et al., 2005; Lehner et al., 2004; Leuschner et al., 2004).

Besides foods, *C. sakazakii* has been isolated from drinking water (Leclerc et al., 2001; Lee and Kim, 2003; Cruz et al., 2004). Drinking water is used for cleaning and rinsing of foods and equipment for food preparation, dilution and reconstituition of infant foods or directly as a beverage. Oger et al. (1981) and Schindler and Metz (1991) found *C. sakazakii* in central and local drinking water supplies. *C. sakazakii* was identified as a bacterium indigenous to the water distribution system by several researchers (Bartolucci et al., 1996; Lee and Kim 2003; Williams and Braun-Howland, 2003). The bacterium was also identified from bottled beverages and mineral water (Leclerc et al., 2001; Lee and Kim, 2003; Cruz et al., 2004). *C. sakazakii* contaminated water from environmental sources (Angles d' Auriac *et al.*, 2000; Emiliani et al., 2001), drinking water (Lee and Kim, 2003), soil (Espeland and Wetzel, 2001), dust (Kandhai et al., 2004b) and air particles (Masaki et al., 2001) are potential sources for contamination of animal and plant based foods throughout the food production chain. In the farm environment, *C. sakazakii* was isolated from dairy farms (Mramba et al., 2006) and a poultry brooder house (Chernaki-Leffer *et al.*, 2002). *C. sakazakii*-colonized insects (Hamilton et al., 2003) and -rats (Gakuya et al., 2001) may also contribute to the contamination of foods under unhygienic conditions of production and management.

Despite the presence of *C. sakazakii* in several types of foods, the bacterium has a closer association with PIF. Clark et al. (1990) were the first to prove, using a combination of typing methods, a clear epidemiological correlation between *C. sakazakii* isolated from patients and that from dried infant formula. Himelright et al. (2002) also reported a clear association between the presence of *C. sakazakii* in a batch of PIF and an outbreak in a hospital. Intrinsic contamination, during the manufacturing process, or extrinsic contamination from utensils such as blenders and spoons, used during reconstitution of powdered infant formula can potentially occur (van Acker et al., 2001; Caubilla-Barron et al., 2007). Since PIF is a non-sterile product, it may be contaminated with *C. sakazakii*, and once reconstituted, the nutrient-rich environment can support the growth of the pathogen to high numbers, thereby leading to infection (Chenu and Cox, 2009).

Muytjens et al. (1988) examined 141 different breast milk substitute powders from 35 countries, and enumerated *C. sakazakii* from 20 samples at levels ranging from 0.36 to 66 CFU/100 gram. Simmons et al. (1989) reported the presence of 8 cells of the pathogen per 100 gram of PIF from an opened can of infant formula, which was linked to an outbreak in a neonatal intensive care unit. In a Canadian survey, Nazarowec-White and Farber (1997) tested 120 cans of infant formula from five different companies and found 6.7% of samples contained *C. sakazakii*. Iversen and Forsythe (2004) reported the presence of *C. sakazakii* in dried baby foods and milk powders. The bacterium was isolated from PIF by numerous other investigators (Postupa and Aldova, 1984; Muytjens et al., 1988; Biering et al., 1989; Simmons et al., 1989; Muytjens and Kollee, 1990). Moreover, there have been many recalls of *C. sakazakii*-contaminated infant formula in the United States. In November 2002, a nationwide recall of more than 1.5 million cans of dry infant formula contaminated with *C. sakazakii* was reported (FSNET, 2002). In general, the level of *C. sakazakii* contamination in infant formula was found to be very low, less than one bacterium per gram. However the bacterium has been reported to survive in the powder for at least 12 months (Caubilla-Barron et al., 2007).

Since intestinal carriage of *C. sakazakii* has not been demonstrated in humans, it is uncertain how contamination of infant formula occurs during preparation. However, it is widely accepted that basic aspects of personnel hygiene are frequently ignored and poor hygienic practice could be the probable source of outbreaks (Smeets et al., 1998; Block et al., 2002). In addition to personnel, the environment of an infant formula processing plant can also serve as a potential source of *C. sakazakii*. Reich et al. (2010) reported the isolation of *C. sakazakii* from different locations in an infant formula processing plant, including fluidized bed, drains, surfaces, filters, mixer, agglomerator, silo, filler, can filler and the basement. Intermittent contamination of the formula may take place during the production process after pasteurization, which is possible either via the addition of contaminated heat labile ingredients such as starch, proteins, lecithin, or via materials originating from the production environment (Mullane et al., 2008). Research has shown that addition of plant-derived supplements potentially contaminated with *C. sakazakii* to powdered formula without an additional heating step can represent potential route of entry for the bacterial pathogen to the production line or the products (Brandl, 2006). It has also been proposed that transient residence of opportunistic bacteria in plants may modulate the pathogenesis and fitness of these organisms, enabling them to be more virulent to humans or better adapted to harsh environmental conditions (Brandl, 2006).

C. sakazakii is also found in the hospital environment. *C. sakazakii* isolated from a contaminated dish brush used for cleaning bottles in a hospital was identical to the isolates from three patients (Smeets et al., 1998). The organism was isolated from a doctor's stethoscope (Farmer et al., 1980). Moreover, *C. sakazakii* has been isolated from a variety of abiotic sources such as the surfaces of utensils and equipment used in infant formula preparation in clinical settings, where *C. sakazakii* infections have been reported (Noreiga et al., 1990; Richards et al., 2005; Kim et al., 2006). Neonatal infections caused by *C. sakazakii* have been associated with contaminated formula preparation equipment such as spoons, blenders and brushes (Bar-Oz et al., 2001; Simmons et al., 1989). There have also been reports of previously healthy infants admitted to hospitals with meningitis caused by *C. sakazakii*, suggesting that infection can also be acquired in the home environment (Kleiman et al., 1981; Adamson and Rogers, 1981).

Outbreaks and Cases of Infections

Cronobacter Sakazakii

The number of documented outbreaks and cases of neonatal *C. sakazakii* infections is limited. A review of cases in infants reported from 1961 to 2008revealedapproximately 323 confirmed cases of *C. sakazakii*-induced illness among infants (NSW Food Authority, 2011). In the U.S., a survey of invasive infections with this organism in infants under 1 year of age indicated an infection rate of1 per 100,000 and 8.7 per 100,000 in normal infants and low-birth-weight neonates, respectively (Anonymous, 2002).

The first two documented cases of neonatal *C. sakazakii* meningitis occurred in 1958 (Urmenyi and Franklin, 1961). At that time, the bacterium was described as an unusual pigmented strain of the *E. cloacae* group. The clinical isolate from these cases produced slightly yellow pigmentation when cultured on nutrient agar at 37°C, but produced a non-diffusible yellow-gold pigment when incubated at room temperature. The second report of neonatal meningitis caused by *C. sakazakii* was documented by Joker et al. (1965), where the patient was a newborn female delivered as a primigravida after 27 h of labor. Two days after birth, the child was suspected of having meningitis, and the pathogen was isolated from three specimens of cerebrospinal fluid. Following aggressive antibiotic administration, the child recovered at about 4 months of age, although experiencing extreme mental impairment. Although it was not known whether the child was fed breast milk or rehydrated powdered infant formula, meningitis was attributed to the prolonged delivery period (Joker et al., 1965).

Monroe and Tift (1979) reported a male, term infant with *C. sakazakii* bacteremia at 7 days of age, where the source of infection was attributed to post-birth due to the 6-day delay in symptoms. This was the first reported case of non-meningital bacteremia caused by *C. sakazakii*. Kleiman et al. (1981) reported a full-term, 5-week-old infant with meningoencephalitis and cerebral ventricular compartmentalization resulting in bulging fontanelles and grand mal seizures. When the isolate was cultured, *C. sakazakii* formed 2-3 mm diameter colonies on chocolate agar during incubation under an atmosphere containing 10% carbon dioxide and 90% air. However, yellow pigmented colonies developed when the culture was incubated anerobically for 48 h at 25°C.

During the period from 1975 to 1981, eight cases of neonatal meningitis involving *C. sakazakii* were reported in The Netherlands, where two of the eight patients experienced necrotizing enterocolitis (Muytjens *et al.*, 1983). The bacterium was isolated from the blood and CSF of all eight patients. Twenty-three Enterobacter isolates were recovered from the CSF of six patients, with eight of these testing positive for *C. sakazakii*. *C. sakazakii* isolates indistinguishable from those from CSF were recovered from prepared infant formula as well as from the utensils used to prepare formula. Muytjens and Kollee (1990) later reported that upon opting for sterile liquid formula in place of powdered formula, no further cases of *C. sakazakii* were reported in the following 8 years.

Arseni et al. (1987) reported a case of neonatal septicemia caused by *C. sakazakii* in the neonatal intensive care unit of a children's hospital in Athens, Greece, where the bacterium was isolated from the umbilical catheter and blood. This isolate was found to be resistant to ampicillin, netilmicin, cefotaxime and amikacin. Three cases of *C. sakazakii* meningitis in full-term male neonates in Iceland were reported by Biering et al. (1989). All affected infants were fed a rehydrated powdered infant formula within 2 h of its preparation. Although freshly prepared formula failed to yield the bacterium,*C. sakazakii* was recovered from five packages of rehydrated formula incubated for 4 h at 36°C. In addition, *C. sakazakii* was isolated from urine as well as groin and anal swabs of a 3-day old asymptomatic male child. Twenty-two of the twenty-three isolates were identical in biotype, antibiotic sensitivity/resistance profile and plasmid profile to the four neonatal strains (Clark et al., 1990). It was concluded that these infections must have originated from the rehydrated infant formula stemming from unknown contributing factors in the infected infants, as many neonates had received the same contaminated infant formula with no detectable disease. One of the causal factors may have been that formula bottles were occasionally left in heaters at 35-37°C for lengthy periods of time.

In yet another outbreak, Willis and Robinson (1988) reported that two infants, 4 weeks and 8 days of age, developed *C. sakazakii*-induced meningitis, which led to cerebral destruction, developmental damage and severe neurologic complications. In the following year, Simmons et al. (1989) reported an outbreak of neonatal *C. sakazakii*-induced septicemia and meningitis clearly linked to PIF which contained *C. sakazakii* at populations of 8 CFU/100 g. This outbreak involved four pre-term neonates demonstrating symptoms of bacteremia, septicemia, urinary tract infection, abdominal distension and bloody diarrhea. Laboratory investigations implicated a blender as the possible source of contamination after testing positive for *C. sakazakii*. This study reported that *C. sakazakii* infections did not occur after the replacement of the contaminated blender with a sterilized blender. The study also revealed that all infant formula isolates and three clinical isolates displayed the same plasmid and multilocus enzyme profile (Clark et al., 1990).

Noriega et al. (1990) reported a case involving a 6-month old female who developed septicemia following small bowel complications associated with an exploratory laprotomy and gastrostomy tube. Blood cultures from the patient and central venous catheter tip were found to be positive for *C. sakazakii*. The authors reported that the blender used to rehydrate the powdered infant formula was heavily contaminated with *C. sakazakii*. Van Acker et al. (2001) reported an outbreak of 12 cases of neonatal necrotizing enterocolitis at a neonatal intensive care unit in Belgium. All 12 patients were fed reconstituted infant formula prior to the illness, and *C. sakazakii* was isolated from blood, swabs and stomach aspirates from patients. A follow-up survey of powdered infant formula yielded 14 *C. sakazakii* isolates. The first report of a pathologically proven brain abscess formation by *C. sakazakii* and its isolation from purulent material of an abscess cavity was presented by Burdette and Santos (2000), while describing a case of neonatal meningitis in a 6-day old infant that occurred in Winston-Salem, North Carolina. These researchers used CT scan and magnetic resonance imaging of the head to identify lesions of cerebritis and intraparenchymal abscess formation. The patient was treated with antibiotics and drainage of the abscess by craniotomy, which resulted in an uneventful recovery.

Two cases of neonatal meningitis were reported by Bar-Oz et al. (2001), where *C. sakazakii* was isolated from the CSF and blood. In addition to the two infected individuals, three additional infants had *C. sakazakii* positive stools for 3, 4 and 8 weeks, demonstrating colonization without infection. Samples from the blender and rehydrated formula from the preparation kitchen were positive for *C. sakazakii*. Himelright et al. (2002) and Weir (2002) described a 2001 outbreak of *C. sakazakii* infections in Tennessee in which 49 infants in a neonatal intensive care unit were screened; 10 infants tested positive for the bacterium and 1 died of meningitis following 9 days of intravenous treatment with antibiotics. The source of the bacterium was traced to a PIF specific for individuals with nutritional and malabsorption problems. In 2008, *Cronobacter* spp. was isolated from two infants in New Mexico, where one of the two infants recovered following hospitalization but suffered severe brain damage while the other succumbed to the infection (CDC, 2009).

Other Relevant Pathogens

Salmonella enterica

Salmonella contamination of infant formula has been responsible for multiple outbreaks in infants (Rowe at al., 1987, Olsen et al., 2001, Bornemann et al., 2002). The earliest known outbreak of salmonellosis attributed to contaminated dried milk powder was in the early 1950's in the United Kingdom and Bulgaria (Marth, 1969). Following this there was a multistate outbreak of *Salmonella* Newbrunswick in the United States in 1966, where the contamination was traced to dried milk produced from one manufacturer. The pathogen was isolated form unopened containers, the manufacturing plant environment and other milk products in the plant (Collins et al., 1968). In 1973, approximately 3000 infants were infected with *Salmonella* Derby in Trinidad. Retrospective investigation and case-controlled studies linked the illness to the consumption of seven brands of powdered milk packaged at a single plant (Weissman et al., 1977).

Although several steps were taken to control *Salmonella* in dried milk products, outbreaks due to the presence of the pathogen in powdered infant formula continue to arise in different parts of the globe. In the 20-year period between 1985 and 2005, there were atleast 6 PIF-associated *Salmonella* outbreaks involving approximately 287 infants. In 1985, 48 infants were affected due to contamination of infant formula contaminated with *S.* Ealing in the UK (Rowe et al., 1987), where the pathogen was traced to the spray driers used in the infant formula manufacturing process. In the United States and Canada, children were infected with a lactose-fermenting strain of *S*. Tennessee in 1993 (CDC, 1993), where again the source of pathogen was traced back to the manufacturing plant. Following this, a similar outbreak was reported in Spain in 1994 in which the implicated pathogen was a lactose-fermenting strain of *S*. Virchow (Usera et al., 1996). In 2000, an infant formula outbreak in Korea was attributed to *S*. London. This outbreak affected 30 children and was traced back to the consumption of a particular brand of PIF. However, further investigation revealed that the pathogen could not be traced back to the manufacturing plant. The pathogen was isolated only from an opened package of formula, highlighting potential contamination by the end user (Park et al., 2004). The potential for formula contamination by the end user was evident in a 2001 *S*. Saintpaul outbreak in the United States. This was a hospital acquired outbreak and the source was traced to formula prepared in the hospital's formula preparation room (Bornemann et al., 2002). This outbreak emphasized the potential for contamination of the reconstituted formula with *Salmonella* even when the PIF is not the source of the pathogen. This outbreak was followed by others in France and Spain caused by *S*. Agona, *S*. Kedougou and *S*. Give in 2005 and 2008 (FAO/WHO, 2006, Soler et al., 2008, Jourdan et al., 2008). In all these cases, the implicated source was powdered infant formula. A common feature in these reported outbreaks was the low levels of *Salmonella* found in the PIF, and their isolation from bulk, storage or retail packaged samples.

Clostridium botulinum / Citrobacter fruendii

In addition to *C. sakazakii* and *Salmonella* sp., the other pathogens associated with PIF outbreaks include *Citrobacter fruendii* and *Clostridium botulinum*. The only known outbreak of PIF associated *C. fruendii* was reported from Germany, which occurred at a neonatal intensive care unit where the pathogen was isolated from the hospital environment (Thurm and Gericke, 1994). A PIF associated outbreak of *C. botulinum* type Bin a 5-month old female was reported from the UK in 2001, which was confirmed by both isolation of the pathogen and detection of the type B botulinum toxin in the rectal washout and feces. An isolate obtained from an open can of infant formula had the same AFLP patterns as that of the clinical isolate. Although the patient's condition improvement, the child had significant global development delay affecting her cognitive and gross motor components (Brett et al, 2005).

Microbiological Criteria for Infant Formula

With the emergence of infections in infants attributed to the consumption of infant formula, the Codex Alimentarius Commission (CAC) criteria within the Code of Hygienic practice for powdered formulae for infants and young children was revised (CAC, 2008). The microbiological criteria for powdered infant formula in the United States include total aerobic plate count (TAPC; $<10^4$ CFU/g); coliforms, fecal coliforms, and *E. coli* (absence based on a 0.1, 0.01 and 0.001 three-tube (most probable number) MPN, < 3.01 MPN/g); *Salmonella* (absence in 60 25-g samples); *Staphylococcus aureus* (<3.01 MPN/g); and *Bacillus cereus* (100 CFU/g; U.S. Food and Drug Administration, 1996). Due to the association of *Cronobacter* with fatal neonatal infections the CAC requires that powdered infant formula to be microbiologically tested for all members of the *Cronobacter* genus (absence based on 333-

g MPN analysis; Masood et al., 2013). Follow up formula (FUP) used for infants greater than six months of age have similar microbiological recommendations. In the European Union, the criteria include *Salmonella enterica*, *Cronobacter* spp., and Enterobacteriaceae for PIF, and *S. enterica* and Enterobacteriaceae for FUF (European Commission, 2009). Similarly the microbiological criteria in Canada include TAPC ($<10^4$ CFU/g), *E. coli* ($<10^1$ CFU/g), *Salmonella* (absence in 20 25-g samples), *S. aureus* ($<10^2$ CFU/g), *B. cereus* ($<10^3$ CFU/g) and *C. perfringens* ($<10^3$ CFU/g).

The microbiological criteria for infant formula in Australia and New Zealand include TAPC ($<10^4$ CFU/g), *Salmonella* (absence in 10 25-g samples), coliforms (<10 MPN/g), *S. aureus* (< 10 CFU/g) and *B. cereus* ($<10^2$ CFU/g; Australia New Zealand Food Safety Authority, 2008). Recently China revised its microbiological criteria for PIF to include TAPC ($<10^4$ CFU/g), coliforms ($<10^2$ CFU/g), *Cronobacter* spp. (absence in three 100-g samples), and *S. enterica* (absence in five 25-g samples). These criteria indicate substantial differences in microbial testing and standards in different countries. Since these differences in criteria can affect international trading, the United States Department of Agriculture set commodity requirements on microbiological standards for infant formula to be used in domestic programs (USDA, 2008). Upon microbiological analysis, the test results of powdered infant formula shall meet the following values to be able to be marketed in the United States: *Salmonella* (negative), *Listeria monocytogenes* (negative), coliforms (not greater than 10 CFU/g), fecal coliforms (< 3 CFU/g), *E. coli* (< 3 CFU/g), Coagulase Positive *S. aureus* (< 3 CFU/g), *B. cereus* (< 50 CFU/g) and aerobic plate count (< 500 CFU/g).

Considerations

PIF-associated bacterial infections in infants have been mainly attributed to two sources that include the manufacturing environment and the end user. Therefore strategies aimed at reducing or preventing infections in infants should target the PIF plant and implementation of guidelines for the preparation and storage of formula. The guidelines for preparation, storage and handling of infant formula were published by the WHO (WHO, 2007b). These guidelines emphasize the need for correct handling, storage and distribution of reconstituted infant formula both at the hospital and home settings. The guidelines encourage the use of hot water of at least 70°C for reconstitution of PIF, followed by storage at 4°C unless consumed within 30 min of preparation. The guidelines also recommend the disposal of any formula that has been refrigerated for 24h. Besides these recommendations for proper preparation, the guidelines also highlight the importance of the use of clean utensils and preparatory area.

The commitment of the manufacturers to ensure the highest level of hygiene in the manufacture of PIF is highly critical. Implementation of environmental monitoring programs such as GMP and HACCP to control microbial hazards in the ingredients, and during the entire processing will help minimize pathogen entry and persistence in PIF (Yan et al., 2012). Industry and regulators have a significant role in reducing the infection risk from consumption of contaminated infant formula (Cahill et al., 2007). Finally it is essential that consumers be aware of the infant formula associated health hazards, and obtain scientific assistance from caregivers, doctors and researchers in order to provide safe feeding for all infants.

References

Adamson D.H., Rogers J. R. 1981. *Enterobacter sakazakii* meningitis with sepsis. *Clinical Microbiology Newsletter.* 3: 19–20.

Angles d'Auriac, M. B., Roberts, H., Shaw, T., Sirevag, R., Hermansen, L. F., Berg, J. D. 2000. Field evaluation of a semiautomated method for rapid and simple analysis of recreational water microbiological quality, *Appl. Environ. Microbiol.* 66: 4401–4407.

Anonymous, 2002. Belgian baby death sparks safety questions. Baby Milk Action Update, 31:4. Available at http://www.babymilkaction.org/update/update31.html#3. Accessed on Sep. 12, 2013.

Arseni, A., Malamou-Ladas, E., Koutsia, C., Xanthou, M., Trikka, E. 1987. Outbreak of colonization of neonates with *Enterobacter sakazakii.* J. Hosp. Infect. 9:143–150.

Australia New Zealand Food Authority. 2008. Australia New Zealand food standards code. Standard 1.6.1. Microbiological limits for food. Accessed on December 1, 2013 at http://www.comlaw.gov.au/Details/F2009C00854.

Baker, R. D. 2002. Infant formula safety. *Pediatrics.* 110:833-835.

Bar-Oz, B., Preminger, A., Peleg, O., Block, C., Arad, I. 2001. *Enterobacter sakazakii* infection in the newborn. *Acta Paediatr.* 90:356–358.

Bartolucci, L., Pariani, A., Westall, F., Gardini, F., Guerzoni, M. E. 1996. A proposed method for determining bacterial colonization in drinking-water pipe networks, *Water Supply* 14: 453–471.

Biering, G., Karlsson, S., Clark, N. C., Jonsdottir, K. E., Ludvigsson, P., Steingrimsson, O. 1989. Three cases of neonatal meningitis caused by *Enterobacter sakazakii* in powdered milk. *J. Clin. Microbiol.* 27:2054-2056.

Block, C., Peleg, O., Minster, N., Bar-Oz, B., Simhon, A., Arad, I., Shapiro, M. 2002. Cluster of neonatal infections in Jerusalem due to unusual biochemical variant of *Enterobacter sakazakii. Eur. J. Clin. Microbiol. Infect. Dis.* 21:613-616.

Bornemann, R., Zerr, D. M., Heath, J., Koehler, J., Grandjean, M., Pallipamu, R. and Duchin, J. 2002. An outbreak of *Salmonella* serotype Saintpaul in a children's hospital. *Infect. Control Hosp. Epidemiol.* 23:671-676.

Bowen, A. B., Braden, C. R. 2006. Invasive *Enterobacter sakazakii* disease in infants. *Emerging Infectious Diseases.* 12: 1185–9.

Brandl, M. J. 2006. Fitness of human enteric pathogens on plants and implications for food safety, *Annu. Rev. Phytopathol.* 44: 367–392.

Brett, M. M., McLauchlin, J., Harris, A., O'Brien, S., Black, N., Forsyth, R. J., Roberts, D. and Bolton, F. J. 2005. A case of infant botulism with a possible link to infant formula milk powder: evidence for the presence of more than one strain of *Clostridium botulinum* in clinical specimens and food. *J. Med. Microbiol.* 54:769-776.

Burdette, J. H., Santos, C. 2000. *Enterobacter sakazakii* brain abscess in the neonate: the importance of neuroradiologic imaging. *Pediatr. Radiol.* 30:33–34.

Cahill, S. M., Wachsmuth, I. K., Costarrica Mde, L., Ben Embarek, P. K. 2008. Powdered infant formula as a source of *Salmonella* infection in infants. *Clin. Infect. Dis.* 46:268-273.

Caubilla-Barron, J., Hurrell, E., Townsend, S. Cheetham, P., Loc-Carrillo, C., Fayet, O., Prère, M. F., Forsythe, S. J. 2007. Genotypic and phenotypic analysis of *Enterobacter sakazakii* strains from an outbreak resulting in fatalities in a neonatal intensive care unit in France. *J Clin Microbiol.* 45(12):3979-85.

Centers for Disease Control and Prevention. 1993. *Salmonella* serotype Tennessee in powdered milk products and infant formula-Canada and the United States, 1993. *MMWR Morb Mortal Wkly Rep.* 42: 516-7.

Centers for Disease Control and Prevention. 2009. *Cronobacter* species isolation in tow infants-New Mexico, 2008. *MMWR Morb Mortal Wkly* Rep. 58: 1179-1183.

Chenu, J. W., Cox, J. M. 2009. *Cronobacter* (*'Enterobacter sakazakii'*): current status and future prospects. *Lett. Appl. Microbiol.* 49(2):153-9.

Chernaki-Leffer, A. M., Biesdorf, S. M., Almeida, L. M., Leffer, E. V., Vigne, F. 2002. Isolation of enteric and litter organisms from *Alphitobius diaperinus* in brooder chicken houses in West of Parana State, Brazil, *Rev. Bras. Cienc. Avic.* 4: 243–247.

Clark, N. C., Hill, B. C., O'Hara, C. M., Steingrimsson, O., Cooksey, R. C. 1990. Epidemiologic typing of *Enterobacter sakazakii* in two neonatal nosocomial outbreaks, *Diagn. Microbiol. Infect. Dis.* 13: 467–472.

Codex Alimentarius Commission. 2008. Code of hygiene practice for powdered infant formulae for infants and young children. CAC/RCP 66-2008. Accessed on December 2, 2013 at http://www.codexalimentarius.net/download/standards/11026/cxp_066e.pdf

Collins, R. N., Treger, M. D., Goldsby, J. B., Boring, J. R. 3rd., Coohon, D. B., Barr, R. N. 1968. Interstate outbreak of *Salmonella* newbrunswick infection traced to powdered milk. *JAMA.* 203:838-844.

Coulin, P., Farah, Z., Assanvo, J., Spillmann, H., Puhan, Z. 2006. Characterization of the microflora of attieke, a fermented cassava product, during traditional small-scale preparation, *Int. J. Food* Microbiol. 106:131–136.

Cruz, A. C., Fernandez, E., Salinas, E., Ramirez, P., Montiel, C., Eslava, C. A. 2004. Characterization of *Enterobacter sakazakii* isolated from different sources, Abstract Q-051, 104th Gen. Mtg., Am., Soc. Microbiol., 23–27 May, New Orleans, LA.

De Clerck, E., Vanhoutte, T., Hebb, T., Geerinck, J., Devos, J., De Vos, P. 2004. Isolation, characterization, and identification of bacterial contaminants in semifinal gelatin extracts, *Appl. Environ. Microbiol.* 70: 3664–3672.

Drudy, D., Mullane, N. R., Quinn T., Wall, P. G., Fanning, S. 2006. *Enterobacter sakazakii*: an emerging pathogen in powdered infant formula. *Clin. Infect. Dis.* 42(7):996-1002.

Emiliani, F., Lajmanovich, R., González, S M. 2001. *Escherichia coli*: biochemical phenotype diversity in freshwaters (Santa Fe Province, Argentina), *Rev. Argent. Microbiol.* 33: 65–74.

Espeland, E. M., Wetzel R.G. 2001. Complexation, stabilisation, and UV photolysis of extracellular and surface-bound glucosidase and alkaline phoshatase: implications for biofilm microbiota. *Microb. Ecol.* 42: 572–585.

European Commission. 2009. Implementation of microbiological criteria to infant formulae, follow-up formulae and baby food. Accessed on November 2, 2013 at http://ec.europa.eu/food/committees/regulatory/scfcah/biosafety/sum_16032010_non_paper.pdf.

Farmer, J. J., Asbury, M. A., Hickman, F. W., Brenner, D. J., and the Enterobacteriaceae Study Group. 1980. *Enterobacter sakazakii*, new species of Enterobacteriaceae isolated from clinical specimens. *Int. J. Syst. Bacteriol.* 30:569–584.

Farmer, J. J., Davis, B. R., Hickman-Brenner, F. W., Mcwhorter, A., Huntley-Carter, G. P., Asbury, M. A., Riddle, C., Wathen-Grady, H. G., Elias, C., G.R. Fanning, G.R., Steigerwalt, A.G., Ohara, C. M., Morris, G. K., Smith, P. B., Brenner, D. J. 1985. Biochemical identification of new species and biogroups of Enterobacteriaceae isolated from clinical specimens, *J. Clin. Microbiol.* 21: 46–76.

Food and Agriculture Organization of the United Nations/World Health Organization. *Enterobacter sakazakii* and *Salmonella* in powdered infant formula; meeting report. *Microbiological Risk Assessment Series*, 2006:10.

Forlani, G., Mantelli, M., Branzoni, M., Nielsen, E., Favilli, F. 1995. Differential sensitivity of plant-associated bacteria to sulfonylurea and imidazolinone herbicides, *Plant Soil.* 176: 243–253.

Forsythe, S. J. 2005. *Enterobacter sakazakii* and other bacteria in powdered infant formula. *Maternal and Child Nutrition.* 1: 44-50.

Friedemann M. 2009. Epidemiology of invasive neonatal *Cronobacter (Enterobacter sakazakii)* infections. *Eur. J. Clin. Microbiol. Infect. Dis.* 28:1297-1304.

FSNET. 8, November 2002. Recalled Baby Formula Found In Colorado Stores. November 6, 2002. Colorado Department of Public Health and Environment Press Release. Accessed on November 21, 2013 at: http://131.104.232.9/fsnet/2002/11-2002/fsnet_november_8-2.htm#RECALLED%20BABY.

Gakuya, F. M., Kyule, M. N., Gathura, P. B., Kariuki, S.. 2001. Antimicrobial resistance of bacterial organisms isolated from rats, *East Afr. Med. J.* 78: 646–649.

Gardner, J. M., Feldman, A. W., Zablotowicz, R. M. 1982. Identity and behavior of xylem-residing bacteria in rough lemon roots of Florida citrus trees, *Appl. Env. Microbiol.* 43: 1335–1342.

Geiges, O., Stählin, B., Baumann, B 1990. The microbiological evaluation of prepared salad vegetables and sprouts, Mitt. Lebensm.unters. *Hyg.* 81: 684–721.

Giovannini, M., Verduci, E., Ghisleni, D., Salvatici, E., Riva, E., Agostoni, C.2008. *Enterobacter sakazakii*: an emerging problem in paediatric nutrition. *J. Int. Med. Res.* 36:394–399.

Goullet, P., Picard, B 1986. Characterization of *Enterobacter cloacae* and *E. sakazakii* by electrophoretic polymorphism of acid phosphatase, esterases, and glutamate, lactate and malate dehydrogenases, *J. Gen. Microbiol.* 132: 3105–3112.

Gurtler, J. B., Kornacki, J. L., Beuchat, L. R. 2005. *Enterobacter sakazakii*: a coliform of increased concern to infant health. *Int. J. Food Microbiol.* 104(1):1-34.

Hamilton, J. V., Lehane, M. J., Braig, H. R. 2003. Isolation of *Enterobacter sakazakii* from midgut of Stomoxys calcitrans. *Emerg. Infect. Dis.* 9:1355–1356.

Healy, B., Cooney, S., O'Brien, S., Iversen, C., Whyte, P., Nally, J., Callanan, J. J., Fanning, S. 2010. *Cronobacter (Enterobacter sakazakii)*: an opportunistic foodborne pathogen. *Foodborne Pathog Dis.* 7(4):339-50.

Himelright, I., Harris, E., Lorch, V., Anderson, M., Jones, T., Craig, A., Kuehnert, W., Forster, T., Arduino, M., Jensen, B., Jernigan, D. 2002. From the Centers for Disease Control and Prevention. *Enterobacter sakazakii* infections associated with the use of powdered infant formula—Tennessee, 2001, *JAMA* 287: 2204–2205.

International Commission on Microbiological Safety of Food. 2002. Microorganisms in foods 7. Microbiological testing in food safety management. Kluwer Academic/Plenum Publishers.

Iversen, C., Forsythe, S. 2003. Risk profile of *Enterobacter sakazakii*, an emergent pathogen associated with infant milk formula. *Trends Food Sci. Technol.* 14:443–454.

Iversen, C., Forsythe, S. 2004. Isolation of *Enterobacter sakazakii* and other Enterobacteriaceae from powdered formula milk and related products. *Food Microbiol.* 21:771–777.

Jacobs, C., Braun, P. and Hammer, P. 2011. Reservoir and routes of transmission of *Enterobacter sakazakii* (*Cronobacter spp.*) in a milk powder-producing plant. *J. Dairy Sci.* 94:3801-3810.

Jaradat, Z. W., Ababneh, Q. O., Saadoun, I. M., Samara, N. A., Rashdan, A. M. 2009. Isolation of *Cronobacter* spp. (formerly *Enterobacter sakazakii*) from infant food, herbs and environmental samples and the subsequent identification and confirmation of the isolates using biochemical, chromogenic assays, PCR and 16S rRNA sequencing. *BMC Microbiol.* 9:225.

Joker, R. N., Norholm, T., Siboni, K. E. 1965. A case of neonatal meningitis caused by a yellow *Enterobacter. Danish Med. Bull.* 12:128–130.

Jourdan, N., Le Hello, S., Delmas, G., Clouzeau, J., Manteau, C., Desaubliaux, B., Chagnon, V., Thierry-Bled, F., Demare, N., Weill, F. and de Valk H. 2008. Nationwide outbreak of *Salmonella enterica* serotype Give infections in infants in France, linked to infant milk formula, September 2008. *Euro Surveill.* 13:18994.

Kandhai, M. C., Reij, M. W., Gorris, L. G., Guillaume-Gentil, O., van Schothorst, M. 2004b. Occurrence of *Enterobacter sakazakii* in food production environments and households. *Lancet.* 363:39-40.

Kandhai, M. C., Reij, M. W., van Puyvelde, K., Guillaume-Gentil, O., Beumer, R. R., van Schothorst. M. 2004a. A new protocol for the detection of *Enterobacter sakazakii* applied to environmental samples. *J. Food. Prot.* 67:1267-1270.

Kanivets, V. I., Pishchur, I. N. 2001. Bacterial microflora on disinfected sugar beet seeds, *Microbiology* 70: 316–318.

Kim, H., Ryu, J. H., Beuchat, L. R. 2006. Attachment of and biofilm formation by *Enterobacter sakazakii* on stainless steel and enteral feeding tubes. *Appl. Environ Microbiol.* 72(9):5846-56.

Kleiman, M. B., Allen, S.D., Neal, P., Reynolds, J. 1981. Meningoencephalitis and compartmentalization of the cerebral ventricles caused by *Enterobacter sakazakii. J. Clin. Microbiol.* 14:352–354.

Kuklinsky-Sobral, J., Araujo, W. L., Mendes, R., Pizzirani-Kleiner, A. A., Azevedo, J. L. 2005. Isolation and characterization of endophytic bacteria from soybean (*Glycine max*) grown in soil treated with glyphosate herbicide, *Plant Soil* 273: 91–99.

Kuzina, L.V., Peloquin, J. J. Vacek, Miller T. 2001, Isolation and identification of bacteria associated with adult laboratory Mexican fruit flies, *Anastrepha ludens* (Diptera: Tephritidae). *Curr. Microbiol.* 42:290–294.

Lai, K. K. 2001. *Enterobacter sakazakii* infections among neonates, infants, children, and adults. Case reports and a review of the literature. *Med.* (Baltimore). 80:113-122.

Leclerc, H., Mossel, D. A. A., Edberg, S. C., Struijk, C. B. 2001. Advances in the bacteriology of the coliform group: their suitability as markers of microbial water safety, *Ann. Rev. Microbiol.* 55: 201–234.

Leclercq, A., Wanegue, C., Baylac, P. 2002. Comparison of fecal coliform agar and violet red bile lactose agar for fecal coliform enumeration in foods. *Appl. Environ. Microbiol.* 68:1631–1638.

Lee, D. G., Kim, S. J. 2003. Bacterial species in biofilm cultivated from the end of the Seoul water distribution system, *J. Appl. Microbiol.* 95: 317–324.

Lehner, A., Riedel, K., Eberl, L., Breeuwer, P., Diep, B., Stephan, R. 2005. Biofilm formation, extracellular polysaccharide production, and cell-to-cell signaling in various *Enterobacter sakazakii* strains: aspects promoting environmental persistence. *J. Food Prot.* 68(11):2287-94.

Lehner, A., Stephan, R. 2004. Microbiological, epidemiological, and food safety aspects of *Enterobacter sakazakii*. *J. Food Prot.* 67(12): 2850-7.

Lehner, A., Tasara, T., Stephan, R. 2004. 16S rRNA gene based analysis of *Enterobacter sakazakii* strains from different sources and development of a PCR assay for identification, *BMC Microbiol.* 4: 43.

Leuschner, R. G. K., Baird, F., Donald, B., Cox, L. J. 2004. A medium for the presumptive detection of *Enterobacter sakazakii* in infant formula, *Food Microbiol.* 21: 527–533.

Liu, Y., Gao, Q., Zhang, X., Hou, Y., Yang, J., Huang, X. 2005. PCR and oligonucleotide array for detection of *Enterobacter sakazakii* in infant formula, *Mol. Cell. Probes* 20: 11–17.

Lucas, A., Cole, T. J. 1990. Breast milk and neonatal necrotising enterocolitis. *Lancet.* 336(8730):1519-23.

Masaki, H., Asoh, N., Tao, M., Ikeda, H., Degawa, S., Matsumoto, K., Inokuchi, K., Watanabe, K., Watanabe, H., Oishi, K., Nagatake, T. 2001. Detection of gram-negative bacteria in patients and hospital environment at a room in geriatric wards under the infection control against MRSA, *J. Jap. Ass. Inf. Dis.* 75: 144–150.

Masood N, Moore K, Farbos A, Hariri S, Paszkiewicz K, Dickins B, McNally A, Forsythe S. 2013. Draft Genome Sequences of Three Newly Identified Species in the Genus *Cronobacter*, *C. helveticus* LMG23732T, *C. pulveris* LMG24059, and *C. zurichensis* LMG23730T. *Genome Announc.* 1:10.1128/genomeA.00783-13.

Mensah, P., Yeboah-Manu, D., Owusu-Darko, K., Ablordey, A. 2002. Street foods in Accra, Ghana: how safe are they?, *Bull.* WHO 80, pp. 546–554.

Miranda, C. D., Kehrenberg, C., Ulep, C., Schwarz, S., Roberts, M. C. 2003. Diversity of tetracycline resistance genes in bacteria from Chilean salmon farms, *Antimicrob. Agents Chemother.* 47: 883–888.

Monroe, P. W., Tift, W. L. 1979. Bacteremia associated with *Enterobacter sakazakii* (yellow, pigmented *Enterobacter cloacae*). *J. Clin. Microbiol.* 10:850–851.

Montgomery, J. M., Gillespie, D., Sastrawan, P., Fredeking, T. M., Stewart, G. L. 2002. Aerobic salivary bacteria in wild and captive Komodo dragons, *J. Wildl. Dis.* 38: 545–551.

Mramba, F., Broce, A., Zurek, L. 2006. Isolation of *Enterobacter sakazakii* from stable flies, *Stomoxys calcitrans* L. (Diptera: Muscidae), *J. Food Prot.* 69: 671–673.

Mullane, N., Healy, B., Meade, J., Whyte, P., Wall, P. G., Fanning, S. 2008. Dissemination of *Cronobacter* spp. (*Enterobacter sakazakii*) in a powdered milk protein manufacturing facility. *Appl. Environ Microbiol.* 74(19):5913-7.

Muytjens, H. L., Kollée, L. A. 1990. *Enterobacter sakazakii* meningitis in neonates: causative role of formula? Pediatr Infect Dis J. 9(5):372-3.

Muytjens, H. L., Roelofs-Willemse, H., Jaspar, G. H. 1988. Quality of powdered substitutes for breast milk with regard to members of the family Enterobacteriaceae, *J. Clin. Microbiol.* 26: 743–746.

Muytjens, H. L., Zanen, H. C., Sonderkamp, H. J., Kolee, L. A., Wachsmuth, I. K., Farmer, J. J. 1983. Analysis of eight cases of neonatal meningitis and sepsis due to *Enterobacter sakazakii*. *J. Clin. Microbiol.* 18:115–120.

Nassereddin, R. A., Yamani, M. I. 2005. Microbiological quality of sous and tamarind, traditional drinks consumed in Jordan, *J. Food Prot.* 68: 773–777.

Nazarowec-White, M., Farber, J. M. 1997. Incidence, survival, and growth of *Enterobacter sakazakii* in infant formula. *J. Food. Prot.* 60:226-230.

New South Wales Food Authority, 2011. Microbiological quality of powdered infant formula. Accessed on November 25, 2013 at http://www. foodauthority.nsw.gov.au/ _Documents/science/Microbiological_quality_powdered_formula.pdf

Nketsia-Tabiri, J., Adu-Gyamfi, A., Montford, K. G., Gbedemah, C. M., Sefa-Dedeh, S. 2003. Optimising processing conditions for irradiated cured fish, *Int. Atomic Energy Agency Techn. Doc.* vol. 1337: 207–216.

Noriega, F. R., Kotloff, K. L., Martin, M. A., Schwalbe, R. S. 1990. Nosocomial bacteremia caused by *Enterobacter sakazakii* and *Leuconostoc mesenteroides* resulting from extrinsic contamination of infant formula. *Pediatr. Infect. Dis.* 9:447–449.

Oger, C., Gavini, F., Delattre, J. M., Leclerc, H. 1981. On the coliform organisms and their count in water-supply analysis, *Ann. Microbiol.* A132:183–189.

Olsen, S. J., Bishop, R., Brenner, F. W., Roels, T. H., Bean, N., Tauxe, R. V. and Slutsker, L. 2001. The changing epidemiology of salmonella: trends in serotypes isolated from humans in the United States, 1987-1997. *J. Infect. Dis.* 183:753-761.

Osterblad, M., Pensala, O., Peterzens, M., Heleniuse, H., Huovinen, P. 1999. Antimicrobial susceptibility of Enterobacteriaceae isolated from vegetables, *J. Antimicrob. Chemother.* 43: 503–509.

Park, J. K., Seok, W. S., Choi, B. J., Kim, H. M., Lim, B. K., Yoon, S. S., Kim, S., Kim, Y. S. and Park, J. Y. 2004. *Salmonella enterica* serovar London infections associated with consumption of infant formula. *Yonsei Med. J.* 45:43-48.

Postupa, R., Aldová, E. 1984. *Enterobacter sakazakii*: a Tween 80 esterase-positive representative of the genus Enterobacter isolated from powdered milk specimens. *J. Hyg., Epidemiol. Microbiol. Immunol.* 28:435–440.

Reich, F., König, R., von Wiese, W., Klein, G. 2010. Prevalence of Cronobacter spp. in a powdered infant formula processing environment. *Int. J. Food Microbiol.* 140(2-3):214-7.

Reij, M. W., Jongenburger, I., Gkogka, E., Gorris, L. G., Zwietering, M. H. 2009. Perspective on the risk to infants in the Netherlands associated with *Cronobacter spp.* occurring in powdered infant formula. *Int. J. Food Microbiol.* 136:232-237.

Restaino, L., Frampton, E. W., Lionberg, W. C., Becker, R. J. 2006. A chromogenic plating medium for the isolation and identification of *Enterobacter sakazakii* from foods, food ingredients, and environmental sources. *J. Food Prot.* 69(2):315-22.

Richards, G. M., Gurtler, J. B., Beuchat, L. R. 2005. Survival and growth of *Enterobacter sakazakii* in infant rice cereal reconstituted with water, milk, liquid infant formula, or apple juice. *J. Appl. Microbiol.* 99:844-850.

Rowe, B., Begg, N. T., Hutchinson, D. N., Dawkins, H. C., Gilbert, R. J., Jacob, M., Hales, B. H., Rae, F. A. and Jepson, M. 1987. *Salmonella* Ealing infections associated with consumption of infant dried milk. *Lancet.* 2:900-903.

Salmon, S. A., Watts, J, L., Aarestrup, F. M., Pankey, J. W., Yancey, R. J. 1998. Minimum inhibitory concentrations for selected antimicrobial agents against organisms isolated from the mammary glands of dairy heifers in New Zealand and Denmark, *J. Dairy Sci.* 81: 570–578.

Sanders, W. E., Sanders, C. C. 1997. *Enterobacter* spp.: pathogens poised to flourish at the turn of the century. *Clin. Microbiol. Rev.* 10:220-241.

Schindler, P. R. G., Metz, H. 1991. Coliform bacteria in drinking water from South Bavaria: identification by the API 20E-system and resistance patterns, *Water Sci. Technol.* 24: 81–84.

Simmons, B. P., Gelfand, M. S., Has, M., Metts, L., Ferguson, J. 1989. *Enterobacter sakazakii* infections in neonates associated with intrinsic contamination of a powdered infant formula. *Infect Control Hosp Epidemiol.* 10(9):398-401.

Skladal, P., Mascini, M., Salvadori, C., Zannoni, G. 1993. Detection of bacterial contamination in sterile UHT milk using and L-lactate biosensor. *Enzyme Microb. Technol.* 15:508–512.

Smeets, L.C., Voss, A., Muytjens, H. L., Meis, J. F. G. M., Melchers, W. J. G. (1998) Genetische karakterisatie van *Enterobacter sakazakii*-isolaten van Nederlandse patiënten met neonatale meningitis. *Nederlands Tijdschrift voor Medische Microbiologie.* 6: 113–115.

Soler, P., Herrera, S., Rodriguez, J., Cascante, J., Cabral, R., Echeita-Sarriondia, A., Mateo, S. 2008. National Surveillance Network of Spain. Nationwide outbreak of *Salmonella enterica* serotype Kedougou infection in infants linked to infant formula milk, Spain, 2008. *Euro Surveill.* 13:18963.

Stoll, B. J., Hansen, N., Fanaroff, A. A. and Lemons, J. A.2004. *Enterobacter sakazakii* is a rare cause of neonatal septicemia or meningitis in VLBW infants. *J. Pediatr.* 144:821-823.

Thurm, V., Gericke, B. 1994. Identification of infant food as a vehicle in a nosocomial outbreak of *Citrobacter freundii*: epidemiological subtyping by allozyme, whole-cell protein and antibiotic resistance. *J. Appl. Bacteriol.* 76:553-558.

U.S Department of Agriculture. 2008. USDA Commodity Requirements. IFD3. Infant formula for use in domestic programs. Accessed on December 2, 2013 at http://www.fsa.usda.gov/Internet/FSA_File/ifd3.pdf

U.S Food and Drug Administration. 2002. FDA warns about possible *Enterobacter sakazakii* infections in hospitalized newborns fed powdered infant formulas. FDA Talk Paper, April 12, 2002. Accessed on December 2, 2013 at http://www. fda.gov/ bbs/topics/ANSWERS/2002/ANS01146.html.

Urmenyi, A. M., Franklin, A. W. 1961. Neonatal death from pigmented coliform infection. *Lancet.* 1:313-315.

Usera, M. A., Echeita, A., Aladuena, A., Blanco, M. C., Reymundo, R., Prieto, M. I., Tello, O., Cano, R., Herrera, D. and Martinez-Navarro, F. 1996. Interregional foodborne salmonellosis outbreak due to powdered infant formula contaminated with lactose-fermenting Salmonella virchow. *Eur. J. Epidemiol.* 12:377-381.

van Acker, J., de Smet, F., Muyldermans, G., Bougatef, A., Naessens, A., Lauwers, S 2001. Outbreak of necrotizing enterocolitis associated with *Enterobacter sakazakii* in powdered milk formula. *J. Clin. Microbiol.* 39:293-297.

Weir, E., 2002. Powdered infant formula and fatal infection with *Enterobacter sakazakii*. *Canadian Medical Association Journal.* 166: 1570.

Weissman, J. B., Deen, A. D., Williams, M., Swanston, N., Ali, S. 1977. An island-wide epidemic of salmonellosis in Trinidad traced to contaminated powdered milk. *West Indian Med. J.* 26:135-143.

Williams, M. M., Braun-Howland, E. B. 2003. Growth of *Escherichia coli* in model distribution system biofilms exposed to hypochlorous acid or monochloramine, *Appl. Env. Microbiol.* 69: 5463–5471.

Willis, J., Robinson, J. E. 1988. *Enterobacter sakazakii* meningitis in neonates. *Pediatr. Infect. Dis. J.* 7:196–199.

World Health Organization. 2007a. *Enterobacter sakazakii* and other microorganisms in powdered infant formula: meeting report, MRA series 6. Accessed on November 12, 2013 at http://www.who.int/foodsafety/publications/micro/mra6/en/.

World Health Organization. 2007b. Guidelines for the safe preparation, storage and handling of powdered infant formula. Department of Food Safety, Zoonoses and Foodborne Diseases, WHO, Geneva. Accessed on September 13, 2013 at http://www.who.int/ foodsafety/publications/micro/pif_guidelines.pdf.

Yan, Q. Q., Condell, O., Power, K., Butler, F., Tall, B. D., Fanning, S. 2012. *Cronobacter* species (formerly known as *Enterobacter sakazakii*) in powdered infant formula: a review of our current understanding of the biology of this bacterium. *J. Appl. Microbiol.* 113:1-15.

Yang, H. L., Sun, X. L., Song, W., Wang, Y. S., Cai, M. Y. 1999. Screening, identification and distribution of endophytic associative diazotrophs isolated from rice plants, *Acta Botan. Sin.* 41: 927–931.

Zogaj, X., Bokranz, W., Nimtz, M., Romling, U. 2003. Production of cellulose and curli fimbriae by members of the family Enterobacteriaceae isolated from the human gastrointestinal tract, *Infect. Immun.* 71: 4151–4158.

In: Advances in Medicine and Biology. Volume 77   ISBN: 978-1-63117-444-5
Editor: Leon V. Berhardt   © 2014 Nova Science Publishers, Inc.

Chapter 2

Spontaneous Bacterial Peritonitis

Sushma Singh, MD[1] and Nancy Khardori, MD,PhD,FIDSA[2]*
[1]Hospitalist, Franklin Hospital, Franklin, Virginia, US
Professor, Division of Infectious Diseases,
Department of Internal Medicine
[2]Professor, Department of Microbiology and Molecular Cell Biology
Eastern Virginia medical School, Norfolk, Virginia, US

Abstract

Spontaneous bacterial peritonitis (SBP) is defined as the primary infection of peritoneum not directly related to an intraabdominal process. It is a frequent and severe complication seen in patients with cirrhosis and ascites. The basic pathophysiology is the translocation of bacterial flora into the peritoneal fluid. Most patients who develop SBP are in Child Pugh C class of liver disease severity. Renal failure following SBP is the most predictive factor for mortality. The most common symptoms and signs of SBP are abdominal pain and fever followed by vomiting, hepatic encephalopathy, gastrointestinal bleeding and renal impairment. The diagnosis is confirmed by cell counts, protein, glucose and microbiological evaluation of ascitic fluid. The pathogens are of enteric origin in more than two-thirds of cases. Antibiotic resistant bacteria including Pseudomonas aeruginosa, methicillin resistant Staphylococcus aureus and extended spectrum betalactamase producing E.coli are seen in hospitalized patients and those with prior antibiotic therapy. Initial presumptive antimicrobial therapy should have a broad spectrum of coverage and includes third generation cephlosporins like cefotaxime and ceftriaxone, extended spectrum penicillin like piperacillin-tazibactam, carbapenems like meropenem and newer fluoroquinolones like moxifloxacin. Patients with risk factors for multiple drug resistant bacteria should receive appropriate therapy based on local microbiology. For long term antibiotic prophylaxis following an episode of SBP fluoroquinolones like norfloxacin and trimethprim/sulfamethoxazole have been used

* Corresponding Author: khardoNM@evms.edu, Suite 572, 825 Fairfax Avenue, Norfolk, Virginia 23507.

resulting in resistance to these agents. Recently, Rifaximin a non-absorbable antibiotic has been shown to cause a significant reduction in the rate of SBP and a transplant-free survival benefit.

Introduction

Inflammation of peritoneal cavity secondary to infective agents or noxious chemicals or both is called peritonitis. Infective peritonitis is classified into primary, secondary and tertiary. Spontaneous Bacterial Peritonitis (SBP) is an example of primary peritonitis which is infection not directly related to an intra-abdominal process. In secondary peritonitis, an intra-abdominal process, such as a ruptured viscus is the underlying etiology. Tertiary peritonitis is a late stage disease, when the local infection along with signs of sepsis and multiorgan failure persist or recur after treatment for secondary peritonitis. In this type of peritonitis no pathogens or only low-grade pathogens of nosocomial nature frequently multidrug-resistant are isolated from the peritoneal exudate. [1,2,3]. In this review, we focus on the diagnosis and management of Spontaneous Bacterial Peritonitis (SBP).

SBP is a frequent and severe complication seen in patients with cirrhosis and ascites. Patients with cirrhosis have altered gastrointestinal tract physiology which favors the translocation of bacterial flora into peritoneal fluid. The most common and life-threatening infection in cirrhosis with ascites is spontaneous bacterial peritonitis followed by urinary tract infections, pneumonia, endocarditis and skin and soft-tissue infections. Prevalence of SBP ranges from 25%-30% in this patient population [4] and results in high mortality rates of 30%-50% [5] with one year mortality as high as 65%-93% [6]. The cumulative mortality after any infection in patients with cirrhosis is 43.5%. Risk factors associated with the development of SBP are severe liver failure, variceal bleeding, low ascetic fluid protein level and prior episodes of spontaneous bacterial peritonitis (SBP). [7]

Pathogenesis

The most significant predisposing factor for SBP is the severity of liver disease, about 70% of the patients who develop SBP are in Child Pugh C class [8] and the most significant predictive factor for mortality after infection is renal failure. The release of inflammatory mediators during infection leads to systemic, renal, and hepatic and hemodynamic impairment, worsening the prognosis even with appropriate treatment of infection. Pharmacologic acid suppression has been found to be associated with a greater risk of SBP in hospitalized patients with cirrhosis. Patients with cirrhosis receiving a proton pump inhibitor have approximately three times the risk of developing SBP compared with those not receiving this medication. [9, 10]

The hallmark of pathogenesis in SBP is the translocation of bacteria from the gut lumen to mesenteric lymph nodes, to the systemic circulation (bacteremia), and then to existing fluids (ascites and/or hydrothorax). [11] This is enhanced by the increased hydrostatic pressure and low oncotic pressure seen in liver disease.

Chronic liver disease is associated with an impaired host defense mechanisms which worsens overtime and with disease progression. Both humoral and cell-mediated immunity are impaired leading to decreased bacterial clearance. This along with structural and functional alterations in the intestinal mucosa lead to an increase in permeability followed by translocation of bacteria/derived products across the mucosa. [12] The alteration of the intestinal mucosal barrier in cirrhosis is caused by increased mucosal permeability (especially in patients with sepsis) because of the oxidative stress, malfunctioning of enterocyte mitochondria, endotoxemia, increased nitric oxide and proinflammatory cytokine levels as well as by structural changes. The intestinal bacterial overgrowth plays a key role in bacterial translocation (BT) in cirrhosis and is secondary to delayed intestinal transit in these patients. The delay in intestinal transit is caused by the sympathoadrenal stimulation leading to increased nitric oxide synthesis and the oxidative stress.

In addition to physical barrier provided by the intestinal mucosa it offers secretory factors that prevent microbial penetration, the most significant being immunoglobulin IgA secreted by plasmocytes in lamina propria. The secretory IgA binds to bacteria preventing their adhesion to the mucosa and bacterial colonization; neutralizes bacterial toxins; and forms complexes with the bacterial antigens. The IgA-antigen complexes are then actively transported from the lamina propria back into the intestinal lumen. The normal constituents of bile contribute to the local defense by decreasing the colonization by enteric bacteria, by neutralization of endotoxin and by inhibition of excessive proliferation of intestinal flora. In addition bile has a trophic effect on the intestinal mucosa and interferes with bacterial adherence. [11] The concentration of bile acids in cirrhosis decreases in the intestinal lumen due to reduced secretion.

The natural antimicrobial peptides molecules secreted by intestinal epithelium are able to decrease the number of microorganisms in the gastrointestinal tract. A major role is played by the α-defensin, synthesized in response to the presence of bacteria or lipopolysaccharides and to a lesser extent by the lysozyme and secretory phospholipase A2. In addition most epithelial cells from small intestine and colon can secrete β-defensin - a peptide involved in the defense against commensal bacteria. [13]

The gut-associated lymphoid tissue (GALT) is the largest and the best known immunological organ which includes Peyer's patches, lymphocytes/dendritic cells, intraepithelial lymphocytes, mesenteric lymph nodes (MLN). This lymphoid tissue continuously reacts to the presence of bacteria by ongoing proliferation and secretion of protective immunoglobulins. Further immunological intervention is offered by the mononuclear cells that carry toll like receptors (TLR), the most important being TLR 2, 4 and 9. The stimulation of these receptors by bacterial ligands (lipopolysaccharides, lipoteichoic acid, and peptidoglycans) activates the cytokine and chemokine synthesis and the antimicrobial gene transcription. The chemokines synthesized by the epithelial cells activate dendritic cells that in turn present antigens to B cells leading to the production of immunoglobulins like IgA. The antigen presentation also leads to production of cytotoxic T lymphocytes from the Peyer's patches. In patients with cirrhosis immunologic impairment is enhanced by qualitative neutrophil dysfunction i.e decreased phagocytosis, low serum complement levels and impaired function of the Fc receptors of the macrophages.

Normally the Kupffer cells in liver collaborate with neutrophils in the process of bacterial extraction from the circulation, followed by their destruction. In patients with cirrhosis, circulant bacteria do not come in contact with Kupffer cells because of intra and extra hepatic shunts due to portal hypertension. This results in poor clearance of bacteria by the liver leading to bacteremia and ascitic fluid infection. Low complement level in the ascitic fluid leading to impaired bactericidal activity adds to the risk of SBP. [14]

A combination of the deficiencies in local and systemic immune mechanisms described above in cirrhosis leads to the translocation of bacteria, their proliferation followed by bacteremia and ascitic fluid infection.

Diagnosis

Most common symptoms and signs of SBP are abdominal pain and fever, followed by vomiting, hepatic encephalopathy, gastrointestinal bleeding and renal impairment. Absence of these signs and symptoms does not rule out SBP and therefore index of suspicion should be high. [15]

The laboratory evaluation of ascetic fluid is the most optimal diagnostic approach. The criterion with high sensitivity is the presence of polymorphoneuclear (PMN) cells at or $250/mm^3$. In patients with hemorrhagic ascites (red blood cell count $> 10\ 000/mm^3$), subtraction of one PMN per 250 red blood cells should be made to account for the presence of blood. Other ascetic fluid parameters that may be helpful are any two of the following: total protein >1 g/dL, lactate dehydrogenase >the upper limit of normal for serum, and glucose <than 50 mg/dL. Unfortunately bacterial cultures are positive only in 40%-70% of infections [16, 17]. In a classic case of SBP, cultures are positive and PMN count is greater than 250/µL. When the cultures are positive and the PMN count is<250/µL, the syndrome is called Bacteriascites. This form of SBP can be self-limited and managed with careful observation and repeat paracentesis after 48 hours. In contrast, ascitic fluid with negative culture but PMN > or = 500/µL, is called culture negative neutrophilic ascites (CNNA). CNNA and classic SBP are managed identically [18, 19]

In an attempt to improve early diagnosis of SBP and reduce morbidity and mortality, a number of biomarkers have been studied. Like in many other infectious processes serum CRP level is elevated as an acute phase reactant. The higher CRP levels have been related to lower response rate to antibiotics, and higher mortality rate in patients with SBP. This prognostic function of elevated CRP is not a surrogate for underlying hepatic dysfunction since it is negatively correlated with the Child Pugh and Model for End-Stage Liver Disease scores [20]. Serum procalcitonin levels have been shown to provide satisfactory diagnostic accuracy in determining bacterial infections in hospitalized patients with all-cause cirrhosis but not in non-cirrhosis related malignant ascites. Seiken el al showed that a cut-off value less than 0.61ng/mL for culture-positive SBP, less than 0.225 ng/mL for culture-negative SBP, less than 1.12 ng/mL for bacterascites and less than 0.42 ng/mL for patients who have either culture-positive SBP or culture-negative SBP (combination group)accurately rules out the diagnosis of bacterial peritonitis for clinical use. [21]. A new marker, ascetic fluid calprotectin has been shown to predict PMN count > 250/µL reliably, and may prove to be useful in the diagnosis of SBP. This would be helpful in resource poor settings because of availability of a bedside testing device. [22]

Presence of hepatocellular carcinoma (HCC), higher serum bilirubin levels (≥3 mg/dl), a prolonged serum prothrombin time (i.e., international normalized ratio >2.3), renal dysfunction (creatinine>1.3 mg/dL), and lower glucose levels in the ascitic fluid (<50 mg/dL) are associated with higher mortality rates in cirrhotic patients with SBP. [23].

Microbiology

In patients with cirrhosis and SBP, > 69% of the pathogens are of enteric origin. Escherichia coli is the most frequently recovered pathogen, followed by Klebsiella pneumoniae, S. pneumoniae, and other streptococcal species and Enterococci. [24]

However the widespread use of fluoroquinolones and other antibiotics, multiple hospitalization and procedures in cirrhosis have favored changes in bacterial flora and the development of antibiotic resistance. Figure 1 A and B show the distribution of pathogens in community acquired and nosocomial SBP. [Figure 1] [25]

A retrospective study done over 4 years (2008-2011) in Greece showed that 55% cases of SBP were due to gram positive cocci. Streptococcus and Enterococcus spp were the most common organisms followed by Escherichia coli, Klebsiella pneumoniae, methicillin-sensitive Staphylococcus aureus and coagulase-negative Staphylococcus spp.

In the same study multiply drug resistant organisms including carbapenamase-producing K. pneumoniae, extended-spectrum beta-lactamase-producing E. coli and Pseudomonas aeruginosa were reported to be responsible for 19% of the cases. These were, understandably, isolated more frequently in healthcare-associated SBP, patients receiving long-term quinolone prophylaxis and patients with advanced liver disease (higher MELD score) compared to community acquired infections. [26]

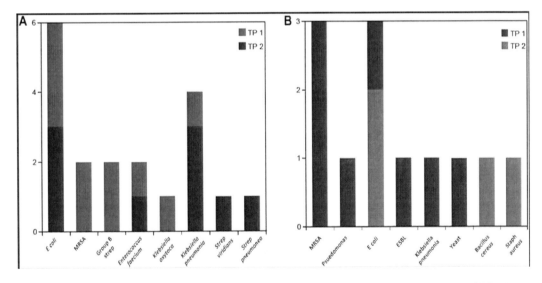

Figure 1. A. Microorganisms seen in community acquired spontaneous bacterial peritonitis (SBP). B. Microorganisms seen in hospital acquired SBP. TP, Treatment period; MRSA, Methicillin-resistant Staphylococcus aureus; ESBL, Extended-spectrum beta-lactamase.[Hasnain M Jafferbhoy, Michael H Miller, W Gashau et al. Spontaneous bacterial peritonitisprophylaxis in the era of healthcare associated infection. Gut. 2012 Mar 22] [With permission].

Treatment

Since Gram-negative aerobic bacteria from the family of *Enterobacteriaceae* and non-enterococcal *Streptococcus* spp. are the most common causative organisms, the initial presumptive antibiotic therapy of SBP should provide activity against these organisms [2]. Third generation cephalosporins like cefotaxime/ceftriaxone have been established as the standard treatment of SBP.

A combination of ampicillin plus an aminoglycoside is as efficacious as the third generation cephalosporins for presumptive therapy in SBP. However the risk of renal impairment from aminoglycoside is high. Other antimicrobial agents, like broad-spectrum penicillins such as ticarcillin or piperacillin, carbapenems (e.g., imipenem, meropenem, doripenem, and ertapenem), β-lactam/β-lactamase combinations (e.g., piperacillin-tazobactam, ticarcillin-clavulanate, and ampicillin- sulbactam), and the newer fluoroquinolones (e.g., levofloxacin and moxifloxacin), are potential alternatives. [1].

The rising incidence of multidrug resistant bacteria in SBP demands a review of the established antibiotic choices. In a retrospective study done in Spain, third-generation cephalosporin resistance occurred in 21.5% and risk of resistance was particularly high in nosocomial-acquired episodes of spontaneous bacterial peritonitis, but also occurred in healthcare system-acquired cases. [28]

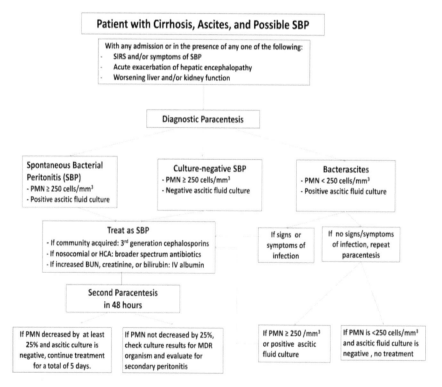

Figure 2. Approach to the patient with ascites and possible SBP. If a patient is admitted with ascites and suspected SBP, diagnostic paracentesis is performed. Based on these results, treatment strategies differ. It is important to stratify the patient based. [29] [Permission pending, to be taken by publishers].

Therefore patients with SBP at risk for multiply drug resistant bacterial infections should receive alternate appropriate agents. The risk factors for MDR pathogens include prior antibiotic treatment, intensive care unit stay and recent hospitalization. Carbapenems other than ertapenem should be chosen for nosocomially acquired SBP in areas with a high prevalence of extended-spectrum β-lactamase-producing Enterobacteriaceae and P. aeruginosa. Tigecycline, as an alternative, has recently been shown to be associated with increased mortality and therefore should not be recommended as first-line therapy. [30] Definitive antimicrobial therapy should be based on culture and sensitivity results if positive. If the cultures are negative and index for suspicion for MDR pathogens is high, agents like polymixin B, colistin with or without linezolid or daptomycin should be tried.

Although 5 days of antibiotics therapy has been reported to be efficacious [31], most patients are treated for 10-14 days as long as improvement is noted.A determination of response is made by a follow-up paracentesis two days after starting antibiotic therapy. A less than 25% reduction in the ascitic fluid PMN countcompared to pretreatment value indicates treatment failure and a need for modifying antibiotic treatment. Albumin is considered adjuvant treatment to antibiotics in patients with SBP and impaired renal or liver function, in order to prevent worsening of renal function. [32] Albumin infusion is effective inpatients with serum bilirubin $\geq$ 4 mg/dL or serum creatinine $\geq$ 1 mg/dL while its use in patients without these criteria remains controversial. [33]

Prevention

The survival rate at 1 year after an episode of SBP is about 30%-50%, with a cumulative recurrence rate at 1year of 70%. [34]. Hence, after first episode of SBP, liver transplantation and long-term antibiotic prophylaxis should be considered. In older studies, the long term antibiotics prophylaxis with norfloxacin (400mg/d), a fluoroquinolones, has been shown to reduce recurrence rate at 1 year from 70% to 20%. When resistance to norfloxacin develops, trimethoprim/sulfamethoxazole has been suggested to be the alternate for long term prophylaxis. However many bacteria causing SBP are already resistant to trimethoprim/sulfamethoxazole. In a recent study of 404 patients, rifaximin, a non-absorbable antibiotic was found to be effective in prophylaxis of SBP. There was a 72% reduction in the rate of SBP in the rifaximin group compared to patients not on any prophylaxis. Patients on rifaximin also demonstrated a transplant-free survival benefit 72% vs. 57% [35, 36].

References

[1] Matthew E. Levison, Larry M. Bush. Peritonitis and intraperitoneal abscesses. Volume 1, Part 2, section F. Mandell textbook of infectious diseases 7th edition.

[2] Nathens AB, Rotstein OD, Marshall JC. Tertiary peritonitis: clinical features of a complex nosocomial infection. *World J. Surg.* 1998;22:158-163.

[3] Malangione MA. Evaluation and management of tertiary peritonitis. *Am Surg.* 2000;66:157-161.

[4]   Fernández J, Navasa M, Gómez J, Colmenero J, Vila J, Arroyo V, Rodés J. Bacterial infections in cirrhosis: epidemiological changes with invasive procedures and norfloxacin prophylaxis. *Hepatology*. 2002;35:140–148.

[5]   Wong F, Bernardi M, Balk R, Christman B, Moreau R, Garcia-Tsao G, Patch D, Soriano G, Hoefs J, Navasa M. Sepsis in cirrhosis: *report on the 7th meeting of the International Ascites Club. Gut.* 2005;54:718–725.

[6]   Cohen MJ, Sahar T, Benenson S, Elinav E, Brezis M, Soares-Weiser K. Antibiotic prophylaxis for spontaneous bacterial peritonitis in cirrhotic patients with ascites, without gastro-intestinal bleeding. *Cochrane Database Syst. Rev.* 2009;(2):CD004791.

[7]   Pleguezuelo M, Benitez JM, Jurado J, Montero JL, De la Mata M. Diagnosis and management of bacterial infections in decompensated cirrhosis. *World J. Hepatol.* 2013 Jan 27;5(1):16-25.

[8]   Cirera I, Bauer TM, Navasa M et al. Bacterial translocation of enteric organisms in patients with cirrhosis. *J. Hepatol.*2001; 34: 32-37.

[9]   Deshpande A, Pasupuleti V, Thota P, Pant C, Mapara S, Hassan S, Rolston DD, Sferra TJ, Hernandez AV.Acid-suppressive therapy is associated with spontaneous bacterial peritonitis in cirrhotic patients: a meta-analysis. *J. Gastroenterol. Hepatol.* 2013 Feb;28(2):235-42.

[10] Siple JF, Morey JM, Gutman TE, Weinberg KL, Collins PD.Proton pump inhibitor use and association with spontaneousbacterialperitonitis in patients with cirrhosis and ascites. *Ann. Pharmacother.* 2012 Oct;46(10):1413-8.

[11] R. Wiest, G. Garcia-Tsao. Bacterial translocation (BT) in cirrhosis. *Hepatology,* 41 (2005), pp. 422–433.

[12] Rajkovic IA, Williams R. Abnormalities of neutrophil phagocytosis, intracellular killing and metabolic activity in alcoholic cirrhosis and hepatitis. *Hepatology.* 1986;6:252–262.

[13] Căruntu FA, Benea L. Spontaneous bacterial peritonitis: pathogenesis, diagnosis, treatment. *J. Gastrointestin Liver. Dis.* 2006 Mar;15(1):51-6.

[14] Such J, Runyon BA. Spontaneous bacterial peritonitis. *Clin. Infect. Dis.* 1998; 27: 669-674.

[15] Chinnock B, Afarian H, Minnigan H, Butler J, Hendey GW. Physician clinical impression does not rule out spontaneous bacterial peritonitis in patients undergoing emergency department paracentesis. *Ann. Emerg. Med.* 2008;52:268–273.

[16] European Association for the Study of the Liver. EASL clinical practice guidelines on the management of ascites, spontaneous bacterial peritonitis, and hepatorenal syndrome in cirrhosis. *J. Hepatol.*, 53 (2010), pp. 397–417.

[17] B.A. Runyon, AASLD. Introduction to the revised American Association for the Study of Liver Diseases Practice Guideline management of adult patients with ascites due to cirrhosis 2012. *Hepatology,* 57 (2013), pp. 1651–1653.

[18] Infectious diseases; The Clinician's Guide to Diagnosis, *Treatment and Prevention.* 2011.

[19] Singh S, Khardori NM.Intra-abdominal and pelvic emergencies. *Med. Clin. North Am.* 2012 Nov;96(6):1171-91.

[20] Cho Y, Lee HS et al. High-sensitivity C-reactive Protein Level is an Independent Predictor of Poor Prognosis in Cirrhotic Patients With Spontaneous Bacterial Peritonitis. *J. Clin. Gastroenterol.* 2013 Sep 16.

[21] Cekin Y, Cekin AH, Duman A, Yilmaz U, Yesil B, Yolcular BO. The role of serum procalcitonin levels in predicting ascitic fluid infection in hospitalized cirrhotic and non-cirrhotic patients. *Int. J. Med. Sci.* 2013 Aug 20;10(10):1367-74.

[22] Burri E, Schulte F, Muser J, Meier R, Beglinger C. Measurement of calprotectin in ascitic fluid to identify elevated polymorphonuclear cell count. *World J. Gastroenterol.* 2013 Apr 7;19(13):2028-36.

[23] Tsung PC, Ryu SH, Cha IH, Cho HW, Kim JN, Kim YS, Moon JS. Predictive factors that influence the survival rates in liver cirrhosis patients with spontaneous bacterial peritonitis. *Clin. Mol. Hepatol.* 2013 Jun;19(2):131-9.

[24] Wilcox CM, Dismukes WE. Spontaneous bacterial peritonitis: a review of pathogenesis, diagnosis and treatment. *Medicine* (Baltimore). 1987;66:447-456.

[25] Hasnain M Jafferbhoy1, Michael H Miller1,W Gashau1 et al. Spontaneous bacterial peritonitis prophylaxis in the era of healthcare associated infection. *Gut.* 2012 Mar 22.

[26] Alexopoulou A, Papadopoulos N, Eliopoulos DG, Alexaki A, Tsiriga A, Toutouza M, Pectasides D. Increasing frequency of gram-positive cocci and gram-negative multidrug-resistant bacteria in spontaneous bacterial peritonitis. *Liver. Int.* 2013 Aug;33(7):975-81.

[27] Rimola A, García-Tsao G, Navasa M, Piddock LJ, Planas R, Bernard B, Inadomi JM. Diagnosis, treatment and prophylaxis of spontaneous bacterial peritonitis: a consensus document. International Ascites Club. *J. Hepatol.* 2000 Jan;32(1):142-53.

[28] Ariza X, Castellote J, Lora-Tamayo J, Girbau A, Salord S, Rota R, Ariza J, Xiol X. Risk factors for resistance to ceftriaxone and its impact on mortality in community, healthcare and nosocomial spontaneous bacterial peritonitis. *J. Hepatol.* 2012 Apr;56(4):825-32.

[29] Nicole Ming-Ming Loo, Fernanda Fernandes Souza, Guadalupe Garcia-Tsao. Non-hemorrhagic acute complications associated with cirrhosis and portal hypertension. Best Practice & Research Clinical Gastroenterology Volume 27, Issue 5 2013 665 - 678

[30] Yahav D, Lador A, Paul M, Leibovici L. Efficacy and safety of tigecycline: a systematic review and meta-analysis. *J. Antimicrob. Chemother.* 2011;66:1963–1971.

[31] Runyon BA, McHutchison JG, Antillon MR, et al. Short-course versus long-course antibiotic treatment of spontaneous bacterial peritonitis: a randomized controlled study of 108 patients. *Gastroenterology.* 1991;100:1737-1742

[32] Follo A, Llovet JM, Navasa M, Planas R, Forns X, Francitorra A, Rimola A, Gassull MA, Arroyo V, Rodés J. Renal impairment after spontaneous bacterial peritonitis in cirrhosis: incidence, clinical course, predictive factors and prognosis. *Hepatology.* 1994;20:1495–1501.

[33] Sort P, Navasa M, Arroyo V, Aldeguer X, Planas R, Ruiz-del-Arbol L, Castells L, Vargas V, Soriano G, Guevara M, et al. Effect of intravenous albumin on renal impairment and mortality in patients with cirrhosis and spontaneous bacterial peritonitis. *N. Engl. J. Med.* 1999;341:403–409.

[34] Rimola A, Navasa M. Infections in liver disease. *Oxford Textbook of Clinical Hepatology. 2nd* ed. 1999. pp. 1861–1876.

[35] Hanouneh MA, Hanouneh IA, Hashash JG, Law R, Esfeh JM, Lopez R, Hazratjee N, Smith T, Zein NN. The role of rifaximin in the primary prophylaxis of spontaneous

bacterial peritonitis in patients with liver cirrhosis. *J. Clin. Gastroenterol.* 2012 Sep;46(8):709-15.

[36] Kalambokis GN, Mouzaki A, Rodi M, Tsianos EV. Rifaximin for the prevention of spontaneous bacterial peritonitis. *World J. Gastroenterol.* 2012 Apr 14;18(14):1700-2.

In: Advances in Medicine and Biology. Volume 77
Editor: Leon V. Berhardt

ISBN: 978-1-63117-444-5
© 2014 Nova Science Publishers, Inc.

Chapter 3

IL-7 in Rheumatoid Arthritis: Pathogenesis, Biomarker and Rationale for Anti-IL-7 Therapy

Frederique Ponchel[1,], Ph.D., Agata Burska[1], Ph.D., Effie Myrthianou[2], Ph.D., and George Goulielmos[2], Asst. Prof.*
[1]Leeds Institute of Rheumatic and Musculoskeletal Medicine & Leeds Musculoskeletal Biomedical Research Unit, The University of Leeds, Leeds, UK
[2]Molecular Medicine and Human Genetics Section, Department of Medicine, University of Crete, Heraklion, Greece

Abstract

Rheumatoid arthritis (RA) is a chronic disease primarily affecting the joints and producing marked inflammatory changes in the synovial membrane and adjacent structures. Although any joint can be affected the disease normally affects the hands, feet, knees and wrists. Disease activity and the rate of progression to involve new joints are variable. The pain and disability associated represent a real burden both for the patients and society and the disease is also associated with premature mortality [1, 2].

There is currently no cure for RA. Historically, treatments which deplete T-cells led to reduction of symptoms supporting the notion of a T cell mediated disease. Today, the pathology is thought to be the product of a series of complex cellular interactions where synovial T-cells orchestrate disease through their interaction with fibroblasts, B-cells, dendritic cells, and macrophages. Modern treatment options include the use of "biological" drugs, which block cytokines such as TNF alpha, IL-1, IL-6, limit co-stimulation between B and T-cells or deplete B-cells. Although their use bring great benefit, a wide range of adverse events have been reported (including infections, cancer, vasculitis, lupus-like and multiple sclerosis, liver disease, hematologic abnormalities (such as aplastic anemia, lymphoma) and aseptic meningitis). In addition resistance to these agents or loss of response, relapse on cessation of treatment, side effects occurs in more than 40% of patients. The cost of these therapies is also major pitfall.

* Corresponding author: Dr. Frederique Ponchel, Email: mmefp@leeds.ac.uk.

The complex cellular interactions in the synovium between stromal cells, T-cells and their subsequent effect on B-cells, macrophages and endothelial cells provide a large panel of alternative targets, both cellular and molecular, for therapeutic intervention in RA. Inhibiting cytokines signalling has proven successful and we (and others) hypothesise that IL-7 may be an appropriate therapeutic target in RA as well as in several other autoimmune diseases. The main rational for targeting IL-7 is that it is (i) over expressed specifically at the disease site, however only in active disease, (ii) not capable of exiting the joint (due to its retention and presentation by extra-cellular matrix) (iii) produced by local resident cells with no mobility (i.e. fibroblasts). In addition, low levels of circulating IL-7 in RA patients suggest that efficient inhibition of IL-7 signalling may only take place in the joint. The role of IL-7 in the disease itself is slowly being dissected and will be reviewed to support this statement.

Abbreviation List

ACPA- anti-citrullinated-peptide antibody
AP1- activator protein 1
ATK- Protein Kinase B
Bcl2- B-cell lymphoma 2
BM-Bone marrow
CD3, 4, 28, 127- cluster of differentiation 3, 4, 28 and 127
CDC25- Cell division cycle 25 phosphatase
CIA- collagen induced arthritis
DAS44- Disease activity score 44 MTX- methotrexate
DCs-dendritic cells
DM1- Diabetes mellitus type 1
DMARD- Disease-modifying anti-rheumatic drugs
EAE- experimental autoimmune encephalomyelitis
ELISA- enzyme-linked immunosorbent assay
GATA1,3 - transcription factors binding "GATA" sequence of DNA
GCs-germinal centres
HLA- Human leukocyte antigens
IFN-gamma- Interferon gamma
IHC-Immunohistochemistry
IL-1,4,5,6,7,11,12,17,23- interleukins 1,4,5,6,7,11,12,17and 23
IL-12R- Interleukin 12 receptor
IL-7R- Interleukin 7 receptor (membrane-bound form)
IMID- Immune mediated inflammatory diseases
IRF1,2,3,7- Interferon regulatory factor 1,2,3 and 7
JAK3- Janus kinase 3
JIA-Juvenile Idiopatic Arthritis
KGF- keratinocyte growth factor
LN-lymph nodes
MBP- myelin basic protein
MHC- Major Histocompatibility Complex
MMP9- Matrix metalloproteinase 9

MS-multiple sclerosis

NFAT- Nuclear factor of activated T-cells

NOD- non-obese diabetic mice

OA-osteoarthritis

p38- p38 mitogen-activated protein kinase

PHA- Phytohaemagglutinin

Pi3K- Phosphoinositide 3-kinase

RANK- Receptor activator of nuclear factor kappa-B

RANKL- Receptor activator of nuclear factor kappa-B ligand

RA-Rheumatoid arthritis

sIL-2R- soluble interleukin 2 receptor

sIL-7R- soluble interleukin-7 receptor

SLE- systemic lupus erythomatosus

SMAD3,4 - small mother against decapentaplegic (MAD) homolog

SNP- single nucleotide polymorphism

STAT3,5- Signal Transducer and Activator of Transcription 3 and 5

TA -tissue architecture

TGF-beta1- Transforming growth factor beta 1

Th1- T helper 1cells

Th17- T helper 17 cells

Th2- T helper 2 cells

TNF alpha- tumour necrosis factor alpha,

Treg- regulatory T-cells

VAS- visual analog scale

VCAM-1- vascular cell adhesion molecule

vWF- Von Willebrand factor

Introduction

Interleukin 7 (IL-7) has emerged as an important factor in the development of autoimmune diseases when a possible role in enhancing reactivity to self-antigens was proposed while levels of IL-7 were increased in response to lymphopenia and may predispose to the development of autoimmunity [3]. Animal models and human studies provided further evidence that IL-7 is involved in perpetuating autoimmune inflammation.

Immune mediated inflammatory diseases (IMID) represent a vast number of disorders of which Rheumatoid Arthritis (RA) is the most prominent affecting approximately 1% of the population. RA is a chronic disease primarily affecting the joints and producing marked inflammatory changes in the synovial membrane and adjacent structures resulting in severe disability and reduced life expectancy [1, 2]. Although any joint can be affected the disease normally affects the hands, feet, knees and wrists. Disease activity and the rate of progression to involve new joints are variable. For some, the disease is mild with little or no progression but for many the disease is progressive with the involvement of new joints within months. The pain and the disability associated with the disease can affect an individual's ability to carry out everyday tasks. The disease may not be confined to the joints and surrounding tissues but become systemic, involving extra-articular tissues throughout the body including the skin, blood vessels, heart, lungs and muscles. Many of those with RA also suffer from anaemia either as a consequence of the disease itself or following gastrointestinal bleeding as a side effect of drugs, especially non-steroidal anti-inflammatory agents used for analgesia. The long-term prognosis for sufferers is poor with severe disability reported in approximately 80% of patients after 20 years.

The exact pathogenesis of RA remains uncertain, however, autoimmune processes are known to play a role as evidenced by Major Histocompatibility Complex (MHC) linkage [4, 5], autoantibody production (with novel specificity recently identified) [6] and lymphocyte infiltration in synovial tissue [7, 8]. These features supported the hypothesis of a T-cell driven disease which was developed in the late 80s [9-11] and following the demonstration that the main genetic risk associated with RA was associated with T-cells related genes, recently regained considerable interest [12] considering the interplay between T-cell activation and immune suppression (naturally occurring regulatory T-cells (Treg)). In addition, immune dysfunctions related to IL-7 are present in RA patients [13-15], some identified by our group [16-19].

1. Evidence for Genetic Association in RA with IL-7 Axis

a. Genetic Studies in Autoimmune Diseases

The IL-7/IL-7R pathway has recently been implicated in large-scale genetic studies. IL-7R is one of the novel putative autoimmune susceptibility loci that was recently associated with multiple autoimmune diseases. Particularly, polymorphisms in *IL7R (alpha subunit)* gene, encoding the specific subunit of the IL7R, were found to be associated with an increased risk of developing multiple sclerosis [20, 21], sarcoidosis [22], ulcerative colitis [23], rheumatoid arthritis [24], type 1 diabetes [25] and primary biliary cirrhosis [26].

All individual nucleotide polymorphisms (SNPs) in the *IL-7R* locus, which have been associated with autoimmunity, are in strong linkage disequilibrium with rs6897932, a functional SNP located in exon 6 of *IL-7R* gene. This is a non-synonymous SNP (corresponding to a rs6897932*C or rs6897932*T genotype) affecting whether amino acid 244 is transcribed as a threonine or an isoleucine, thus. The rs6897932 SNP has a functional effect on protein expression by influencing the amount of soluble (sIL-7R) and membrane-bound (IL-7R) isoforms of the receptor, through a disruption of an exonic splicing silencer.

The SNP rs6897932 of the *IL-7R* gene was first associated with susceptibility to multiple sclerosis (MS) independently confirmed in various studies [20, 21, 27-32]. Although, it is worth noting that in a study conducted in Norway no association between the SNP rs6897932 and MS was found [33]. The rs6897932 SNP was suggested to explain only 0.2% of the variance in the risk of development of MS [34]. A genome-wide analysis offered evidence of Diabetes type 1 (DM1) association with the rs6897932 [25, 35] as well as showed evidence of DM1 association with rs3194051 SNP, another SNP in the *IL-7R* [25]. The frequency of TT-rs6897932 genotype was significantly reduced in the young patients and was confirmed to have protective effect [36]. In an analysis of 27 new ulcerative colitis risk loci, an increased susceptibility to the disease was found with the rs3194051 SNP of the *IL-7R* gene only but not to rs6897932 [23]. Finally, the same "C" allele of rs6897932 SNP was very recently associated with an increased risk for SLE [37]. Therefore, a modest influence on disease susceptibility appeared in most diseases studies so far, the overall data suggesting a possible role of the IL-7R polymorphism in the development of human autoimmune diseases.

In RA more specifically, an initial tendency for association of the rs6897932 SNP of *IL7R* gene was reported [24] followed by a few studies which did not achieve statistical significance at the corrected p-value threshold probably due to an inadequate power. Plant et al failed to detect any association of the same SNP with RA [38] but, Hinks et al [39] found a weak trend toward association of the same SNP with Juvenile Idiopathic Arthritis (JIA) probably because of the very low power (18%) of the study. In a study combining RA and JIA patients no allelic association was found between these diseases and any of the 13 SNPs analysed; however, an association between the diseases and the TT genotype of rs6897932 SNP appeared [40]. In various European RA patient's populations (Table 1, data kindly provided by our collaborators Prof Javier Martín Ibañez, Dr María Teruel form Spain, Prof Rene Toes, Dr FinaKurreeman from the Netherlands and Prof Jane Worthington, Dr Stephen Eyre from the UK) showed again low levels of significance for this particular SNP. Data form a Cretan population (provided by Dr Effie Myrthianou and Prof George Goulielmos (Greece)) also did not show particular association. Data in RA therefore appear quite negative across the range despite the initial association. An interesting observation was however made when refining the analysis to anti-citrullinated-peptide antibody (ACPA) negative disease in patients from the Netherlands (Table 1) although this was not verified in other populations.

Interestingly, the association detected in a few studies reporting association is RA patients was opposite to that seen in MS, associating the "C" allele (not the "T") with disease. If confirmed, these studies would substantiate diverging roles for the IL-7/IL-7RA axis in RA pathogenesis compared to other autoimmune disease.

b. Exploring the Functional Significance of the IL-7R-alpha rs6897932 Polymorphism

Numerous studies in several autoimmune diseases demonstrated an association between the *IL-7R* gene polymorphism and the development of the disease. However, the precise mechanism by which the SNP leads to altered risk has not been elucidated so far. A possible role of the rs6897932 SNP in the pathogenesis of MS has been suggested. This SNP may be involved in the alternative splicing of exon 6, which subsequently may have potential consequences for the function of the receptor [41]. SNP rs6897932 changes a threonine to isoleucine at amino acid position #244 and the disease-associated allele leads to decreased inclusion of exon 6 [20]. This exon codes for a transmembrane domain of the receptor [42]. When exon 6 is included splicing produces a membrane-bound isoform (IL-7R). A soluble isoform of the receptor (sIL-7R) results from alternative splicing where exon 6 is lacking [43, 44]. Both isoforms are able to bind IL-7 with high affinity [45, 46]. The presence of the SNP therefore results in a modified IL-7R/ sIL7R ratio [20, 28, 47]. As a consequence, IL-7 levels were significantly decreased in MS patients compared with healthy individuals, while levels of the soluble sIL-7R were increased in patients with the C (risk) allele of the rs6897932 SNP [31, 48]. Moreover, the higher mRNA levels of both IL-7R and IL-7 detected in the cerebrospinal fluid of patients with MS compared to those found in non-inflammatory neurological diseases, emphasizes the putative involvement of IL-7/IL-7R in the pathogenesis of MS [27].

Table 1. IL7R SNP rs6897932 form different European cohorts

Population	group	MAF (controls)	n Cases	n Controls	effect estimate/ OR	95% CI	p-value	regression/ association	method
UK* [156]	RA	0.29	3943	3505	0.91	0.84-0.97	0.007	association	GWA
Northern Ireland [40]	RA+JIA	0.264	532	368	1.19	0.96-1.46	0.110	association	GWA
UK [39]	JIA	0.29	943	3505	0.90	0.80-1.01	0.060	association	GWA
Spanish	total		838	1940	1.039	0.91-1.19	0.572	logistic (additive)	immunochip
	ACPA+	0.2597			1.097	0.92-1.29	0.2783		
	ACPA-				1.037	0.83-1.28	0.7436		
English	ACPA+	0.2719	2406	8430	0.9991	0.92-1.074	0.9803	logistic regression	immunochip
	ACPA-		1000	8430	0.966	0.86-1.075	0.5248		
Dutch	total		648	1085	1.146	0.98-1.33	0.083	logistic (additive)	immunochip
	ACPA+	0.2654	332	1085	0.9904	0.81-1.21	0.923		
	ACPA-		330	1085	1.275	1.04-1.56	0.016		
Greek (Crete)	total	0.18	600	600	1.028	0.83-1.26	0.79	association	TaqMann

* Another SNP in the IL-7 was also showing association.

In RA, levels of IL-7 are also reduced however, in absence of clear association with the rs6897932 SNP, an alternative mechanism may be responsible for this reduction. As such, increased expression of the sIL-7R was associated with direct stimulation of pro-inflammatory cytokine on the IL-7R gene promoter [49, 50].

2. Regulation of IL-7 Expression

The regulation of IL-7 expression is not fully elucidated and is likely to be cell-type specific. Loops in cytokine networks of regulation are probably involved. To date, one transcriptional mechanism has been well characterised but post-transcriptional regulation may also be relevant. INF-gamma is a known positive regulator of IL-7 [51] whereas TGF-beta1 is a negative regulator [52]. Both the mouse and human IL-7 promoters have been sequenced and present large region of high homology. They are unusual promoters, lacking definitive initiation signals (such as TATA box). Transcriptional initiation is nevertheless highly regulated and different regions of the promoter are used to nucleate a transcriptional machinery complex (transcriptional initiators) [51, 53]. These are either used for spontaneous expression or in response to IFN-gamma. Response to INF-gamma, TGF-beta1 and other stimuli use transcription factors such as IRF1,2,3,7; SMAD3,4 or NFAT, AP1, GATA1,3. TGF-beta1 and IL-7 actually share a close reciprocal relationship where one is capable of down-regulating the other at the mRNA level [52, 54]. We exemplified this close relationship at the protein levels following therapeutic lymphodepletion in cancer patients and importantly showed that it is lost in RA [55]. Further regulation has been established in response to TNF-alpha [56] and by the keratinocyte growth factor (KGF) [57] or IL-6 [58].

3. IL-7 and RA

a. IL-7 Expression in the Joint

IL-7 is highly expressed in the joints of RA patients [15, 59, 60] in contrast to the circulation where levels are reduced compared to health [61, 62]. IL-7 was consistently detected in the synovial fluid and tissue of RA patients in higher amounts compare to a non-inflammatory form of arthritis, osteoarthritis (OA) [15, 59]. In the RA synovial membrane IL-7 expression was also reported in the late 1990s as an activator of cells now identified as osteoclasts [56, 59, 63, 64]. IL-7 is known to be expressed by stromal cells (bone marrow (BM), thymus, soft tissue), epithelial cells (liver, gut), endothelial cells, fibroblasts, smooth muscle cells and keratinocytes but not by immune cells with the exception of dendritic cells (DCs) however, only following activation [65-70]. Accordingly, its' expression was not detected in synovial immune cells (T, B or macrophages) but mRNA was found in RA chondrocytes, but not in OA [63, 71]. Immunohistochemistry (IHC) analysis associated IL-7 expression with one of the OMERACT biomarkers [15], an antibody clone which reacts with several cell types (macrophages and fibroblasts) [72] and is a surrogate measure of disease activity [73]. We also showed that the expression of IL-7 in the synovium of patients was directly related to a measure of local inflammation (Arthroscopic VAS) [60] and was lowered when they went into remission [60]. Expression was however difficult to analyse due to heterogeneity of the patterns. Some tissues showed diffuse, "patchy" expression with scattered positive single cells and other showed more consistent staining around blood vessels or associated with lymphocyte aggregates and more complex tissue architecture (Figure 1). The expression of IL-7 in RA tissue was therefore associated with fibroblasts and endothelial cells but was also largely extracellular [74].

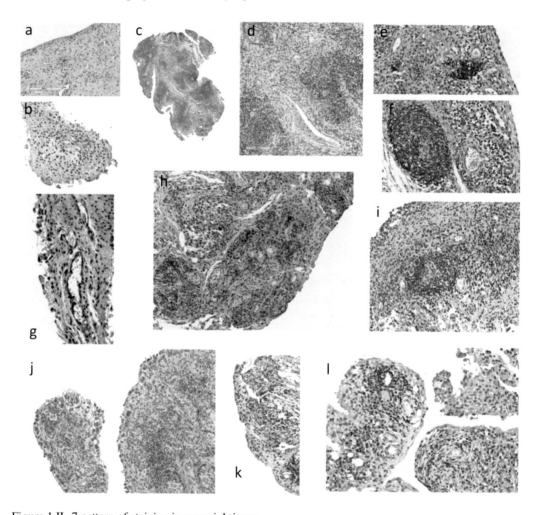

Figure 1.IL-7 pattern of staining in synovial tissue.

Paraffin embedded sections were cut from RA synovial biopsies, dewaxed (Access Super solution Menarini diagnostics), then stained using standard protocols (X-Cell plus staining kit, Menarini diagnostics), blocking solution, HRP reagent and 3, 3'-Diaminobenzidine (DAB) and counterstained in haematoxylin. The primary antibody anti- IL7 was a mouse monoclonal (R&D labs MAB207 1: 200 dilution) a) and b) isotype control. c) Low magnification view of a biopsy with staining surrounding lymphocyte aggregates). Higher magnification of IL-7 positive region surrounding lymphocyte d,e,f,i,h) blood vessel, g) blood vessel endothelium staining, j,k) positive and negative lining layer staining.

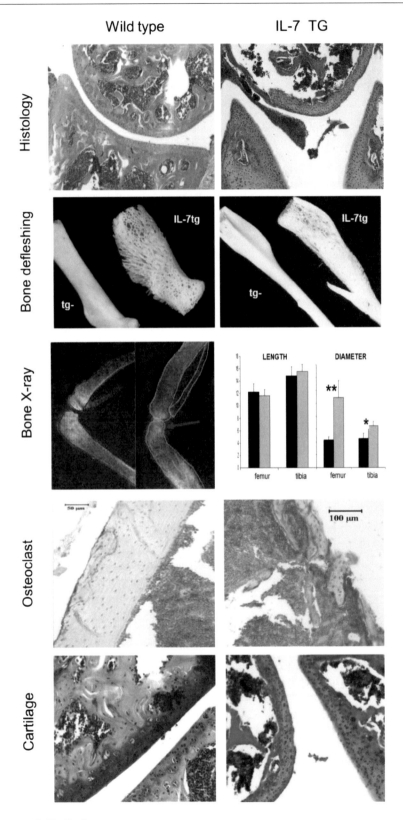

Figure 2.Transgenic IL-7 mice.

Thanks to a gift from Dr Daniela Finke, we were able to examine mouse legs from a transgenic IL-7/CIITA mouse (TG), which has been shown to have elevated basal levels of IL-7 in all tissues. Histology (H&E) staining of the paw showed inflammatory infiltrate in TG mice (right) and an outgrowth of the synovial membrane compared to the wild type (WT) littermates. In the TG mice cartilage surface damage was also observed. Upon dissection, clear phenotypic differences were observed in the femur and tibia of the TG mice compared to the WT. Following further and boiling, the femur and tibia of the TG mice lacked a smooth cortical bone and were spongy in nature. X-ray analysis demonstrated disorganised bone architecture within the femur and proximal tibia of TG mice. X-rays of the TG mice also proved a narrowing of the joint cavity (red arrow). TG mice had a similar bone length but a significantly greater bone diameter in the femur and tibia than WT mice. Osteoblast and osteoclast activity was analysed using alkaline phosphatase and tartrate resistant acid phosphatase (TRAP) methods. Histological analysis verified that the bone architecture was disorganised, with little compact cortical bone and the bone marrow cavity was exposed to the surrounding muscle and large numbers of osteoblasts and osteoclasts throughout the bone architecture. Larger numbers of osteoclasts were noted in TG bones compared to WT littermates Fast Green/Safranin 'O' staining was used to examine cartilage. Articular surface was damaged and lower Safranin 'O' staining, indicative of lower proteoglycan content, was evident in cartilage of TG mice compared to WT littermates. Fast Green/Safranin 'O' staining also confirmed that the bone architecture was disorganised with little compact cortical bone and trabecular bone invading the marrow cavity in the TG micef.

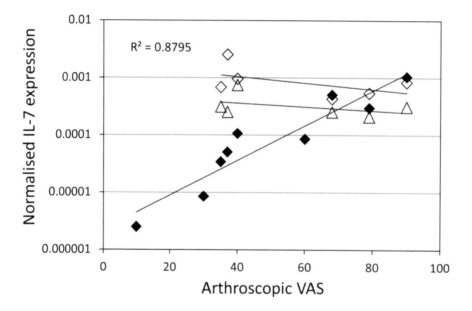

Figure 3. Synovial IL-7 mRNA expression.

 Synovial biopsy were digested and cell grown in tissue culture for 3 passages (157). Cell cultures were then stimulated with IFN-gamma or TNF-alpha for 8 hours. RNA was extracted and IL-7 mRNA measured using qPCR (55) as previously described (158). The direct relationship between IL-7 mRNA expression and local levels of inflammation measure during arthroscopic knee inspection (VAS) is displaued (black diamonds, n=9, rho=0.937 p<0.0001) (55). Stimulation with IFN-gamma (open diamonds) or TNF-alpha (open triangles) increased the levels of IL-7 expression to its maximum however no more than what *in vivo* exposure to high levels of inflammation would have produced.

Using a transgenic IL-7 mice model whereby IL-7 expression is increased in all but particularly in stromal cells (generous gift of Prof Danielle Finke, Zurich, Switzerland) we investigated the effect of increased IL-7 expressing in joints (Figure 2). Histology analysis revealed infiltration in the transgenic mice, absent in the WT, suggesting that the mere presence of more IL-7 in the synovial membrane was sufficient to create an environment allowing tissue infiltration by lymphocytes.

The regulation of IL-7 expression in the synovial tissue however remains elusive. Primary cells from RA biopsy expressed more IL-7 mRNA in RA compared with OA [59]. Synovial fibroblasts grown from RA biopsies spontaneously produce detectable amounts of IL-7 at both the transcriptional and protein levels [59]. In synovial fibroblast cultures from RA patients this effect was directly dependent on *in vivo* exposure to local levels of inflammation (measured during arthroscopic joint inspection) at the time of tissues resection [55] importantly demonstrating an effect maintained over 3 passage in culture.

Expression in expanded synovial fibroblasts was significantly increased by stimulation with different cytokines such as TNF and IL-1 [59]. We confirmed these data and further showed that maximum stimulation was achieved in all cultures independently of the degree of previous activation of IL-7 expression in relation with inflammation (Figure 3). In contrast, TGF-beta-1 and 3 had lost their inhibiting activity in these synovial fibroblast cultures compared to BM cells (data not shown).

b. IL-7 in the Circulation

The discrepancy between low systemic but high synovial expression has been difficult to explain and has brought confusion. Therefore the idea that RA can co-exist as a systemic and a synovial disease is attractive [75]. The origin of circulating IL-7 remains to be fully elucidated. Several tissues including the BM, lymph node, skin, gut and liver are all capable of producing IL-7. Under normal conditions, IL-7 was thought to be released from stromal cells in lymphoid organs, although this was not formally proven. Furthermore, IL-7 expressed in tissue is presented at the surface of stromal cells by extracellular matrix protein (fibronectin and heparan sulphate) [76-78] and signal in a cell-to-cell fashion. These potential tissue origins are therefore unlikely to be the source of circulating IL-7 with the exception of the liver which is capable of producing large amount of protein when needed. Recent data demonstrated that indirect TLR-ligand activation of an unknown cell intermediate, promoted IL-7 production from hepathocytes using IFN-gamma as mediator [79]. Our own experiments [55] confirmed that primary BM stromal cells and hepathocyte cultures, liver and colon cell lines, synovial fibroblast from RA and OA patients but not skin fibroblasts all spontaneously produced IL-7 and released additional amounts (3–30 fold) when stimulated with IFN-gamma, but only synovial fibroblast when stimulated with TNF-alpha and IL-1beta.

Following lymphodepletion, a prolonged CD4+T-cell lymphopenia is observed in RA patients [80-82]. We showed that the thymus in RA patients has a similar reserve to that of disease controls (solid tissue cancer patients and RA patients in clinical remission) although, thymic rebound response to lymphopenia is delayed in RA by several months or does not occur [61]. This was associated with a reduced amount of BM expression of IL-7 available to support progenitors and by extension low thymic IL-7 and absence of *de novo* mature T-cell generation. Furthermore we showed an absence of circulating IL-7 rebound in response to lymphopenia and no homeostatic proliferation of T-cells, notably CD4+T-cells. The mechanism that controls IL-7 levels in the circulation remain unknown but several hypotheses have been proposed to explain how IL-7 in turn controls T-cell homeostasis. IL-7 controls a key-molecular point between two pathways: survival (JAK3/STAT5/Bcl2) and cell cycle progression (p38/CDC25) as well as provides energy to sustain these critical cellular activities (Pi3K/ATK/metabolism) [83]. In the absence of external control over the levels of circulating IL-7, the rate of IL-7 consumption by T-cells determines its levels [84]. IL-7 and T-cells are in equilibrium most of the time. When T-cells are depleted (due to disease or therapy) they will encounter abundant IL-7 leading to homeostatic proliferation. When T-cells proliferate (following activation), overconsumption of IL-7 will reduce its circulating levels and T-cells will die. The lack of rebound in circulating IL-7 in RA [61] does not support such a mechanism in this disease. Altruism has been proposed as an alternative hypothesis: some T-cells having satisfied their IL-7 need to survive and proliferate will abstain from consuming IL-7 by down-regulating their expression of CD127/IL-7R in turn allowing other T-cells to acquire IL-7 signalling [85, 86]. No changes in levels of IL-7R expression on T-cells (detected by flow-cytometry) were found following therapeutic lymphodepletion (F Ponchel unpublished observations) to support this hypothesis. We proposed a possible role for TGF-beta as a negative regulator of IL-7 [55]; however we have not been able to verify this proposition in RA patients. The most promising hypothesis may however be that levels of circulating IL-7 are regulated through a decoy sIL-7R. Circulating sIL-7R is expressed as an active regulation of alternative splicing of the IL-7 mRNA rather than through cell surface shedding [45]. The affinity of IL-7 is equivalent for both forms of receptor. Inflammatory cytokines such as IL-17 and TNF-alpha synergise to increase the expression of IL-7 as well as IL-7R in synovial fibroblast (personal communication from Prof Pierre Miossec, gene expression microarray). Neutralization of IL-7 by its sIL-7R may therefore represent an important level of regulation. A similar role for the sIL-2R has long been recognised in RA [87, 88] and investigation need to be performed as it was reported at the American College of Rheumatology annual conference in 2011 that sIL-7R levels are high in SLE [49], and furthermore, that inflammation triggers the expression of the sIL-7R by fibroblasts [89]. Available ELISA for the IL-7 protein recognize full length IL-7 (as well as 2 shorter forms of the protein [90]) but are not able to make the difference between free IL-7 and IL-7/sIL-7R complexes. An ELISA for the sIL-7R has now been developed (Human sIL-7R ELISA Kit, CUSABIO) and it need to be used to investigate if this is indeed the mechanism by which inflammation may exert some control over IL-7 levels in the circulation.

c. IL-7 Effect on T-Cells

The ability of IL-7 to affect synovial T-cells in RA was examined a long time ago and compared to the effect of IL-7 on circulating T-cells [59]. Purified synovial macrophages and T-cell did not spontaneously released IL-7 in contrast to fibroblasts. The proliferation of synovial tissue T-cells from RA patients was stimulated by IL-7 however less than by IL-15 another cytokine of the same family. CD4+ T-cells and macrophages isolated from SF were hyper-responsive to IL-7 when compared with peripheral blood cells [15] but IL7-stimulated lymphocyte responses were not inhibited by TNF-alpha blockade [91]. The cell-cell contact dependent activation of T-cells by macrophages was also enhanced by IL-7, resulting in IL-7 driven expression of TNF-alpha from such co-cultures [91]. IL7 and TNF-alpha levels in RA synovial fluid and synovial tissue were therefore directly correlated.

Considering the role of IL-7 driving the Th1/Th2 balance [92-94] it was hypothesized that IL-7 may affect such balance in the RA synovium [14]. Naïve circulating CD4+ T-cells stimulated by CD3/CD28 in the presence of IL-7 spontaneously produced twice as much IFN-gamma but little more IL-4. Stimulation under Th2 polarisation conditions (in the presence of IL-4) did reduced slightly the production of IFN-gamma but Th2 polarisation in the presence of IL-7 abolished the Th1 bias [14]. Synovial T-cells stimulated with IL-7 produced twice as much TNF-alpha and IL-4 but 3 time more IFN-gamma showing clear Th1 engagement and little effect on Th2 [13]. The activity of IL-7 was mediated by induction of the IL-12R expression for Th1 polarisation (IFN-gamma) but not for Th2 or the pro-inflammatory activation of T-cells (TNF-alpha).

Prolonged and profound CD4+T-cell lymphopenia is a hallmark of RA patients treated with different lymphocyte-depleting therapy [95-97] and we showed that poor reconstitution result from a lack of IL-7 mediated homeostatic proliferation as well as poor progenitor support and thymic rebound [61]. The response of RA patients circulating CD4+ T-cells to IL-7 was not different to that of healthy control; however it is the absence of IL-7 rebound itself that appears to be the main limiting factor in the BM and thymus for the generation of new T-cells and in the circulation for the lack of homeostatic proliferation.

Taking advantage of a remission RA clinic where 50% of patients achieving clinical remission also recovered normal levels of circulating IL-7 [61], we examined the fine-tuning role that IL-7 exerts on T-cells in the circulation (activation and regulation) and compared it with exogenously provided IL-7 mimicking the situation in the joint [98]. Reduced levels of circulating IL-7 [61] probably underlie the dysfunctions associated with circulating T-cells in RA as evidenced by the direct relationship between circulating levels of IL-7 and T-cell responses to stimuli such PHA, CD3/CD28 as well as recall antigen [60] and may provide a mechanism for some of the anergic characteristics of T-cells in the disease. Similarly, synovial regulatory T-cell were affected by the presence of IL-7 in RA [99] and suppression in the presence of IL-7 was shown to be abolished [100-102]. We confirmed these findings in RA [98]. In contrast the effect of additional stimulation provided by IL-7 (like in the joint) had the potential to modify T-cells' role towards sustaining the vicious circle, enhancing proliferation and responsiveness to stimulation, altogether contributing to perpetuating inflammation [98].

d. IL-7 and Cellular Networking

Analysis at the disease sites (synovium) may actually provide additional information. The cellular composition of rheumatoid synovial membrane is relatively consistent amongst patients including resident cells, fibroblasts, macrophages and endothelial cells. The inflammatory cell infiltrate consists mostly of T and B-cells, dendritic cells (DCs) and plasma cells. Any direct effect of IL-7 on B-cells is unlikely as human B-cells do not express the IL-7R which was confirmed on RA synovial B-cells [103]. Monocytes in RA were shown to express high levels of IL-7R [104] possibly closing a loop between TNF and IL-7 co-activation with fibroblasts in relation with chronic inflammation.

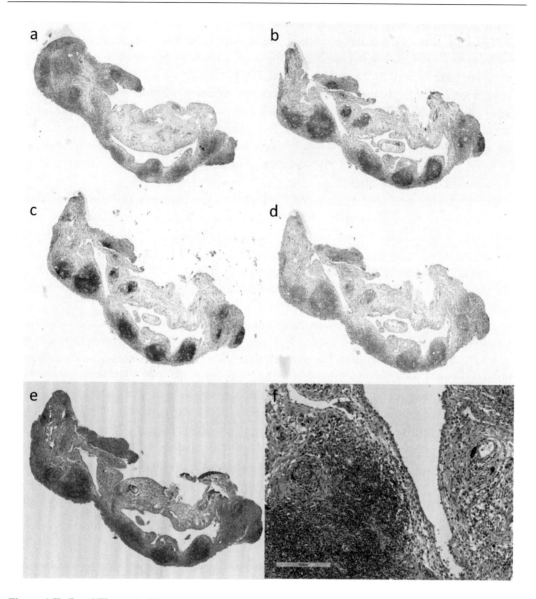

Figure 4.IL-7 and Tissue Architecture.

A synovial biopsy with clear TA including GCL structure (a) (H&E) was stained with anti IL-7 (e and f) and lineage marker (as described in figure 1) using (b) anti CD3 (rabbit monoclonal clone SP7 Abcam ab16669, 1:200) (c) anti CD20 (M-20 Goat polyclonal Santa Cruz sc-7735, 1:200) and (d) anti CD68 (Rat monoclonal Abcam ab53444,1:100).

The tissue architecture (TA) of the synovial membrane in RA is complex and sometimes highly organized. A diffuse infiltration in which T cells, B cells and macrophages are scattered among resident fibroblasts with no higher level of organization is observed in a third of tissues [8]. In the remaining patients, B and T cells organize themselves into defined structures: lymphoid aggregates formed around blood vessels, or structures showing clear features of ectopic formation of lymphoid tissue germinal centres (GCs) (Figure 4), with separated T- and B -cell zones, [105, 106]. Colocalisation of IL-7 with T-cells but interestingly also with B-cells was observed in the RA synovium [74]. Therefore, the hypothesis that IL-7 can orchestrate the synovial cellular network leading to chronic inflammation and joint destruction was put forward [60]. IL-7 stimulation of DC *in vitro* results in their DC1 polarisation and IL-7 also induce the expression of IL-12R on T-cells [92]. Whether synovial IL-7 can activate local DC in RA remains to be investigated.

The role of IL-7 in the formation of lymph nodes (LN) and Peyer's patch has long been known (for review see [107, 108]) in addition to a critical role in driving T-cell homeostasis in LN [109]. No evidence of a sequential relationship with time or location between these different forms of TA has been reported. Similar structures were identified in several other IMID (Crohn's disease, multiple sclerosis, gastritis, hepatitis, thyroiditis and Sjorgren's syndrome). Gene expression analysis in RA synovial tissue, confirmed IL-7 signalling to be highly associated with structures resembling GCs [74].

e. IL-7 and Bone in RA

IL-7 is a recognised regulator of bone turnover (for review see [110]). Bone mass results from a complex equilibrium between bone formation (activation of osteoblasts) and resorption (activation of osteoclasts), the later mediated by IL-7 [56, 111]. IL-7 deficient mice present a significant increase in bone mass [112], which is directly related to the absence of IL-7-driven expression of RANK ligand (RANKL) by T-cells [56]. On the other hand, a clear bone mass deficit is associated with over expression of IL-7 and such transgenic IL-7 mice are usually unable to survive very long in addition to other immune phenotype [110, 113]. Using the IL-7 transgenic mice model (see above), we confirmed that bone shape was altered in these animals (Figure 2) associated with evidence of reduced thickness of bone and increased presence of osteoclasts, further associated with cartilage proteoglycan loss. This was also observed in collagen induced arthritis where the intra-peritoneal administration of IL-7 exacerbated arthritis leading to a more severe destructive phenotype [114]. The mechanism by which Il-7 mediate this bone destruction has been related to stromal cells expression of IL-7, enhancing the expression of RANKL by T-cells and inducing the differentiation of CD14 monocytes into multi-nucleated, giant, bone-resorbing, tartrate resistant acid phosphatase (TRAP)-positive cells [115].

4. IL-7 as Biomarker in RA

We previously reviewed existing data published for the detection of IL-7 [60]. It is not one of cytokines known to need particular pre-analytical precautions during blood collection (related to stress, cachexia, diurnal rhythm or diet, delay in possessing, storage temperature (-20 acceptable) and 1 to 2 freeze thaw cycle) that may influence its measurement; although there are several ELISAs and other types of assay (cytometric beads assay or Luminex assay) commercially available. Importantly, levels of IL-7 reported in 17 publications in healthy controls using 5 different kits were quite similar (reviewed in [60]). In RA however, the use of multiplex Luminex beads assay yielded false positive results as this method is sensitive to heterophilic antibody interferences such as RF [116, 117].

a. Diagnostic

We demonstrated [62] that low serum IL-7 can identify patients with very early inflammatory joint symptoms who will progress to RA over the next 2 years (sensitivity 30% and specificity 83%, independently of ACPA status) using a cut-off value of 10 pg/mL. Our data also suggested that IL-7 would be the second best diagnostic biomarker of RA after ACPA however, it was the best one for the sub-group of ACPA(-) patients for which such novel biomarker is of utter most importance.

One of the issues discussed in this original report of the IL-7 diagnostic potential [62] was the need to look into factors that can influence IL-7 measurements in addition to donor variability in both health and disease. Reports of the presence of sIL-7R responsible for reducing circulating levels of IL-7 in HIV-infected patients have recently been published [118, 119]. More work is ongoing to validate IL-7 as a diagnostic biomarker.

b. Prognostic

In patients with recent onset of joint inflammatory symptoms and a confirmed RA diagnosis, disease progression over the next 2 years (evaluated using an increase in DAS44-Ritchie at 1 and 2 year) was associated with ACPA(+) disease and longer symptom duration at baseline [62]. Using a different cut-off from diagnostic (upper quartile of the distribution >17.0 pg/ml), higher IL-7 levels at baseline were associated with low levels of disease activity (DAS<1.6) at 1 year. Using multivariate logistic regression, absence of disease progression was clearly associated with lack of reduction in IL-7 above ACPA-negativity (n=108) and was even more predictive in the ACPA(-) subgroup (n=67). A regression analysis of the development of novel erosion over 2 years, showed that only reduced levels of IL-7 (using a low level cut-off <10 pg/ml at baseline) was predictive.

The effect of TNF-alpha blockade on circulating IL7 levels was studied [91]. Baseline levels were not investigated with respect to prediction of response but IL7 levels were reduced in patients who successfully responded to anti-TNF-alpha treatment and persisted in non-responders. Our own data in early RA treated with methotrexate (MTX) or MTX combined with TNF-alpha blocking agent as 1st line treatment suggests that there is no predictive value for IL-7 at baseline with respect to response to treatment (n=50, p=0.749).

c. Remission and Relapse

In established RA, we have showed that circulating levels of IL-7 that remained low (<10pg/ml) in clinical remission on DMARDs (DAS<2.6), were predictive of relapse over the next 12 months [98]. In patients with early RA achieving remission on DMARDs pilot data suiggest that low IL-7 was also associated with relapse over the next 12 month (n=10, p=0.03). The main parameters allowing the prediction of safe discontinuation of anti-TNF drug was actually duration of disease before biologics treatment and T-cell subset phenotyping [120]. Nevertheless, lack of IL-7 recovery in established RA in clinical remission post anti-TNF treatment was again associated with relapse in the next few months (n=21, p=0.05); however in patients treated early, no difference in IL-7 levels were observed between those destined to relapse or not (n=14, p=0.533). The absence of IL-7 recovery in clinical remission could indicate low levels of disease activity, however we could not establish any relationship between IL-7 levels and residual disease activity using advanced ultrasound and MR imaging technique [121, 122]. Further associations with smoking and early disease onset were also observed and discussed [98], notably as associations between IL-7 and smoking have been reported but the mechanisms behind these observations remains to be clarified.

5. Rationale for Blocking IL-7 in RA

RA is one of the most common autoimmune diseases and is the main cause of potentially treatable disability in the western world [123, 124]. Uncontrolled inflammation over time imposes a significant patient and health economic burden which is expected to continue to increase due to population ageing, and changes in lifestyle (increased obesity and lack of physical activity) [123]. The worldwide incidence of RA is about 1-2% with the disease being more common in women than men and most often starts between the ages of 30 and 40. There is an increased incidence in those with a family history and an association with HLA-specific alleles. In the UK the RA annual incidence is ~36/100,0000 in women and ~14/100,000 in men with a prevalence of 0.8% in the adult population. The current impact of RA in terms of resource usage is considerable, somewhere in the region of £400 million annually for healthcare services, £60 million in laboratory tests, and £40 million in medicines costs. Add to this the costs of the social services, the loss of income and the benefits to be paid, brings the overall annual costs to almost to £1 billion per year.

Optimal management of such chronic condition is therefore a priority. DMARDs remain the cornerstone of management of RA although it is clear that sub-optimal response limits the potential of conventional therapies. The need however to intervene at the earliest opportunity and aim for maximal disease control to minimise the impact of disease is now well-established [125-127].The development of modern biologic therapies has made the treatment aim of achieving long-term remission an attainable target [128]. However, differences in response to therapy between early and established RA have been observed that remain to be explained. Response to anti-TNF therapies in early RA is qualitatively and quantitatively superior [129], with virtually complete suppression of inflammation in most patients [128-130] compared to classic DMARDs. In comparison, in late RA TNF-alpha blockade produces only partial control over inflammation [131] and it is clear that response is neither complete nor universal [132, 133]. These findings have suggested the existence of a critical therapeutic window during which optimal control of inflammation can be obtained.

RA is a very heterogeneous disease, notably recently highlighted by difference in the genetic contribution to ACPA(+/−) disease [134-136], illustrating two divergent pathogenic models, with different rates of progression [137-139] and response to treatment [138, 140]. Although an improved understanding of RA pathogenesis has identified TNF-alpha and IL-6 as pivotal in driving inflammation, the spectrum of clinical responses to these cytokine-blockade suggest that they may play a particularly important role in the early phases of disease, with the development of a more heterogeneous disease drive and notably independency towards TNF and IL-6 later. The need for alternative treatments for RA therefore remains high; however the cost of developing new biologicals as well as their side effects and resistance suggest that alternative approaches may be more successful.

We proposed the IL-7/IL-7R signalling axis as a potential candidate for therapeutic intervention for RA [60] in agreement with others [141] and with the general interest for IL-7 as therapeutic target in several other autoimmune diseases. In support of this hypothesis MS autoreactive T-cells against MBP were increased by IL-7 however only in MS patients with active disease [142]. A transgenic mouse model with a mutant form of the IL-6 receptor gp130-subunit (F759) with enhanced signal transduction and activation of STAT-3, spontaneously developed a RA-like joint disease (Table 2) [58]. The mutation was sufficient and necessary only in non-haemtopoietic cells and resulted in specific increased production of IL-7 by stromal cells.

Similarly, administration of IL-7 in the CIA model (at the time of disease development day 21 to 31) exacerbated disease (increased clinical severity and radiological scores) [143, 144] with no major other side effect on T and B-cells. Our own findings in transgenic mice showed that the sole over-expression of IL-7 in stromal cells was sufficient to increased cellular infiltration (Figure 2). In the F759 model, a blocking IL-7 antibody completely abolished the development of arthritis when injected intra-peritoneally into 7-day-old thymectomised neonatal mice every 2 days for 2 weeks [58]. Thymectomy was necessary to overcome the difficulty to maintain enough anti–IL-7 antibodies in vivo over 1 year. However, a cross-over between an IL-7R-KO and the F759 mice showed reduced incidence of arthritis (11% of mice developing disease) over more than 1 year compared to the F795 animals (85%). Following these data a prophylactic protocol using an IL-7R blocking antibody showed reduced severity of arthritis (clinical and radiologic scores) in the CIA model as well as delayed the appearance of diseases by a few days [145]. Similarly, a receptor blocking antibody used in a proteoglycan induced disease in BalbC mice, showed reduced incidence (from 92% to 58%) and less severe disease [144]. Using IL-7R blocking antibody in a therapeutic protocol in the CIA model, more limited effect were observed with mostly reduced severity score [145]. Investigating the mechanism by which IL-7 inhibition may prevent disease progression has not been fully elucidated in RA animal models, however a mild reduction in T-cell number (splenic and thymic cell counts, both CD4 and CD8 as well as both naïve and memory CD4) and no difference in B-cell, monocyte or DC numbers were observed in the CIA model treated with an IL-7R blocking antibody [145]. The anti-collagen antibody titres were not affected but T-cell cytokine secretion was reduced (IFN-gamma, IL-5, IL-17). Local levels of several cytokines (IL-1beta, IL-11, TNF-alpha, IL-6) chemokines (IP10, MCP-5), tissue factors (RANKL, MMP9) and vascular factors (vWF, VCAM-1) were reduced. Furthermore, a prophylactic protocol using IL-7R blockade in the CIA model considerably reduced monocyte recruitment into the joint [104] as well as their differentiation into osteoclast. This also resulted in clear inhibition of bone erosions as well as suppressed vascularisation mediated by a loss of the MIP2 chemokine expression.

Additional insight may be provided by experiments in the non-obese diabetic mice (NOD) [146-148]. Using an IL-7R receptor blockade, disease was reversed in new onset diabetic mice.Pathogenic T-cell were not depleted but specifically suppressed in their expression of IFN-gamma and conversely expressed more receptor Programmed Death-1. Cells from animals treated with the IL-7R antibody were no longer able to transfer the disease suggesting that the IL-7R blockade induced T-cell tolerance. The balance between regulatory and pathogenic T-cells was also altered. These data provide strong evidence that in T-cell dependent (phases of) autoimmune disease, IL-7 signalling inhibition represent an important target for therapy.

Table 2. Animal model testing IL-7/IL-7R signalling inhibition

Disease	Animal model	treatment	results	ref
RA	F759 mutation in the gp130 IL-6R subunit enhanced signal transduction activation of STAT-3	Anti-IL-7 antibody (M25 hybridoma culture supernatant) injection intraperitoneally into 7-day-old thymectomised neonatal mice	– Spontaneous arthritis by 6-7 months of age – Disease is CD4+T-cell dependent – Increased IL-7 expression restricted to stromal cells – Blocking antibody fully prevent the development of arthritis – A cross over between an IL-7R-KO and the F759 mice showed reduced incidence of arthritis	[58].
	BalbC proteoglycan induced arthritis	IL-7Rblocking Antibody	– Reduced incidence – Less severe disease	EWRR Warsaw 2009 [144]
	DBA/1J mice CIA model	IL-7 Injection at the time of disease development (day 21 to31)	– Exacerbation of disease: increased clinical severity and radiological scores – No major side effect on T and B-cells.	EWRR Warsaw 2009 [143]
	DBA/1J mice CIA	IL-7Rblocking Antibody (M595, Amgen) prophylactic protocol	– Reduced severity of arthritis (clinical and radiologic scores) – Delayed the appearance of diseases by a few days	[145]
	DBA/1J mice CIA	Blocking Antibody (M595, Amgen) therapeutic protocol	– Used when arthritis score >2 – Reduced the arthritis score	[145]
	DBA/1J mice CIA	Anti-IL-7R antibody (R&D Systems) Therapeutic protocol	– Reduced synovial inflammation (40%), joint lining thickness (45%), and erosion (40%) – Reduced joint TNF-a – Reduced serum levels of MCP-1 – Reduced synovial fluid mediated monocyte migration	[104]
	Transgenic mice		– Over-expression of IL-7 in stromal cells – Increased cellular infiltration	Own unpublished observation

Table 2. (Continued)

Disease	Animal model	treatment	results	ref
colitis	TCR alpha-chain knockout (TCRα−/−) mice	anti–IL-7R mAb (A7R34) therapeutic protocol	– Selective depletion of IL-7Rα high CD4+ LPLs completely ameliorated established colitis	[153]
	TCRα−/− mice.	anti–IL-7R mAb (A7R34) intraperitoneal injection. Prophylactic protocol	– Inhibits the development of colitis – Decrease expansion of memory CD4+ LPLs	[149]
	bacterial-induced colitis in Mdr1a−/− mice 9T Rag2−/− mice	anti–IL-7Rα (M595) therapeutic protocol	– Colitis model involving T cells but also innate immune cells (macrophages, DC, and NK cells). – Inhibition of colitis was associated with decreases in T-cell (especially reduced pool of naïve T-cells) and non-T-cell population) – Reduction of inflammatory cytokines and chemokines.	[154]
NOD,	NOD mice,	anti–IL-7Rα mAb prophylactic and therapeutic protocols	– Efficacy in the prevention of diabetes – Reverses established DM1 by modulating effector T-cell function – Induces durable disease remission in newly established DM1 cases	[146]
	NOD mice,	Anti–IL-7Rα (clone A7R34) prophylactic and therapeutic protocols	– Prevents and – Reverses Autoimmune Diabetes	[148]
MS/EAE	MOG immunized mice with EAE	Anti–IL-7Rα(SB/14; BD Biosciences) in-house clone 28G9 prophylactic and therapeutic protocols	– Treatment before or after onset of paralysis exhibited reduced clinical signs of EAE – Reduction in peripheral naïve and activated T cells, – Central memory T, regulatory T, B, and natural killer cell populations were largely spared. – Treatment markedly reduced lymphocyte infiltration into the central nervous system in mice with EAE.	[41]

Disease	Animal model	treatment	results	ref
	Egfp-transgenic C57BL/6 (B6) mice *Ifng*$^{-/-}$ and *Il6*$^{-/-}$ mice EAE induced with MOG peptide	Anti–IL–7Rα(SB/14; BD Biosciences), –antiIL–7 (AB-407-NA; R&D systems) prophylactic and therapeutic protocols	– IL–7–IL–7R signalling is required for survival and expansion of committed Th17 cells in both mouse and human experimental systems. – Disease development dependent ondifferentiation of Th17 cells – Prophylactic treatment before EAE onset is not sufficient to alter the severity of the disease, – Treatment administered after onset markedly affect the clinical course of EAE. – IL–7 is crucial for Th17 survival and expansion through STAT5 signalling in establisheddisease – This unique effect of IL–7 is independent of IL–6	[150]
SLE	T cell-deficient TCRb–/– MRL-Fas^{lpr} mice (lupus-predisposed mice)	Anti–IL–7Rα(clone A7R34) prophylactic and therapeutic protocols	– Prophylactic treatmentinducessignificant reductions in dermatitis, lymphadenopathy, splenomegaly and total serum – Marginal reduction in anti-chromatin IgG2a autoantibodies, – Reduced numbers of CD4+, CD8+, as well as immature (T1) and follicular (T2-F0) B cells – Treatment of established disease (14 weeks old mice),inducessignificantly reduction in proteinuria, glomerulonephritis, and lymphocyte infiltrates in the kidneys – All antibody treated mice were alive at 24 weeks of age compared to .50% mortality in the control group	[151]
primary Sjögren`s syndrome	C57BL/6.NOD-*Aec1Aec2*	anti–IL–7Ralpha prophylactic protocol	– Almost completely abolished the development of pSjS (based on salivary gland inflammation and apoptosis, autoantibody production and secretory dysfunction	[152]

Several other models of auto-immune disease were also effectively controlled by anti-IL-7R therapies. In several animal models of autoimmune diseases the use of prophylactic protocols with either anti-IL-7 or receptor-inhibition allowed prevention or complete inhibition of disease development (Table 2) [41, 145, 148-152]. Therapeutic protocols showed important effects as well in many models [41, 104, 145, 146, 148, 150, 153, 154] notably with abrogation of established colitis, MS and diabetes. Therefore, animal studies have clearly demonstrated that IL-7-signalling blockade can prevent the development and ameliorate or reverse established autoimmune diseases.

The previously un-described mechanism of action of IL-7/IL-7R signalling in T_H17 cells survival and expansion [150] may provide powerful explanations for the treatment efficacy of IL-7R antagonism in EAE and therapeutic implications for human autoimmune diseases such as multiple sclerosis. The IL-7 signalling blockade offered the selectivity that distinguishes pathogenic Th1 and Th17 cells from Treg and unrelated immune cells. Additional therapeutic advantages of IL-7R antagonism involve its selective effect on survival and expansion of effector Th17 cells versus Th17 cell differentiation. In contrast, IL-6 or IL-23 antagonism given as prevention protocol when Th17 cells still undergo differentiation is effective during EAE, whereas the same regimen administered once EAE is established showed no efficacy [155]. IL-7 antagonism mainly targeting committed Th17 cells [150 therefore has unique therapeutic advantages.

Altogether, these data suggest that the best window of opportunity for anti-IL-7 therapy is in the early phases of the disease when T-cells are more likely to be essential however good result may also be obtained in established diseases. In RA they may also indicate that the best time to use anti-IL-7 therapy maybe in preventing progression to RA from very early symptom or even in pre-clinical phases such as ACPA+ arthralgia.

This work has been partly supported by a European Union funded FP7-integrated project Masterswitch No. 223404 and the IMI funded project BeTheCure *No 115142-2.*

References

[1]   Wolfe F, Mitchell DM, Sibley JT, Fries JF, Bloch DA, Williams CA, et al. The Mortality of Rheumatoid-Arthritis. *Arthritis Rheum.* 1994;37(4):481-94.

[2]   Sokka T, Abelson B, Pincus T. Mortality in rheumatoid arthritis: 2008 update. *Clin. Exp. Rheumatol.* 2008;26(5 Suppl 51):S35-61.

[3]   Ernst B, Lee D-S, Chang JM, Sprent J, Surh CD. The peptide ligands mediating positive selection in the thymus control T cell survival and homeostatic proliferation in the periphery. *Immunity.* 1999;11(2):173-81.

[4]   Winchester R. The Molecular-Basis of Susceptibility to Rheumatoid-Arthritis.*Advances in Immunology*1994. p. 389-466.

[5]   Gregersen PK, Silver J, Winchester RJ. The Shared Epitope Hypothesis - an Approach to Understanding the Molecular-Genetics of Susceptibility to Rheumatoid- Arthritis. *Arthritis and Rheumatism.* 1987;30(11):1205-13.

[6]   Strollo R, Ponchel F, Malmström V, Rizzo P, Bombardieri M, Wenham CY, et al. Auto-antibodies to post translationally modified type II collagen as potential biomarkers for rheumatoid arthritis. *Arthritis & Rheumatism.* 2013.

[7] Feldmann M, Brennan FM, Maini RN. Role of cytokines in rheumatoid arthritis. *Annu. Rev. Immunol.* 1996;14:397-440.

[8] Goëb V, Walsh C, Reece R, Emery P, Ponchel F. Potential role of arthroscopy in the management of inflammatory arthritis. *Clinical and Experimental Rheumatology.* 2012;30(3):429-35.

[9] Panayi GS, Lanchbury JS, Kingsley GH. The Importance of the T-Cell in Initiating and Maintaining the Chronic Synovitis of Rheumatoid-Arthritis. *Arthritis and Rheumatism.* 1992;35(7):729-35.

[10] Salmon M, Gaston J. The role of lymphocytes in rheumatoid arthritis. *Br. Med. Bull.* 1995;51:332-45.

[11] Lanchbury JS, Pitzalis C. Cellular Immune-Mechanisms in Rheumatoid-Arthritis and Other Inflammatory Arthritides. *Current Opinion in Immunology.* 1993;5(6):918-24.

[12] Ponchel F, Vital E, Kingsbury SR, El-Sherbiny YM. CD4+ T-cell subsets in rheumatoid arthritis. *International Journal of Clinical Rheumatology.* 2012;7(1):37-53.

[13] Van Roon J, Glaudemans C, Bijlsma J, Lafeber F. Differentiation of naive CD4+ T cells towards T helper 2 cells is not impaired in rheumatoid arthritis patients. *Arthritis Res. Ther.* 2003;5(5):R269-R76.

[14] van Roon JAG, Glaudemans K, Bijlsma JWJ, Lafeber F. Interleukin 7 stimulates tumour necrosis factor alpha and Th1 cytokine production in joints of patients with rheumatoid arthritis. *Annals of the Rheumatic Diseases.* 2003;62(2):113-9.

[15] van Roon JAG, Verweij MC, Wenting-van Wijk M, Jacobs KMG, Bijlsma JWJ, Lafeber F. Increased intraarticular interleukin-7 in rheumatoid arthritis patients stimulates cell contact-dependent activation of CD4+T cells and macrophages. *Arthritis And Rheumatism.* 2005;52(6):1700-10.

[16] Emery P, Panayi GS, Nouri AME. Interleukin-2 Reverses Deficient Cell-Mediated Immune-Responses in Rheumatoid-Arthritis. *Clin Exp Immunol.* 1984;57(1):123-9.

[17] Ponchel F, Morgan A, Bingham S, Quinn M, Buch M, Verburg R, et al. Dysregulated lymphocyte proliferation and differentiation in patients with rheumatoid arthritis. *Blood.* 2002;100:4550-6.

[18] Lawson CA, Brown AK, Bejarano V, Douglas SH, Burgoyne CH, Greenstein AS, et al. Early rheumatoid arthritis is associated with a deficit in the CD4(+)CD25(high) regulatory T cell population in peripheral blood. *Rheumatology.* 2006;45(10):1210-7.

[19] Burgoyne C, Field S, AK Brown, Hensor E, English A, Bingham S, et al. Abnormal T-cell differentiation persists in rheumatoid arthritis patients in clinical remission and predicts relapse. *Ann. Rheum. Diseases.* 2008;67;:750-7.

[20] Gregory SG, Schmidt S, Seth P, Oksenberg JR, Hart J, Prokop A, et al. Interleukin 7 receptor α chain (IL7R) shows allelic and functional association with multiple sclerosis. *Nature genetics.* 2007;39(9):1083-91.

[21] Haas J, Korporal M, Schwarz A, Balint B, Wildemann B. The interleukin-7 receptor α chain contributes to altered homeostasis of regulatory T cells in multiple sclerosis. *Eur. J. Immunol.* 2011;41(3):845-53.

[22] Heron M, Grutters J, van Moorsel C, Ruven H, Huizinga T, van der Helm-van Mil A, et al. Variation in IL7R predisposes to sarcoid inflammation. *Genes and Immunity.* 2009;10(7):647-53.

[23] Anderson CA, Boucher G, Lees CW, Franke A, D'Amato M, Taylor KD, et al. Meta-analysis identifies 29 additional ulcerative colitis risk loci, increasing the number of confirmed associations to 47. *Nature genetics*. 2011;43(3):246-52.

[24] Barton A, Eyre S, Ke X, Hinks A, Bowes J, Flynn E, et al. Identification of AF4/FMR2 family, member 3 (AFF3) as a novel rheumatoid arthritis susceptibility locus and confirmation of two further pan-autoimmune susceptibility genes. *Human Molecular Genetics*. 2009;18(13):2518-22.

[25] Todd JA, Walker NM, Cooper JD, Smyth DJ, Downes K, Plagnol V, et al. Robust associations of four new chromosome regions from genome-wide analyses of type 1 diabetes. *Nature genetics*. 2007;39(7):857-64.

[26] Mells GF, Floyd JA, Morley KI, Cordell HJ, Franklin CS, Shin S-Y, et al. Genome-wide association study identifies 12 new susceptibility loci for primary biliary cirrhosis. *Nature genetics*. 2011;43(4):329-32.

[27] Lundmark F, Duvefelt K, Hillert J. Genetic association analysis of the interleukin 7 gene (< i> IL7</i>) in multiple sclerosis. *J. Neuroimmunol*. 2007;192(1):171-3.

[28] McKay F, Swain L, Schibeci S, Rubio J, Kilpatrick T, Heard R, et al. Haplotypes of the interleukin 7 receptor alpha gene are correlated with altered expression in whole blood cells in multiple sclerosis. *Genes and Immunity*. 2007;9(1):1-6.

[29] Weber F, Fontaine B, Cournu-Rebeix I, Kroner A, Knop M, Lutz S, et al. IL2RA and IL7RA genes confer susceptibility for multiple sclerosis in two independent European populations. *Genes and Immunity*. 2008;9(3):259-63.

[30] Zuvich RL, McCauley JL, Oksenberg JR, Sawcer SJ, De Jager PL, Aubin C, et al. Genetic variation in the IL7RA/IL7 pathway increases multiple sclerosis susceptibility. *Hum. Genet*. 2010;127(5):525-35.

[31] Evsyukova I, Somarelli JA, Gregory SG, Garcia-Blanco MA. Alternative splicing in multiple sclerosis and other autoimmune diseases. *RNA biology*. 2010;7(4):462-73.

[32] Evsyukova I. Investigating Alternative Splicing and Polyadenylation of the Interleukin 7 Receptor Exon 6: Implications for Multiple Sclerosis. 2012.

[33] Lundström W, Greiner E, Lundmark F, Westerlind H, Smestad C, Lorentzen ÅR, et al. No influence on disease progression of non-HLA susceptibility genes in MS. *J. Neuroimmunol*. 2011;237(1):98-100.

[34] The International Multiple Sclerosis Genetics Consortium. Risk Alleles for Multiple Sclerosis Identified by a Genomewide Study. *New England Journal of Medicine*. 2007;357(9):851-62.

[35] Monti P, Brigatti C, Krasmann M, Ziegler AG, Bonifacio E. Concentration and activity of the soluble form of the Interleukin-7 Receptor alpha in type I diabetes identifies an interplay between hyperglycemia and immune function. *Diabetes*. 2013.

[36] Santiago J, Alizadeh B, Martinez A, Espino L, de la Calle H, Fernandez-Arquero M, et al. Study of the association between the CAPSL-IL7R locus and type 1 diabetes. *Diabetologia*. 2008;51(9):1653-8.

[37] Wang X-S, Wen P-F, Zhang M, Hu L-F, Ni J, Qiu L-J, et al. Interleukin-7 Receptor Single Nucleotide Polymorphism rs6897932 (C/T) and the Susceptibility to Systemic Lupus Erythematosus. *Inflammation*. 2013:1-6.

[38] Plant D, Thomson W, Lunt M, Flynn E, Martin P, Eyre S, et al. The role of rheumatoid arthritis genetic susceptibility markers in the prediction of erosive disease in patients

with early inflammatory polyarthritis: results from the Norfolk Arthritis Register. *Rheumatology.* 2011;50(1):78-84.

[39] Hinks A, Eyre S, Ke X, Barton A, Martin P, Flynn E, et al. Association of the AFF3 gene and IL2/IL21 gene region with juvenile idiopathic arthritis. *Genes and immunity.* 2010;11(2):194-8.

[40] O'Doherty C, Alloza I, Rooney M, Vandenbroeck K. IL7RA polymorphisms and chronic inflammatory arthropathies. *Tissue antigens.* 2009;74(5):429-31.

[41] Lee L-F, Axtell R, Tu GH, Logronio K, Dilley J, Yu J, et al. IL-7 Promotes TH1 Development and Serum IL-7 Predicts Clinical Response to Interferon-β in Multiple Sclerosis. *Science translational medicine.* 2011;3(93):93ra68-93ra68.

[42] Pleiman C, Gimpel S, Park L, Harada H, Taniguchi T, Ziegler S. Organization of the murine and human interleukin-7 receptor genes: two mRNAs generated by differential splicing and presence of a type I-interferon-inducible promoter. *Molecular And Cellular Biology.* 1991;11(6):3052-9.

[43] Goodwin RG, Friend D, Ziegler SF, Jerzy R, Falk BA, Gimpel S, et al. Cloning of the human and murine interleukin-7 receptors: demonstration of a soluble form and homology to a new receptor superfamily. *Cell.* 1990;60(6):941-51.

[44] Korte A, Köchling J, Badiali L, Eckert C, Andreae J, Geilen W, et al. Expression analysis and characterization of alternatively spliced transcripts of human IL-7Rα chain encoding two truncated receptor proteins in relapsed childhood ALL. *Cytokine.* 2000;12(11):1597-608.

[45] Rose T, Lambotte O, Pallier C, Delfraissy J-F, Colle J-H. Identification and biochemical characterization of human plasma soluble IL-7R: lower concentrations in HIV-1-infected patients. *The Journal of Immunology.* 2009;182(12):7389-97.

[46] Kreft K, Verbraak E, Wierenga-Wolf A, van Meurs M, Oostra B, Laman J, et al. Decreased systemic IL-7 and soluble IL-7Rα in multiple sclerosis patients. *Genes and Immunity.* 2012.

[47] Hoe E, McKay FC, Schibeci SD, Gandhi K, Heard RN, Stewart GJ, et al. Functionally Significant Differences in Expression of Disease-Associated IL-7 Receptor α Haplotypes in CD4 T Cells and Dendritic Cells. *The Journal of Immunology.* 2010;184(5):2512-7.

[48] Evsyukova I, Bradrick SS, Gregory SG, Garcia-Blanco MA. Cleavage and polyadenylation specificity factor 1 (CPSF1) regulates alternative splicing of interleukin 7 receptor (IL7R) exon 6. *RNA.* 2013;19(1):103-15.

[49] Houssiau F, Lauwerys B, Badot V, Depresseux G. sIL-7R Is a Novel Marker of Disease Activity in Systemic Lupus Erythematosus Nephritis, Which Reflects Target Organ Involvement. [abstract]. *Arthritis Rheum* 2011 63:DOI.:2258.

[50] Badot V, Durez P, Van den Eynde B, Nzeusseu-Toukap A, Houssiau F, Lauwerys B. Rheumatoid arthritis synovial fibroblasts produce a soluble form of the interleukin-7 receptor in response to pro-inflammatory cytokines. *J. Cell Mol. Med.* 2011;15(11):2335-42.

[51] Ariizumi K, Meng Y, Bergstresser PR, Takashima A. IFN-gamma-dependent IL-7 gene regulation in keratinocytes. *The Journal of Immunology.* 1995;154(11):6031-9.

[52] Tang JH, Nuccie BL, Ritterman I, Liesveld JL, Abboud CN, Ryan DH. TGF-beta down-regulates stromal IL-7 secretion and inhibits proliferation of human B cell precursors. *Journal of Immunology.* 1997;159(1):117-25.

[53] Oshima S, Nakamura T, Namiki S, Okada E, Tsuchiya K, Okamoto R, et al. Interferon regulatory factor 1 (IRF-1) and IRF-2 distinctively up-regulate gene expression and production of interleukin-7 in human intestinal epithelial cells. *Molecular And Cellular Biology*. 2004;24(14):6298-310.

[54] Fry TJ, Mackall CL. Interleukin-7: from bench to clinic. *Blood*. 2002;99(11):3892-904.

[55] Ponchel F, Cuthbert RJ, Goëb V. IL-7 and lymphopenia. *Clinica Chimica Acta*. 2011;412(1):7-16.

[56] Weitzmann MN, Cenci S, Rifas L, Brown C, Pacifici R. Interleukin-7 stimulates osteoclast formation by up-regulating the T-cell production of soluble osteoclastogenic cytokines. *Blood*. 2000;96(5):1873-8.

[57] Min D, Taylor PA, Panoskaltsis-Mortari A, Chung B, Danilenko DM, Farrell C, et al. Protection from thymic epithelial cell injury by keratinocyte growth factor: a new approach to improve thymic and peripheral T-cell reconstitution after bone marrow transplantation. *Blood*. 2002;99(12):4592-600.

[58] Sawa S, Kamimura D, Jin GH, Morikawa H, Kamon H, Nishihara M, et al. Autoimmune arthritis associated with mutated interleukin (IL)-6 receptor gp130 is driven by STAT3/IL-7-dependent homeostatic proliferation of CD4(+) T cells. *J. Exp. Med*. 2006;203(6):1459-70.

[59] Harada S, Yamamura M, Okamoto H, Morita Y, Kawashima M, Aita T, et al. Production of interleukin-7 and interleukin-15 by fibroblast-like synoviocytes from patients with rheumatoid arthritis. *Arthritis And Rheumatism*. 1999;42(7):1508-16.

[60] Churchman S, Ponchel F. Interleukin-7 in rheumatoid arthritis. *Rheumatology*. 2008;47(6):753-9.

[61] Ponchel F, Verburg R, Bingham S, Brown A, Moore J, Protheroe A, et al. Interleukin-7 deficiency in rheumatoid arthritis: consequences for therapy-induced lymphopenia. *Arthritis Res. Ther*. 2005;7(1):R80 - R92.

[62] Goëb V, Aegerter P, Parmar R, Fardellone P, Vittecoq O, Conaghan PG, et al. Progression to rheumatoid arthritis in early inflammatory arthritis is associated with low IL-7 serum levels. *Annals of the Rheumatic Diseases*. 2013;72(6):1032-6.

[63] Shimaoka Y, Attrep JF, Hirano T, Ishihara K, Suzuki R, Toyosaki T, et al. Nurse-like cells from bone marrow and synovium of patients with rheumatoid arthritis promote survival and enhance function of human B cells. *J. Clin. Invest*. 1998;102(3):606-18.

[64] Colucci S, Brunetti G, Cantatore F, Oranger A, Mori G, Quarta L, et al. Lymphocytes and synovial fluid fibroblasts support osteoclastogenesis through RANKL, TNFα, and IL-7 in an in vitro model derived from human psoriatic arthritis. *The Journal of pathology*. 2007;212(1):47-55.

[65] Golden-Mason L, Kelly AM, Traynor O, McEntee G, Kelly J, Hegarty JE, et al. Expression of interleukin 7 (IL-7) mRNA and protein in the normal adult human liver: implications for extrathymic T cell development. *Cytokine*. 2001;14(3):143-51.

[66] Madrigal-Estebas L, McManus R, Byrne B, Lynch S, Doherty DG, Kelleher D, et al. Human small intestinal epithelial cells secrete interleukin-7 and differentially express two different interleukin-7 mRNA Transcripts: implications for extrathymic T-cell differentiation. *Human immunology*. 1997;58(2):83-90.

[67] Kröncke R, Loppnow H, Flad HD, Gerdes J. Human follicular dendritic cells and vascular cells produce interleukin-7: a potential role for interleukin-7 in the germinal center reaction. *Eur. J. Immunol*. 1996;26(10):2541-4.

[68] Watanabe M, Ueno Y, Yajima T, Iwao Y, Tsuchiya M, Ishikawa H, et al. Interleukin 7 is produced by human intestinal epithelial cells and regulates the proliferation of intestinal mucosal lymphocytes. *J. Clin. Invest*. 1995;95(6):2945.

[69] Sorg RV, McLellan AD, Hock BD, Fearnley DB, Hart DN. Human dendritic cells express functional interleukin-7. *Immunobiology*. 1998;198(5):514-26.

[70] de Saint-Vis B, Fugier-Vivier I, Massacrier C, Gaillard C, Vanbervliet B, Aït-Yahia S, et al. The cytokine profile expressed by human dendritic cells is dependent on cell subtype and mode of activation. *The Journal of Immunology*. 1998;160(4):1666-76.

[71] Leistad L, Ostensen M, Faxvaag A. Detection of cytokine mRNA in human, articular cartilage from patients with rheumatoid arthritis and osteoarthritis by reverse transcriptase polymerase chain reaction. *Scand. J. Rheumatol*. 1998;27(1):61-7.

[72] Kunisch E, Fuhrmann R, Roth A, Winter R, Lungershausen W, Kinne R. Macrophage specificity of three anti-CD68 monoclonal antibodies (KP1, EBM11, and PGM1) widely used for immunohistochemistry and flow cytometry. *Annals of the Rheumatic Diseases*. 2004;63(7):774-84.

[73] Bresnihan B, Baeten D, Firestein GS, Fitzgerald OM, Gerlag DM, Haringman JJ, et al. Synovial tissue analysis in clinical trials. *J. Rheumatol*. 2005;32(12):2481-4.

[74] Timmer TCG, Baltus B, Vondenhoff M, Huizinga TWJ, Tak PP, Verweij CL, et al. Inflammation and ectopic lymphoid structures in rheumatoid arthritis synovial tissues dissected by genomics technology: Identification of the interleukin-7 signaling pathway in tissues with lymphoid neogenesis. *Arthritis & Rheumatism*. 2007;56(8):2492-502.

[75] Goronzy JJ, Weyand CM. Rheumatoid arthritis. *Immunological Reviews*. 2005;204:55-73.

[76] Borghesi LA, Yamashita Y, Kincade PW. Heparan Sulfate Proteoglycans Mediate Interleukin-7–Dependent B Lymphopoiesis. *Blood*. 1999;93(1):140-8.

[77] Clarke D, Katoh O, Gibbs R, Griffiths S, Gordon M. Interaction of interleukin 7 (IL-7) with glycosaminoglycans and its biological relevance. *Cytokine*. 1995;7(4):325-30.

[78] Kimura K, Matsubara H, Sogoh S, Kita Y, Sakata T, Nishitani Y, et al. Role of glycosaminoglycans in the regulation of T cell proliferation induced by thymic stroma-derived T cell growth factor. *The Journal of immunology*. 1991;146(8):2618-24.

[79] Sawa Y, Arima Y, Ogura H, Kitabayashi C, Jiang J-J, Fukushima T, et al. Hepatic Interleukin-7 Expression Regulates T Cell Responses. *Immunity*. 2009;30(3):447-57.

[80] Isaacs JD, Greer S, Sharma S, Symmons D, Smith M, Johnston J, et al. Morbidity and mortality in rheumatoid arthritis patients with prolonged and profound therapy-induced lymphopenia. *Arthritis & Rheumatism*. 2001;44(9):1998-2008.

[81] Bingham S, Veale D, Fearon U, Reece R, Isaacs J, McGonagle D, et al. Long-term follow-up of highly selected autologous stem cell transplantation in severe rheumatoid arthritis with studies of peripheral blood reconstitution and macroscopic and histological arthroscopic appearances. *Arthiritis and Rheumatism*. 2000;43(9):S290-S.

[82] Verburg RJ, Kruize AA, van den Hoogen FH, Fibbe WE, Petersen EJ, Preijers F, et al. High-dose chemotherapy and autologous hematopoietic stem cell transplantation in patients with rheumatoid arthritis: Results of an open study to assess feasibility, safety, and efficacy. *Arthritis & Rheumatism*. 2001;44(4):754-60.

[83] Kittipatarin C, Khaled AR. Interlinking interleukin-7. *Cytokine*. 2007;39(1):75-83.

[84] Mazzucchelli R, Durum SK. Interleukin-7 receptor expression: intelligent design. *Nature Reviews Immunology*. 2007;7(2):144-54.

[85] Park J-H, Yu Q, Erman B, Appelbaum JS, Montoya-Durango D, Grimes HL, et al. Suppression of IL7Rα transcription by IL-7 and other prosurvival cytokines: a novel mechanism for maximizing IL-7-dependent T cell survival. *Immunity.* 2004;21(2):289-302.

[86] Fluur C, Rethi B, Thang PH, Vivar N, Mowafi F, Lopalco L, et al. Relationship between serum IL-7 concentrations and lymphopenia upon different levels of HIV immune control. *Aids.* 2007;21(8):1048-50.

[87] Witkowska AM. On the role of sIL-2R measurements in rheumatoid arthritis and cancers. *Mediators Inflamm.* 2005;14(3):121-30.

[88] Klimiuk PA, Sierakowski S, Latosiewicz R, Cylwik JP, Cylwik B, Skowronski J, et al. Interleukin-6, soluble interleukin-2 receptor and soluble interleukin-6 receptor in the sera of patients with different histological patterns of rheumatoid synovitis. *Clin. Exp. Rheumatol.* 2003;21(1):63-9.

[89] Badot V, Durez P, Van den Eynde BJ, Nzeusseu-Toukap A, Houssiau FA, Lauwerys BR. Rheumatoid arthritis synovial fibroblasts produce a soluble form of the interleukin-7 receptor in response to pro-inflammatory cytokines. *J. Cell Mol. Med.* 2011;15(11):2335-42.

[90] Vudattu N, Magalhaes I, Hoehn H, Pan D, Maeurer M. Expression analysis and functional activity of interleukin-7 splice variants. *Genes and immunity.* 2008;10(2):132-40.

[91] van Roon JAG, Hartgring SAY, Wijk MWV, Jacobs KMG, Tak PP, Bijlsma JWJ, et al. Persistence of interleukin 7 activity and levels on tumour necrosis factor alpha blockade in patients with rheumatoid arthritis. *Annals of the Rheumatic Diseases.* 2007;66(5):664-9.

[92] Mehrotra P, Grant AJ, Siegel JP. Synergistic effects of IL-7 and IL-12 on human T cell activation. *The Journal of Immunology.* 1995;154(10):5093-102.

[93] Borger P, Kauffman HF, Postma DS, Vellenga E. IL-7 differentially modulates the expression of IFN-gamma and IL-4 in activated human T lymphocytes by transcriptional and post-transcriptional mechanisms. *The Journal of Immunology.* 1996;156(4):1333-8.

[94] Gringhuis SI, de Leij LF, Verschuren EW, Borger P, Vellenga E. Interleukin-7 Upregulates the Interleukin-2–Gene Expression in Activated Human T Lymphocytes at the Transcriptional Level by Enhancing the DNA Binding Activities of Both Nuclear Factor of Activated T Cells and Activator Protein-1. *Blood.* 1997;90(7):2690-700.

[95] Isaacs J, Hale G, Cobbold S, Waldmann H, Watts R, Hazleman B, et al. Humanised monoclonal antibody therapy for rheumatoid arthritis. *The Lancet.* 1992;340 (8822):748-52.

[96] Moreland L, Bucy R, Knowles R, Wacholtz M, Haverty T, Koopman W. Treating Rheumatoid-Arthritis with a Non-Depleting Anti-CD4 Monoclonal-Antibody (Mab). *Arthritis and Rheumatism.* 1995;38:199-.

[97] Brett SJ, Baxter G, Cooper H, Rowan W, Regan T, Tite J, et al. Emergence of CD52−, glycosyiphosphatidylinositol-anchor deficient lymphocytes in rheumatoid arthritis patients following Campath-1H treatment. *International immunology.* 1996;8(3):325-34.

[98] Churchman S, El-Jawhari, J, Parmar, R, Burska, A, Goëb V,El-Sherbiny, Y.M, Shires, M,Brown, A,Lawson C. A,, Hull M, Conaghan, P. G, Emery P & Ponchel, F.,.

Circulating levels of Interleukin-7 correlate with peripheral T-cell responsiveness. *submitted*2013.

[99] van Amelsfort JM, van Roon JA, Noordegraaf M, Jacobs KM, Bijlsma JW, Lafeber FP, et al. Proinflammatory mediator–induced reversal of CD4+, CD25+ regulatory T cell–mediated suppression in rheumatoid arthritis. *Arthritis & Rheumatism*. 2007;56(3):732-42.

[100] Di Caro V, D'Anneo A, Phillips B, Engman C, Harnaha J, Lakomy R, et al. Interleukin-7 matures suppressive CD127+ forkhead box P3 (FoxP3)+ T cells into CD127-CD25high FoxP3+ regulatory T cells. *Clinical & Experimental Immunology*. 2011;165(1):60-76.

[101] Li C-R, Deiro MF, Godebu E, Bradley LM. IL-7 uniquely maintains FoxP3+ adaptive Treg cells that reverse diabetes in NOD mice via integrin-β7-dependent localization. *Journal of autoimmunity*. 2011;37(3):217-27.

[102] Katzman SD, Hoyer KK, Dooms H, Gratz IK, Rosenblum MD, Paw JS, et al. Opposing functions of IL-2 and IL-7 in the regulation of immune responses. *Cytokine*. 2011;56(1):116-21.

[103] Hartgring SAY, van Roon JAG, Wijk MW, Jacobs KMG, Jahangier ZN, Willis CR, et al. Elevated expression of interleukin-7 receptor in inflamed joints mediates interleukin-7–induced immune activation in rheumatoid arthritis. *Arthritis & Rheumatism*. 2009;60(9):2595-605.

[104] Chen Z, Kim S-j, Chamberlain ND, Pickens SR, Volin MV, Volkov S, et al. The Novel Role of IL-7 Ligation to IL-7 Receptor in Myeloid Cells of Rheumatoid Arthritis and Collagen-Induced Arthritis. *The Journal of Immunology*. 2013;190(10):5256-66.

[105] Schröder AE, Greiner A, Seyfert C, Berek C. Differentiation of B cells in the nonlymphoid tissue of the synovial membrane of patients with rheumatoid arthritis. *Proceedings of the National Academy of Sciences*. 1996;93(1):221-5.

[106] Wagner UG, Kurtin PJ, Wahner A, Brackertz M, Berry DJ, Goronzy JJ, et al. The role of CD8+ CD40L+ T cells in the formation of germinal centers in rheumatoid synovitis. *The Journal of Immunology*. 1998;161(11):6390-7.

[107] Mebius RE. Organogenesis of lymphoid tissues. *Nature Reviews Immunology*. 2003;3(4):292-303.

[108] Yoshida H, Naito A, Inoue J, Satoh M, Santee-Cooper SM, Ware CF, et al. Different cytokines induce surface lymphotoxin-alpha beta on IL-7 receptor-alpha cells that differentially engender lymph nodes and Peyer's patches. *Immunity*. 2002;17(6):823-33.

[109] Link a, Vogt T, Favre S, Britschgi M, Acha-Orbea H, Hinz B, et al. Fibroblastic reticular cells in lymph nodes regulate the homeostasis of naive T cells. *Nature immunology*. 2008;8:1255-65.

[110] Lee S-K, Surh CD. Role of interleukin-7 in bone and T-cell homeostasis. *Immunological reviews*. 2005;208(1):169-80.

[111] Teitelbaum SL, Ross FP. Genetic regulation of osteoclast development and function. *Nature Reviews Genetics*. 2003;4(8):638-49.

[112] Lee SK, Kalinowski JF, Jacquin C, Adams DJ, Gronowicz G, Lorenzo JA. Interleukin-7 Influences Osteoclast Function In Vivo but Is Not a Critical Factor in Ovariectomy-Induced Bone Loss. *Journal of Bone and Mineral Research*. 2006;21(5):695-702.

[113] Weitzmann MN, Roggia C, Toraldo G, Weitzmann L, Pacifici R. Increased production of IL-7 uncouples bone formation from bone resorption during estrogen deficiency. *J. Clin. Invest.* 2002;110(11):1643-50.

[114] Hartgring SA, Willis CR, Bijlsma JW, Lafeber FP, van Roon JA. Interleukin-7-aggravated joint inflammation and tissue destruction in collagen-induced arthritis is associated with T-cell and B-cell activation. *Arthritis Research & Therapy.* 2012;14(3):R137.

[115] Toyosaki-Maeda T, Takano H, Tomita T, Tsuruta Y, Maeda-Tanimura M, Shimaoka Y, et al. Differentiation of monocytes into multinucleated giant bone-resorbing cells: two-step differentiation induced by nurse-like cells and cytokines. *Arthritis Res.* 2001;3(5):306-10.

[116] Churchman S, Geiler J, Parmar R, Horner E, Church L, Emery P, et al. Multiplexing immunoassays for cytokine detection in the serum of patients with rheumatoid arthritis: lack of sensitivity and interference by rheumatoid factor. *Clinical and Experimental Rheumatology.* 2012;30:in press.

[117] Stabler T, Piette JC, Chevalier X, Marini-Portugal A, Kraus VB. Serum cytokine profiles in relapsing polychondritis suggest monocyte/macrophage activation. *Arthritis And Rheumatism.* 2004;50(11):3663-7.

[118] Faucher S, Crawley A, Decker W, Sherring A, Bogdanovic D, Ding T, et al. Development of a Quantitative Bead Capture Assay for Soluble IL-7 Receptor Alpha in Human Plasma. *PLoS One.* 2009;4:e6690.

[119] Crawley AM, Faucher S, Angel JB. Soluble IL-7R alpha (sCD127) inhibits IL-7 activity and is increased in HIV infection. *J. Immunol.* 2010;184(9):4679-87.

[120] Saleem B, Keen H, Goeb V, Parmar R, Nizam S, Hensor EM, et al. Patients with RA in remission on TNF blockers: when and in whom can TNF blocker therapy be stopped? *Ann. Rheum. Dis.* 2010;69(9):1636-42.

[121] Brown A, Conaghan P, Karim Z, Quinn M, Ikeda K, Peterfy C, et al. An explanation for the apparent dissociation between clinical remission and continued structural deterioration in rheumatoid arthritis. *Arthritis & Rheumatism.* 2008;58(10):2958-67.

[122] Brown AK, Quinn MA, Karim Z, Conaghan PG, Peterfy CG, Hensor E, et al. Presence of significant synovitis in rheumatoid arthritis patients with disease-modifying antirheumatic drug–induced clinical remission: Evidence from an imaging study may explain structural progression. *Arthritis & Rheumatism.* 2006;54(12):3761-73.

[123] Harris EJ. Rheumatoid arthritis. Pathophysiology and implications for therapy. *NEJM.* 1990;322(18):1277-89.

[124] Lee DM, Weinblatt ME. Rheumatoid arthritis. *The Lancet.* 2001;358(9285):903-11.

[125] Quinn M, Emery P. Window of opportunity in early rheumatoid arthritis: possibility of altering the disease process with early intervention. *Clin. Exp. Rheumatol.* 2003;21:154-7.

[126] Quinn MA, Emery P. Potential for altering rheumatoid arthritis outcome. *Rheumatic Disease Clinics of North America.* 2005;31(4):763-72.

[127] Goëb V, Smolen J, Emery P, Marzo-Ortega H. Early inflammatory clinics. Experience with early arthritis/back pain clinics. *Clinical and Experimental Rheumatology.* 2009;27(4):S74.

[128] Dhir V, Singh A, Aggarwal A, S N, Misra R. Increased T-lymphocyte apoptosis in lupus correlates with disease activity and may be responsible for reduced T-cell frequency: a cross-sectional and longitudinal study. *LUPUS*2009;18:785-91

[129] Chen I-H, Lai Y-L, Wu C-L, Chang Y-F, Chu C-C, Tsai I-F, et al. Immune impairment in patients with terminal cancers: influence of cancer treatments and cytomegalovirus infection. *Cancer Immunology, Immunotherapy*. 2010;59(2):323-34.

[130] Tikly M, Navarra S. Lupus in the developing world: is it any different? *Best Pract. Res. Clin. Rheumatol*. 2008;22:643-55.

[131] Di Carlo E, D'Antuono T, Pompa P, Giuliani R, Rosini S, Stuppia L, et al. The lack of epithelial interleukin-7 and BAFF/BLyS gene expression in prostate cancer as a possible mechanism of tumor escape from immunosurveillance. *Clinical Cancer Research*. 2009;15(9):2979-87.

[132] Yilmaz-Demirdag Y, Wilson B, Lowery-Nordberg M, Bocchini JJ, Bahna S. Interleukin-2 treatment for persistent cryptococcal meningitis in a child with idiopathic CD4(+) T lymphocytopenia. *Allergy Asthma Proc* 2008 29:421-4.

[133] Puri V, Chaudhry N, Gulati P, Patel N, Tatke M, Sinha S. Progressive multifocal leukoencephalopathy in a patient with idiopathic CD4+T lymphocytopenia. *Neurol India*2010 58:118-21.

[134] Klareskog L, Catrina AI, Paget S. Rheumatoid arthritis. *The Lancet*. 2009;373 (9664):659-72.

[135] Viatte S, Barton A. The Role of Rheumatoid Arthritis Genetic Susceptibility Markers in the Prediction of Erosive Disease. 2012.

[136] Kurreeman F, Liao K, Chibnik L, Hickey B, Stahl E, Gainer V, et al. Genetic basis of autoantibody positive and negative rheumatoid arthritis risk in a multi-ethnic cohort derived from electronic health records. *The American Journal of Human Genetics*. 2011;88(1):57-69.

[137] Berglin E, Johansson T, Sundin U, Jidell E, Wadell G, Hallmans G, et al. Radiological outcome in rheumatoid arthritis is predicted by presence of antibodies against cyclic citrullinated peptide before and at disease onset, and by IgA-RF at disease onset. *Annals of the rheumatic diseases*. 2006;65(4):453-8.

[138] Del Amo NDV, Bosch RI, Manteca CF, Polo RG, Cortina EL. Anti-cyclic citrullinated peptide antibody in rheumatoid arthritis: relation with disease aggressiveness. *Clinical and experimental rheumatology*. 2006;24(3):281-6.

[139] van der Helm-vanMil AHM, le Cessie S, van Dongen H, Breedveld FC, Toes REM, Huizinga TWJ. A prediction rule for disease outcome in patients with Recent-onset undifferentiated arthritis: How to guide individual treatment decisions. *Arthritis & Rheumatism*. 2007;56(2):433-40.

[140] van Dongen H, van Aken J, Lard LR, Visser K, Ronday HK, Hulsmans HMJ, et al. Efficacy of methotrexate treatment in patients with probable rheumatoid arthritis: A double-blind, randomized, placebo-controlled trial. *Arthritis & Rheumatism*. 2007;56(5):1424-32.

[141] Hartgring SAY, Bijlsma JWJ, Lafeber F, van Roon JAG. Interleukin-7 induced immunopathology in arthritis. *Annals Of The Rheumatic Diseases*. 2006;65:69-74.

[142] Traggiai E, Biagioli T, Rosati E, Ballerini C, Mazzanti B, Ben Nun A, et al. IL-7-enhanced T-cell response to myelin proteins in multiple sclerosis. *J. Neuroimmunol*. 2001;121(1-2):111-9.

[143] Hartgring S WC, Bijlsma J, Lafeber F, van Roon J. A71. Il-7 receptor ligands Il-7 and thymic stromal lymphopoietin promote collagen-induced arthritis in the absence of T-cell expansion*Annals of the Rheumatic Diseases*. 2009;68(Suppl 1):A 25.

[144] van Roon J, Hartgring,S.,Broere, F., van Eden, W., Bijlsma, J., Willis C., Lafeber F.,. A64. Blockade of the high affinity Il-7 receptor inhibits proteoglycan-induced arthritis. *Annals of the Rheumatic Diseases*. 2009;68(Suppl 1):A25.

[145] Hartgring SAY, Willis CR, Alcorn D, Nelson LJ, Bijlsma JWJ, Lafeber FPJG, et al. Blockade of the Interleukin-7 Receptor Inhibits Collagen-Induced Arthritis and Is Associated With Reduction of T Cell Activity and Proinflammatory Mediators. *Arthritis and Rheumatism*. 2010;62(9):2716-25.

[146] Lee LF, Logronio K, Tu GH, Zhai W, Ni I, Mei L, et al. Anti-L-7 receptor-alpha reverses established type 1 diabetes in nonobese diabetic mice by modulating effector T-cell function. *Proceedings of the National Academy of Sciences*. 2012;109 (31):12674-9.

[147] Boettler T, von Herrath M. IL-7 receptor Œ± blockade, an off-switch for autoreactive T cells. *Proceedings of the National Academy of Sciences*. 2012;109(31):12270-1.

[148] Penaranda C, Kuswanto W, Hofmann J, Kenefeck R, Narendran P, Walker LSK, et al. IL-7 receptor blockade reverses autoimmune diabetes by promoting inhibition of effector/memory T cells. *Proceedings of the National Academy of Sciences*. 2012;109(31):12668-73.

[149] Okada E, Yamazaki M, Tanabe M, Takeuchi T, Nanno M, Oshima S, et al. IL-7 exacerbates chronic colitis with expansion of memory IL-7Rhigh CD4+ mucosal T cells in mice. *American Journal of Physiology - Gastrointestinal and Liver Physiology*. 2005;288(4):G745-G54.

[150] Liu X, Leung S, Wang C, Tan Z, Wang J, Guo TB, et al. Crucial role of interleukin-7 in T helper type 17 survival and expansion in autoimmune disease. *Nature medicine*. 2010;16(2):191-7.

[151] Gonzalez-Quintial R, Lawson BR, Scatizzi JC, Craft J, Kono DH, Baccala R, et al. Systemic autoimmunity and lymphoproliferation are associated with excess IL-7 and inhibited by IL-7Ralpha blockade. *PLoS One*. 2011;6(11):e27528. Epub 2011/11/22.

[152] Jin JO, Kawai T, Cha S, Yu Q. Interleukin-7 enhances Th1 response to promote the development of Sjögren's Syndrome-Like autoimmune exocrinopathy. *Arthritis & Rheumatism*. 2013.

[153] Yamazaki M, Yajima T, Tanabe M, Fukui K, Okada E, Okamoto R, et al. Mucosal T cells expressing high levels of IL-7 receptor are potential targets for treatment of chronic colitis. *The Journal of Immunology*. 2003;171(3):1556-63.

[154] Willis CR, Seamons A, Maxwell J, Treuting PM, Nelson L, Chen G, et al. Interleukin-7 receptor blockade suppresses adaptive and innate inflammatory responses in experimental colitis. *Journal of Inflammation*. 2012;9(1):39.

[155] Chen Y, Langrish CL, Mckenzie B, Joyce-Shaikh B, Stumhofer JS, McClanahan T, et al. Anti–IL-23 therapy inhibits multiple inflammatory pathways and ameliorates autoimmune encephalomyelitis. *J. Clin. Invest*. 2006;116(5):1317-26.

[156] Barton A, Eyre S, Ke X, Hinks A, Bowes J, Flynn E, et al. Identification of AF4/FMR2 family, member 3 (AFF3) as a novel rheumatoid arthritis susceptibility locus and confirmation of two further pan-autoimmune susceptibility genes. *Human molecular genetics*. 2009;18(13):2518-22.

[157] Jones E, Churchman S, English A, Buch M, Horner E, Burgoyne C, et al. Mesenchymal stem cells in rheumatoid synovium: enumeration and functional assessment in relation to synovial inflammation level. *Annals of the Rheumatic Diseases*. 2010;69(2):450-7.

[158] Ponchel F, Toomes C, Bransfield K, Leong F, Field S, Douglas S, et al. Real-time PCR based on SYBR-green fluorescence: An alternative to the TaqMan assay for a relative quantification of gene rearrangements, gene amplifications and micro gene deletions. *BMC Biotechnology*. 2003;3(1):18.

In: Advances in Medicine and Biology. Volume 77
Editor: Leon V. Berhardt

ISBN: 978-1-63117-444-5
© 2014 Nova Science Publishers, Inc.

Chapter 4

Spontaneous Bacterial Peritonitis: From Risk Factors to Prevention

Eduardo Rodrigues-Pinto, Pedro Pereira† and Guilherme Macedo‡*

Gastroenterology Department, Centro Hospitalar São João, Porto, Portugal

Abstract

Peritonitis is a pathologic inflammation of the serosal membrane that lines the abdominal cavity and can be classified as primary, secondary or tertiary. Primary peritonitis, most often spontaneous bacterial peritonitis (SBP), is a common and severe complication in patients with advanced cirrhosis. Additional risk factors have been identified, as an ascitic fluid total protein <1.5 g/dL with Child-Pugh score ≥9 points and serum bilirubin ≥3 mg/dL or serum creatinine ≥1.2 mg/dL, blood urea nitrogen ≥25 mg/dL or plasma sodium ≤130 mEq/L. SBP is defined as an ascitic fluid infection without an evident intra-abdominal surgically treatable source.

The clinical presentation is non-specific and may range from abdominal pain to subtle changes of mental status, or even, no symptoms. Diagnosis is established with a diagnostic paracentesis, when the number of polymorphonuclear leucocytes in the ascitic fluid exceeds 250 cells/mm3. Antibiotics should be started at diagnosis and adjusted, if necessary, according with the ascitic fluid cultural results. Considering Gram-negative bacteria are the most frequent pathogens involved, the first-line antibiotic treatment is often a third-generation cephalosporin, however, the reports of resistance cases to first-line antibiotics are increasing. Intravenous albumin should be given together at day 1 and day 3. Patients with prior SBP, acute gastrointestinal haemorrhage and patients with low total protein concentration in ascitic fluid should be on a prophylaxis antibiotherapy due to a higher risk of SBP. Approximately half of all deaths in patients with SBP occur after

*   Corresponding author: Eduardo Rodrigues-Pinto, MD. E-mail: edu.gil.pinto@gmail.com. Affiliation: Gastroenterology Department, Centro Hospitalar São João, Porto. Al. Prof. Hernâni Monteiro 4200 - 319 Porto, Portugal. Phone number: +351 919657386. Fax number: +351 22 551 3601.
†   Co-author: Pedro Pereira, MD. E-mail: pedro.pedroreispereira@gmail.com. Affiliation: Gastroenterology Department, Centro Hospitalar São João, Porto. Al. Prof. Hernâni Monteiro 4200 - 319 Porto, Portugal.
‡   Guilherme Macedo, MD, PhD. E-mail: guilhermemacedo59@gmail.com. Affiliation: Gastroenterology Department, Centro Hospitalar São João, Porto. Al. Prof. Hernâni Monteiro 4200 - 319 Porto, Portugal.

the resolution of the infection, usually as a result of gastrointestinal hemorrhage, liver or renal failure. Given the complex nature of SBP, it is not surprising that it heralds increased morbidity and mortality in cirrhotic patients and increased cost-utilization upon the health-care system. This review will detail the risk factors, diagnosis and preventive care of cirrhotic patients with SBP.

Introduction

Peritonitis is an inflammation of the serosal membrane that lines the abdominal cavity and the organs contained therein. The peritoneum, otherwise a sterile environment, reacts to various pathologic stimuli with a fairly uniform inflammatory response. It is most often caused by an infection of the peritoneum; however, it may also be a sterile process, resulting from stimulation by irritants. Peritoneal infections are classified as primary, most often spontaneous bacterial peritonitis (SBP), secondary (related to a pathologic process in a visceral organ), or tertiary (persistent or recurrent infection after adequate initial therapy) [1]. This review article focuses on the diagnosis, risk factors and preventive care of ascitic fluid infection, namely, SBP.

Ascitic fluid infection can be classified into two categories (spontaneous or secondary), subsequently subdivided in a total of five categories, based on ascitic culture results, polymorphonuclear (PMN) count and presence or absence of a surgical source of infection. An abdominal paracentesis must be performed, with ascitic fluid analysis for the distinction of the different entities [2]. SBP, the prototype of spontaneous ascitic fluid infection, was first described as a way to distinguish it from surgical peritonitis [3]. It is the most frequent and life-threatening infection in patients with liver cirrhosis, requiring prompt recognition and treatment. The diagnosis is made when there is a positive ascitic fluid culture and an elevated ascitic fluid absolute PMN count (> 250 cells/mm^3) in the absence of an intra-abdominal source of infection or malignancy [4]. Ascites culture is negative in as many as 60% of patients with clinical manifestations suggestive of SBP and increased ascites neutrophil count, being named bacterascites culture-negative [2, 5]. No other explanation should be identified for the elevated ascitic PMN count (haemorrhage into ascites, peritoneal carcinomatosis, tuberculosis, pancreatitis) [6]. Some patients have bacterascites in which cultures are positive but ascitic fluid neutrophil count is < 250/mm^3, being named monomicrobial non-neutrocytic bacterascites [5, 7]. Secondary bacterial peritonitis is diagnosed in patients with elevated ascitic fluid absolute PMN count (> 250 cells/mm^3), positive ascitic fluid culture (usually for multiple organisms) and an intra-abdominal surgically treatable primary source of infection [8]. Secondary bacterial peritonitis and polymicrobial bacterascites can develop with ascites of any type [8]; the latter may result from a needle penetration into the bowel during attempted paracentesis [9].

The spontaneous variants of ascitic fluid infection occur almost exclusively in the setting of severe liver disease, usually in the stage of cirrhosis, however it may also occur in an acute (fulminant hepatic failure) or sub-acute setting (alcoholic hepatitis). Essentially all patients with SBP have an elevated serum bilirubin level and abnormal prothrombin time due to advanced cirrhosis [4] and ascites appears to be a prerequisite for the development of spontaneous bacterial peritonitis. Peritonitis is unlikely to precede the development of ascites and usually, the infection develops when the volume of ascites is at its maximum [10].

Epidemiology

SBP is the most frequent bacterial infection in cirrhosis. Early, mostly retrospective studies, described SBP in about 8% of patients with ascites; later prospective trials revealed SBP in 10%-30% of patients with ascites admitted to hospital [4, 11-12]. SBP is found in 3.5-5% of outpatients [13], but increases to 8-36% in the nosocomial setting [4].

Lethality is very high, with in-hospital mortality for the first episode of SBP ranging from 10% to 50%, depending on various risk factors [14-18]. One-year mortality after a first episode of SBP has been reported to be 31% and 93% [19-21], once the occurrence of SBP markedly worsens the prognosis of cirrhosis [22]. The high lethality is not primarily associated with the severity of the infection and patients usually, do not die of sepsis. Infections worsen already impaired blood supply and renal function of cirrhotic patients [23], increasing splanchnic vasodilatation, decreasing effective arterial blood volume, with renal function damage and hepatorenal syndrome. Patients with higher levels of urea and higher portal pressure at the time of SBP have a higher risk of renal failure and associated mortality [24]. Predictive factors for poor prognosis include age [16, 20], Child-Pugh score [18, 20, 25], intensive care [16, 18], nosocomial SBP [26], hepatic encephalopathy [27], elevated serum creatinine and bilirubin [28, 29], lack of infection resolution/need to escalate treatment, culture positivity [30-32] as well as the presence of bacteraemia [33] and CARD15/NOD2 variants as a genetic risk factor [34]. The only factors that are modifiable are timely diagnosis and effective first-line treatment.

Pathophisiology

The interface between the bowel, intestinal microbiota and ascitic fluid is dynamic [35, 36], with a constant translocation of bacteria across bowel wall. The wall integrity is variable due to host genetics, nutritional status and local bacterial interactions. Invading bacteria are usually cleared by immune system after surveillance and capture by neutrophils and macrophages with assisted opsonic molecules [37, 38]. SBP thus likely is a manifestation of bacterial type and burden, gut integrity, volume status and local and global immune function [37-39]. Bacterial translocation (BT), the key mechanism in the pathogenesis of SBP, is only possible because of the concurrent failure of defensive mechanisms in cirrhosis [35, 40-43]. BT consists in the active/passive penetration of living microorganisms and their toxic products through the mucosal epithelial layer to the lamina propria *mucosae*. From there, microorganisms migrate to mesenteric lymph nodes (MLN) and/or extra-intestinal sites. Only a few intestinal bacteria are able to translocate into MLN, including *Escherichia coli*, *Klebsiella pneumoniae* and other *Enterobacteriaceae* [44]. The route of pathological BT leading to SBP is largely lymphatic and three factors have been implicated in the development of BT in liver cirrhosis [45] – gut microbiota, increased intestinal permeability and impaired immunity.

Microbiota

Liver cirrhosis is associated with distinct changes in faecal microbial composition [46, 47], with an increased prevalence of potentially pathogenic bacteria such as *Escherichia coli*, *Proteus spp.*, *Klebsiella pneumoniae* and other *Enterobacteriaceae*, as well as *pseudomonas aeruginosa, enterococci, streptococci* and *staphylococci* in immunocompromised patients. Moreover, small intestinal bacterial overgrowth (SIBO) is frequently present in advanced stages of liver cirrhosis and has been linked with pathological BT and SBP [39, 42, 48]. In cirrhosis, the main reasons for SIBO may be deficiencies in paneth cell defensins [39], reduced intestinal motility, abnormalities in bile secretion, portal-hypertensive enteropathy, hypochlorhydria, abnormalities in IgA production and malnutrition [38]. However, BT does not occur in all patients with SIBO and, thus, SIBO is necessary but not sufficient for BT to occur.

Intestinal Permeability

Cirrhosis is associated with structural and functional alterations in the intestinal mucosa that increase permeability to bacteria and bacterial products. The increased intestinal permeability and thus impaired function of the intestinal barrier are mainly due to portal hypertension. The consequences are dilated vessels in the intestinal mucosa, oedema of the lamina propria mucosae, fibromuscular proliferation, hypertrophy of the lamina muscularis mucosae and compromised integrity of the intestinal mucosa. Increased intestinal permeability is likely to be proportional to the degree of portal hypertension, but independent of the severity and etiology of liver disease [49, 50].

Impaired Immunity

Patients with liver cirrhosis have decreased phagocytic activity of neutrophilic granulocytes and the mononuclear phagocytic system, deteriorated humoral immunity and decreased opsonin activity of ascitic fluid [51]. Neutrophilic granulocytes show a decrease in their phagocytic activity, a decreased intracellular destruction of bacteria, deteriorated metabolic activity, frequent apoptosis and considerably reduced chemotaxis. They adhere to the vascular endothelium in a greater extent, thus, their trans-endothelial migration is decreased [52]. Decreased chemotaxis is probably due to the presence of inhibitors of chemotaxis in the blood plasma. The opsonic activity of ascitic fluid correlates with the concentration of immunoglobulins, complement, fibronectin and total protein in ascitic fluid [53].

Clinical Manifestations

SBP is particularly revealed in patients with more severe liver functional damage, often after bleeding from the upper gastrointestinal tract due to portal hypertension. The clinical picture is non-specific (table 1), quite often asymptomatic, frequently manifested only by the occurrence or deepening of symptoms that accompany the course of liver cirrhosis (increased ascites, failure of diuretic therapy, deteriorated encephalopathy, vomiting, deteriorated renal function). Without prompt paracentesis, the diagnosis and treatment of infected ascites may be delayed, often resulting in the death of the patient. Diagnostic paracentesis with leukocyte count is recommended in all patients with ascites admitted to hospital, in cirrhotics with worsened ascites, with signs of abdominal or systemic infection (abdominal pain or tenderness, disturbed intestinal passage, fever, acidosis, peripheral leukocytosis), with encephalopathy or worsened renal function [5].

Table 1. symptoms and signs of spontaneous bacterial peritonitis

Symptoms or signs	Frequency (%)
fever	68
abdominal pain	49
abdominal tenderness	39
rebound tenderness	10
altered mental status	54
diarrhea	32
paralytic ileus	30
hypotension	21
hypothermia	17

data from references 8, 9 and 110.

Risk Factors

Cirrhosis is a form of acquired immunodeficiency. Markers of advanced liver dysfunction have been identified as independent risk factors for a first episode of SBP.

Bilirubin levels higher than 3.2mg/dL and platelets count lower than 98 000/mm^3 significantly increase the likelihood of SBP [54]. Each model for end-stage liver disease (MELD) point increases the risk of SBP by about 11% [55].

The total protein content in ascitic fluid also mirrors opsonic activity and has been shown to be predictive of the development of SBP [56]. The incidence rate of SBP in patients with ascitic fluid protein levels higher than 1.5g/dL has been consistently reported to be lower than 1%. In contrast, protein levels lower than 1.5g/dL correlate with a higher risk of SBP, paralleling the decrease in protein content and reaching incidence rates of 27-41% at levels lower than 1.0g/dL [57-58].

Furthermore, genetic variants influencing host defense mechanisms such as TLR2 polymorphisms and NOD2 variants seem to represent supplementary risk factors [59].

Medication can also affect the chances of developing SBP. Proton pump inhibitors (PPI) have been implicated in SIBO and thus contribute to pathological BT. In contrast, non-selective b-blockers (NSBB) may prevent SBP [60, 61].

Paracentesis itself has been proposed as a risk factor for ascitic fluid infection, however, this theoretical risk has not been substantiated in prospective studies of paracentesis-related complications [62], once SBP is statistically more likely to be diagnosed on the first paracentesis than on subsequent taps [62]. Needle-induced ascitic fluid infections do not occur unless the bowel is penetrated by the paracentesis needle [9, 62], however, this occurs in 1/1000 taps. Iatrogenic peritonitis is most likely to occur when the paracentesis needle enters the bowel during a difficult paracentesis. Gastrointestinal haemorrhage is an under-recognized risk factor for the development of SBP.

The cumulative probability of infection during a single hospitalization for bleeding is approximately 40% [63] and the risk appears to peak 48 hours after the onset of haemorrhage. Urinary tract infections also constitute an under-recognized risk factor for SBP [63], as well as prior SBP episodes and malnutrition [17, 19, 57, 65].

Diagnosis of SBP

Timely diagnosis of ascitic fluid infection requires a high index of suspicion and a low threshold for performing a paracentesis. Diagnosis is based on a fixed defined cut-off PMN count in the ascitic fluid [66-69]. If the ascitic fluid PMN count is elevated, the working diagnosis is ascitic fluid infection until proved otherwise. Although peritoneal carcinomatosis, pancreatitis, haemorrhage into ascites, and tuberculosis can lead to an elevated ascitic fluid PMN count, most cases of neutrocytic ascites are caused by bacterial infection. In patients with haemorrhagic ascites (red blood cell count higher than $10\ 000/mm^3$), subtraction of one PMN per 250 red blood cells should be made to adjust for the presence of blood in ascites [5]. Differential diagnoses of predominant lymphocytosis in ascitic fluid include tuberculosis peritonitis, neoplasias, congestive heart failure, pancreatitis and myxedema, but not usually SBP. PMN are therefore used to define SBP, and the greatest sensitivity is reached at a cut-off value of $250\ PMN/mm^3$, although the best specificity has been reported with a cut-off of $500\ PMN/mm^3$ [70-73]. Nonetheless, this upper limit has been set quite arbitrarily since it was tested in the setting of culture-positive peritonitis. Moreover, SBP caused by Gram-positive cocci has been reported to have a PMN count below the threshold of $250/mm^3$ [74]. Interestingly, bacterial DNA (bactDNA) from Gram-negative bacteria in ascitic fluid is associated with a higher ascitic PMN count than bactDNA from Gram-positive bacteria [75].

Secondary peritonitis should, however, be considered in any patient with neutrocytic ascites, once clinical symptoms and signs do not distinguish secondary peritonitis from SBP [8]. Even with free perforation of the colon into ascitic fluid, a classic surgical abdomen does not develop. Peritoneal signs require contact of inflamed visceral and parietal peritoneal surfaces, and such contact does not occur when there is a large volume of fluid separating these surfaces. Intestinal perforation should be suspected if ascites is neutrocytic and meets two of three criteria (total protein higher than 1 g/dL, glucose less than 50 mg/dL and lactate dehydrogenase greater than the upper limit of normal for serum [8, 76]. The sensitivity of these criteria is, however, less than 68% [76, 77]. In addition, alkaline phosphatase higher than 240U/L or carcinoembryonic antigen higher than 5ng/mL in the ascitic fluid reflects secondary peritonitis in 80% of cases [78]. In secondary peritonitis, cultures nearly always disclose multiple organisms, except in gallbladder rupture, which is usually monomicrobial [79]. Brown ascitic fluid with a bilirubin concentration greater than 6 mg/dL and greater than the serum level is suggestive of biliary or proximal small intestinal perforation [79]. An ascitic fluid amylase level higher than five times of the serum level may also be indicative of intestinal rupture (not gallbladder rupture) [8].

Ascitic PMN cell counts can be determined either by a traditional haematological method using a light microscope and a manual counting chamber or by automated cell counters [80-82]. The manual count is laborious and, in many instances, subjective. Current guidelines have produced clinical evidence that manual and automated PMN counting are equally effective [81, 82]. None of the recent guidelines recommends the use of reagent test strips to assess leukocyte esterase activity of activated PMNs for the diagnosis of SBP owing to unacceptable rates of false negative results [83].

Although only a few species and genera are found to cause SBP, more than 70 different microbial species have been isolated from the ascitic fluid of patients with bacteriological confirmed SBP [84]. Classical culture techniques fail to grow bacteria in up to 60% of neutrocytic ascites. Bedside inoculation of ascites into blood culture bottles has been shown to increase the sensitivity to nearly 80% [84, 85]. Separate and simultaneous blood cultures should be collected since 30-58% of SBP cases are associated with bacteraemia [86].

Detection of bactDNA in the ascitic fluid has recently been proposed [87, 88], however, its detection in ascites or serum was not associated with an enhanced incidence of SBP and does not appear to predict the development of bacterial infections [89].

Other markers previously tested as indicative of SBP included ascitic pH, lactate dehydrogenase and lactate. Although initially attractive [72], they are not sufficiently predictive or discriminative [90] and may be increased in malignancy-related ascites [71, 73, 91, 92]. Procalcitonin, the pro-hormone of calcitonin, has been hailed as an index of inflammation, however, initial interest in SBP (95% sensitivity and 98% specificity with a cut-off of 0.75ng/mL) [93] was dampened a year later, possibly due to the absence of systemic inflammatory response syndrome [94]. Lactoferrin seems far more promising as a rapid and reliable screening tool for SBP, with 95.5% of sensitivity and 97% specificity with a cut-off of 242ng/mL [95]. Confirmation is required in multicentre trials including assessment of its accuracy in haemorrhagic and coexisting malignant ascites.

A second paracentesis should be performed 48 hours after the first one to assess response to therapy. At this time, the ascitic PMN count should be lower than the pre-treatment value and the ascitic culture will be negative in essentially every patient with SBP who has been treated with an appropriate antibiotic [8].

Treatment of SBP

Treatment should be started immediately after diagnosis of SBP, being therefore empirical. The epidemiology of bacterial infections differs between community-acquired and nosocomial infections [7], with different rates of bacterial multi-resistance and mortality [26]. None of the international guidelines differentiates between nosocomial and community-acquired SBP with regard to the type of antibiotic regimen to use.

Historically, Gram-negative bacteria have caused most of community-acquired SBP, mainly *Enterobacteriaceae*. More recently, several studies have found an increasing rate of infections with Gram-positive bacteria and resistant microorganisms [26]. However, in patients with no previous hospitalizations and no prior antibiotic treatment, third-generation cephalosporins (cefotaxime 2g twice daily or ceftriaxone 2g/day for 5 days [96]), amoxicillin/clavulanic acid 1/0.2g/day [97], ofloxacin 400mg twice daily for 7-10 days [98] or quinolones (intravenous ciprofloxacin 200mg twice daily for 2 days followed by oral ciprofloxacin, 500mg twice daily for 5 days [99]) may be used with similar efficacy. Nosocomial SBP has lower rates of resolution with the antibiotics recommended above [100], with 23-44% resistance to third-generation cephalosporins and 38-50% to quinolones [100, 101]. Besides that, there is an increasing incidence of extended-spectrum β-lactamase (ESBL)-producing bacteria and multiresistant Gram-positive bacteria, resistant to first-line antibiotics [102]. Nosocomial SBP due to multi-resistant bacteria is often associated with failure of first-line empirical antibiotic treatment [103, 104] and need of treatment escalation is predictive of in-hospital mortality [26, 32]. Choice of antibiotics needs to be stratified by the risk of resistant bacteria, with previous hospitalization (particularly within 3 months, intensive care treatment), prior prophylactic or therapeutic antibiotic treatment being recognized as independent risk factors for multi-resistance [26, 32, 105, 106]. Therefore, patients with risk factors who develop nosocomial SBP should be started on a broader spectrum antibiotic, namely carbapenems, with de-escalation if microbiological results reveal non-resistant treatable microorganisms.

Albumin

As previously stated, the high lethality of SBP is not primarily associated with the severity of the infection, but rather with deterioration of volemia and renal function. Renal impairment occurs in 33% of episodes of SBP [14]. SBP increases intraperitoneal nitric oxide production, which further increases systemic vasodilatation and promotes renal failure [107]. Therefore, the efforts of expansion of intravascular volume could be beneficial; adjuvant administration of high-dose albumin (1.5g/kg on day 1 [during the first 6 hours] and 1g/kg on day 3) with antibiotic treatment prevented worsening of renal function with a concomitant improvement in in-hospital and 3-month survival [108, 109]. This regimen is mainly effective in high-risk patients characterized by serum bilirubin higher than 4 mg/dL, serum creatinine higher than 1 mg/dL or blood urea nitrogen higher than 30 mg/dL.

Bacterascites

The decision to begin empirical antibiotic treatment in patients with bacterascites must be individualized. Many episodes resolve without treatment [110], however, the hospital mortality rate of 32% in patients with monomicrobial non-neutrocytic bacterascites is attributable, at least, in part, to infection [110].

Therefore, treatment appears to be warranted in many patients. Patients with cirrhosis and ascites who have convincing symptoms or signs of infection should receive treatment regardless of the ascitic fluid PMN count. Empirical treatment can be discontinued after only two to three days if the culture demonstrates no growth. Asymptomatic patients may not need treatment [110].

Paracentesis should be repeated for cell count and culture in patients without clinical evidence of infection, as soon as it is known that the initial culture result is positive. If the PMN count has risen to at least 250/mm^3 or if symptoms or signs of infection have developed, treatment should be started. Culture results usually are negative in patients without a rise in the ascitic fluid PMN count on repeat paracentesis and without clinical evidence of infection, and these persons do not require treatment [110] because colonization has been eradicated by host immune defenses. Empirical antibiotic treatment should be started in patients with culture-negative neutrocytic ascites once culture results are not known. A dramatic decline in PMN count at 48 hours (frequently a reduction of more than 80%) confirms a response to treatment [8] and therapy should be continued for a few days more. A stable ascitic fluid PMN count, especially with a predominance of lymphocytes and monocytes, suggests a nonbacterial (or mycobacterial) cause.

Prevention of SBP

The long-term prognosis of patients with cirrhosis who have had a prior episode of SBP is poor, with one-year mortality after a first episode of SBP between 31% and 93% [19-21]. This is largely a result of the advanced stage of liver cirrhosis in these patients, along with the associated complications [111]. The recurrence rate of SBP following a first episode is up to 70% at 1 year [111].

Patients with variceal hemorrhage, patients who have survived an episode of SBP and patients with ascitic fluid protein concentration less than 1.0g/dL have a higher risk of SBP. Given the high recurrence rate, it seems sensible to recommend prophylaxis to this group of patients and referral for transplant assessment. This therapy is backed up by evidence showing a reduction in recurrence of SBP from 68% to 20% in one study [112].

However, distinction should be made between secondary (prior episode of SBP) and primary prophylaxis (gastrointestinal bleeding setting). For secondary prophylaxis, the evidence is strongest for norfloxacin (400mg/day) [112]. Oral ciprofloxacin (750mg once weekly) [66] or trimethoprim/ sulfamethoxazole (1g/day for 5 days/week) [68] have also been shown to prevent SBP, however, the use of intermittent ciprofloxacin has been associated with a higher rate of quinolone-resistant organisms [113] and data supporting trimethoprim/sulfamethoxazole are weak [114], with potentially dangerous side effects. For primary prophylaxis, quinolones (ciprofloxacin or norfloxacin) are most frequently used, decreasing the incidence of severe infections and mortality, however, in advanced cirrhosis (ascites, severe malnutrition, encephalopathy, bilirubin higher than 3mg/dL) third generation cephalosporin intravenously are superior to oral quinolones [115]. In the setting of low protein ascites (less than 1.5g/dL), quinolones (norfloxacin 400mg/day or ciprofloxacin 500mg/day) are effective in the primary prevention of SBP [66-68]. Trimethoprim/ sulfamethoxazole (1g/day for 5 days/week) may represent an alternative regimen. Despite this evidence, most expert panels do not recommend the routine use of antibiotics in every patient with low protein ascites unless additional risk factors are present. They may be justified if present together with a serum creatinine higher than 1.2mg/dL, blood urea nitrogen higher than 25mg/dL, serum sodium lower than 130mEq/L or Child-Pugh higher than 9 points with bilirubin higher than 3mg/dL [69]. The survival advantage of norfloxacin in these highly selected patients is however most marked during the first 3 months of treatment and decreases over time [66, 116]. Recent studies support the use of rifaximin (1200mg/day for a 4-week regimen) due to the significantly reduced 5-year possibility of SBP [117].

A limitation of antibiotic prophylaxis is the risk of selection of resistant strains, so the continuous use of a single antibiotic is not the optimal solution. They should be used until liver transplantation, disappearance of ascites [67, 68] or improvement of liver disease. Strong efforts should focus on effective prophylactic measures with low or zero risk for development of bacterial resistance including use of antibiotic cycling, rifaximin or non-antibiotic treatments.

Conflicts of Interest Disclosure and Funding Declaration

None declared.

References

[1] Pavlidis TE. Cellular changes in association with defense mechanisms in intra-abdominal sepsis. *Minerva Chir.* Dec 2003;58(6):777-81.
[2] Hoefs JC. Diagnostic paracentesis. A potent clinical tool. *Gastroenterology.* 1990;98:230-6.
[3] Correia JP, Conn HO: Spontaneous bacterial peritonitis in cirrhosis: Endemic or epidemic?. *Med. Clin. North Am.* 1975; 59:963-81.
[4] Runyon BA. Management of adult patients with ascites caused by cirrhosis. *Hepatology* 2004; 39:841-56.
[5] Rimola A, García-Tsao G, Navasa M, Piddock LJ, Planas R, Bernard B, Inadomi JM. Diagnosis, treatment and prophylaxis of spontaneous bacterial peritonitis: a consensus document. International Ascites Club. *J. Hepatol.* 2000; 32: 142-153.
[6] Runyon BA, Hoefs JC. Culture-negative neutrocytic ascites: A variant of spontaneous bacterial peritonitis. *Hepatology* 1984; 4:1209-11.
[7] Lata J, Stiburek O, Kopacova M. Spontaneous bacterial peritonitis: a severe complication of liver cirrhosis. *World Journal of Gastroenterology* 2009; 15:5505-10.
[8] Akriviadis EA, Runyon BA: The value of an algorithm in differentiating spontaneous from secondary bacterial peritonitis. *Gastroenterology* 1990; 98:127-33.
[9] Runyon BA, Canawati HN, Hoefs JC. Polymicrobial bacterascites: A unique entity in the spectrum of infected ascitic fluid. *Arch. Intern. Med.* 1986; 146:2173-5.
[10] Feldman M, Friedman LS, Brandt LJ. *Sleisenger and Fordtran's Gastrointestinal and Liver Disease* – 2 Volume Set, 9th Edition.
[11] Thanopoulou AC, Koskinas JS, Hadziyannis SJ. Spontaneous bacterial peritonitis (SBP): clinical, laboratory, and prognostic features. A single-center experience. *Eur. J. Intern. Med.* 2002; 13:194-198.
[12] Lata J, Fejfar T, Krechler T, Musil T, Husová L, Senkyrík M, Dolina J, Vanasek T. Spontaneous bacterial peritonitis in the Czech Republic: prevalence and aetiology. *Eur. J. Gastroenterol. Hepatol.* 2003; 15: 739-743].
[13] Evans LT, Kim WR, Poterucha JJ, Kamath PS. Spontaneous bacterial peritonitis in asymptomatic outpatients with cirrhotic ascites. *Hepatology* 2003; 37: 897-901.

[14] Follo A, Llovet JM, Navasa M, Planas R, Forns X, Francitorra A, Rimola A, Gassull MA, Arroyo V, Rodés J. Renal impairment after spontaneous bacterial peritonitis in cirrhosis: incidence, clinical course, predictive factors and prognosis. *Hepatology* 1994; 20:1495-501.

[15] Nobre SR, Cabral JE, Gomes JJ, Leitão MC. In-hospital mortality in spontaneous bacterial peritonitis: a new predictive model. *Eur. J. Gastroenterol. Hepatol.* 2008; 20:1176-81.

[16] Thuluvath PJ, Morss S, Thompson R. Spontaneous bacterial peritonitis-in-hospital mortality, predictors of survival, and health care costs from 1988 to 1998. *Am. J. Gastroenterol.* 2001;96:1232-6.

[17] Titó L, Rimola A, Ginès P, Llach J, Arroyo V, Rodés J. Recurrence of spontaneous bacterial peritonitis in cirrhosis: frequency and predictive factors. *Hepatology* 1988;8:27-31.

[18] Toledo C, Salmerón JM, Rimola A, Navasa M, Arroyo V, Llach J, Ginès A, Ginès P, Rodés J. Spontaneous bacterial peritonitis in cirrhosis: predictive factors of infection resolution and survival in patients treated with cefotaxime. *Hepatology* 1993;17:251-7.

[19] Andreu M, Sola R, Sitges-Serra A, Alia C, Gallen M, Vila MC, Coll S, Oliver MI. Risk factors for spontaneous bacterial peritonitis in cirrhotic patients with ascites. *Gastroenterol.* 1993;104:1133-8.

[20] Silvain C, Besson I, Ingrand P, Mannant PR, Fort E, Beauchant M. Prognosis and long-term recurrence of spontaneous bacterial peritonitis in cirrhosis. *J. Hepatol.* 1993;19:188-9.

[21] Terg R, Levi D, Lopez P, Rafaelli C, Rojter S, Abecasis R, Villamil F, Aziz H, Podesta A. Analysis of clinical course and prognosis of culture-positive spontaneous bacterial peritonitis and neutrocytic ascites. Evidence of the same disease. *Dig. Dis. Sci.* 1992; 37:1499-504.

[22] Arvaniti V, D'Amico G, Fede G, Manousou P, Tsochatzis E, Pleguezuelo M, Burroughs AK. Infections in patients with cirrhosis increase mortality four-fold and should be used in determining prognosis. *Gastroenterology* 2010; 139:1246-56, 1256.e1e5.

[23] Coral G, Mattos A. Renal impairment after spontaneous bacterial peritonititis: incidence a prognosis. *J. Gastroent. Hepatol.* 2002; 17 Suppl: A915.

[24] Ruiz-del-Arbol L, Urman J, Fernández J, González M, Navasa M, Monescillo A, Albillos A, Jiménez W, Arroyo V. Systemic, renal, and hepatic hemodynamic derangement in cirrhotic patients with spontaneous bacterial peritonitis. *Hepatology* 2003; 38: 1210-1218.

[25] Altman C, Grangé JD, Amiot X, Pelletier G, Lacaine F, Bodin F, Etienne JP. Survival after a first episode of spontaneous bacterial peritonitis. Prognosis of potential candidates for orthotopic liver transplantation. *J. Gastroenterol. Hepatol.* 1995; 10:47-50.

[26] Cheong HS, Kang CI, Lee JA, Moon SY, Joung MK, Chung DR, Koh KC, Lee NY, Song JH, Peck KR. Clinical significance and outcome of nosocomial acquisition of spontaneous bacterial peritonitis in patients with liver cirrhosis. *Clin. Infect. Dis.* 2009; 48:1230-6.

[27] Almdal TP, Skinhoj P. Spontaneous bacterial peritonitis in cirrhosis. Incidence, diagnosis, and prognosis. *Scand. J. Gastroenterol.* 1987; 22: 295-300.

[28] Terg R, Gadano A, Cartier M, Casciato P, Lucero R, Muñoz A, Romero G, Levi D, Terg G, Miguez C, Abecasis R. Serum creatinine and bilirubin predict renal failure and mortality in patients with spontaneous bacterial peritonitis: a retrospective study. *Liver Int.* 2009; 29:415-19.

[29] Rodrigues-Pinto E, Freitas-Silva M. Hepatorenal syndrome, septic shock and renal failure as mortality predictors in patients with spontaneous bacterial peritonitis. *GE J. Port. Gastrenterol.* 2012; 19(6):278-283.

[30] França AV, De Souza JB, Silva CM, Soares EC. Long-term prognosis of cirrhosis after spontaneous bacterial peritonitis treated with ceftriaxone. *J. Clin. Gastroenterol.* 2001; 33: 295-8.

[31] Kamani L, Mumtaz K, Ahmed US, Ali AW, Jafri W. Outcomes in culture positive and culture negative ascitic fluid infection in patients with viral cirrhosis: cohort study. *BMC Gastroenterol.* 2008; 8:59.

[32] Umgelter A, Reindl W, Miedaner M, Schmid RM, Huber W. Failure of current antibiotic first-line regimens and mortality in hospitalized patients with spontaneous bacterial peritonitis. *Infection* 2009; 37:2-8.

[33] Cho JH, Park KH, Kim SH, Bang JH, Park WB, Kim HB, Kim NJ, Oh MD, Lee HS, Choe KW. Bacteremia is a prognostic factor for poor outcome in spontaneous bacterial peritonitis. *Scand. J. Infect. Dis.* 2007; 39:697-702.

[34] Appenrodt B, Grünhage F, Gentemann MG, Thyssen L, Sauerbruch T, Lammert F. Nucleotid-binding oligomerization domain containing 2 (NOD2) variants are genetic risk factors for death and spontaneous bacterial peritonitis in liver cirrhosis. *Hepatology* 2010; 51:1327-33.

[35] Garcia-Tsao G, Lee FY, Barden GE, Cartun R, West AB. Bacterial translocation to mesenteric lymph nodes is increased in cirrhotic rats with ascites. *Gastroenterology* 1995; 108: 1835-1841.

[36] Woodcock NP, Robertson J, Morgan DR, Gregg KL, Mitchell CJ, MacFie J. Bacterial translocation and immunohistochemical measurement of gut immune function. *J. Clin. Pathol.* 2001; 54: 619-623.

[37] Garcia-Tsao G, Albillos A, Barden GE, West AB. Bacterial translocation in acute and chronic portal hypertension. *Hepatology* 1993; 17: 1081-1085.

[38] Ramachandran A, Balasubramanian KA. Intestinal dysfunction in liver cirrhosis: Its role in spontaneous bacterial peritonitis. *J. Gastroenterol. Hepatol.* 2001; 16: 607-612.

[39] Pardo A, Bartolí R, Lorenzo-Zúñiga V, Planas R, Viñado B, Riba J, Cabré E, Santos J, Luque T, Ausina V, Gassull MA. Effect of cisapride on intestinal bacterial overgrowth and bacterial translocation in cirrhosis. *Hepatology* 2000; 31: 858-863.

[40] Runyon BA, Squier S, Borzio M. Translocation of gut bacteria in rats with cirrhosis to mesenteric lymph nodes partially explains the pathogenesis of spontaneous bacterial peritonitis. *J. Hepatol.* 1994; 21: 792-796.

[41] Llovet JM, Bartolí R, Planas R, Cabré E, Jimenez M, Urban A, Ojanguren I, Arnal J, Gassull MA. Bacterial translocation in cirrhotic rats. Its role in the development of spontaneous bacterial peritonitis. *Gut.* 1994; 35: 1648-1652.

[42] Guarner C, Runyon BA, Young S, Heck M, Sheikh MY. Intestinal bacterial overgrowth and bacterial translocation in cirrhotic rats with ascites. *J. Hepatol.* 1997; 26: 1372-1378.

[43] Cirera I, Bauer TM, Navasa M, Vila J, Grande L, Taurá P, Fuster J, García-Valdecasas JC, Lacy A, Suárez MJ, Rimola A, Rodés J. Bacterial translocation of enteric organisms in patients with cirrhosis. *J. Hepatol.* 2001; 34: 32-37.

[44] Wells CL. Relationship between intestinal microecology and the translocation of intestinal bacteria. *Antonie Van Leeuwenhoek* 1990; 58:87-93.

[45] Wiest R, Garcia-Tsao G. Bacterial translocation (BT) in cirrhosis. *Hepatology* 2005; 41:422-33.

[46] Chen Y, Yang F, Lu H, Wang B, Chen Y, Lei D, Wang Y, Zhu B, Li L. Characterization of fecal microbial communities in patients with liver cirrhosis. *Hepatology* 2011; 54:562-72.

[47] Yan AW, Fouts DE, Brandl J, Stärkel P, Torralba M, Schott E, Tsukamoto H, Nelson KE, Brenner DA, Schnabl B. Enteric dysbiosis associated with a mouse model of alcoholic liver disease. *Hepatology* 2011; 53:96-105.

[48] Bauer TM, Steinbrückner B, Brinkmann FE, Ditzen AK, Schwacha H, Aponte JJ, Pelz K, Kist M, Blum HE. Small intestinal bacterial overgrowth in patients with cirrhosis: prevalence and relation with spontaneous bacterial peritonitis. *Am. J. Gastroenterol.* 2001; 96:2962-7.

[49] Ersöz G, Aydin A, Erdem S, Yüksel D, Akarca U, Kumanlioglu K. Intestinal permeability in liver cirrhosis. *Eur. J. Gastroenterol. Hepatol.* 1999; 11: 409-412.

[50] Goulis J, Patch D, Burroughs AK. Bacterial infection in the pathogenesis of variceal bleeding. *Lancet* 1999; 353: 139-142.

[51] Cereto F, Molina I, González A, Del Valle O, Esteban R, Guardia J, Genescà J. Role of immunosuppression in the development of quinolone-resistant Escherichia coli spontaneous bacterial peritonitis and in the mortality of E. coli spontaneous bacterial peritonitis. *Aliment. Pharmacol. Ther.* 2003; 17: 695-701.

[52] Fiuza C, Salcedo M, Clemente G, Tellado JM. Granulocyte colony-stimulating factor improves deficient in vitro neutrophil transendothelial migration in patients with advanced liver disease. *Clin. Diagn. Lab. Immunol.* 2002; 9: 433-439.

[53] Deschénes M, Villeneuve JP. Risk factors for the development of bacterial infections in hospitalized patients with cirrhosis. *Am. J. Gastroenterol.* 1999; 94: 2193-2197.

[54] Guarner C, Sola R, Soriano G, et al. Risk of a first community acquired spontaneous bacterial peritonitis in cirrhotics with low ascitic fluid protein levels. *Gastroenterology* 1999; 117:414-19.

[55] Obstein KL, Campbell MS, Reddy KR, Yang YX. Association between model for end-stage liver disease and spontaneous bacterial peritonitis. *Am. J. Gastroenterol.* 2007; 102:2732-6.

[56] Runyon BA. Low-protein-concentration ascitic fluid is predisposed to spontaneous bacterial peritonitis. *Gastroenterol.* 1986; 91:1343-6.

[57] Llach J, Rimola A, Navasa M, Ginès P, Salmerón JM, Ginès A, Arroyo V, Rodés J. Incidence and predictive factors of first episode of spontaneous bacterial peritonitis in cirrhosis with ascites: relevance of ascitic fluid protein concentration. *Hepatology* 1992; 16:724-7.

[58] Novella M, Solà R, Soriano G, Andreu M, Gana J, Ortiz J, Coll S, Sàbat M, Vila MC, Guarner C, Vilardell F. Continuous versus inpatient prophylaxis of the first episode of spontaneous bacterial peritonitis with norfloxacin. *Hepatology* 1997; 25:532-6.

[59] Nischalke HD, Berger C, Aldenhoff K, Thyssen L, Gentemann M, Grünhage F, Lammert F, Nattermann J, Sauerbruch T, Spengler U, Appenrodt B. Toll-like receptor (TLR) 2 promotor and intron 2 polymorphisms are associated with increased risk for spontaneous bacterial peritonitis in liver cirrhosis. *J. Hepatol.* 2011; 55:1010-16.

[60] Senzolo M, Cholongitas E, Burra P, Leandro G, Thalheimer U, Patch D, Burroughs AK. beta-Blockers protect against spontaneous bacterial peritonitis in cirrhotic patients: a meta-analysis. *Liver Int.* 2009; 29: 1189-93.

[61] Krag A, Wiest R, Albillos A, et al. Reduced mortality with nonselective betablockers (NSBB) compared to banding is not related to prevention of bleeding or bleeding related mortality: a hypothesis for non-hemodynamic effects of NSBB. *J. Hepatol.* 2011; 54:S72.

[62] Runyon BA. Paracentesis of ascitic fluid: A safe procedure. *Arch. Intern. Med.* 1986; 146:2259-61.

[63] Bernard B, Cadranel JF, Valla D, Escolano S, Jarlier V, Opolon P. Prognostic significance of bacterial infection in bleeding cirrhotic patients: A prospective study. *Gastroenterology* 1995; 108:1828-34.

[64] Cadranel JF, Denis J, Pauwels A, Barbare JC, Eugène C, di Martino V, Poquet E, Medini A, Coutarel P, Latrive JP, Lemaître P, Devergie B. Prevalence and risk factors of bacteriuria in cirrhotic patients: A prospective case-control multicenter study in 244 patients. *J. Hepatol.* 1999; 31:464-8.

[65] Rimola A, Bory F, Teres J, Perez-Ayuso RM, Arroyo V, Rodes J. Oral, nonabsorbable antibiotics prevent infection.

[66] Fernández J, Navasa M, Planas R, Montoliu S, Monfort D, Soriano G, Vila C, Pardo A, Quintero E, Vargas V, Such J, Ginès P, Arroyo V. Primary prophylaxis of spontaneous bacterial peritonitis delays hepatorenal syndrome and improves survival in cirrhosis. *Gastroenterology* 2007; 133:818-24.

[67] Grangé JD, Roulot D, Pelletier G, Pariente EA, Denis J, Ink O, Blanc P, Richardet JP, Vinel JP, Delisle F, Fischer D, Flahault A, Amiot X. Norfloxacin primary prophylaxis of bacterial infections in cirrhotic patients with ascites: a double-blind randomized trial. *J. Hepatol.* 1998; 29:430-6.

[68] Terg R, Fassio E, Guevara M, Cartier M, Longo C, Lucero R, Landeira C, Romero G, Dominguez N, Muñoz A, Levi D, Miguez C, Abecasis R. Ciprofloxacin in primary prophylaxis of spontaneous bacterial peritonitis: a randomized, placebo-controlled study. *J. Hepatol.* 2008; 48: 774-9.

[69] Runyon BA. Management of adult patients with ascites due to cirrhosis: an update. *Hepatology* 2009; 49:2087-107.

[70] Albillos A, Cuervas-Mons V, Millán I, Cantón T, Montes J, Barrios C, Garrido A, Escartín P. Ascitic fluid polymorphonuclear cell count and serum to ascites albumin gradient in the diagnosis of bacterial peritonitis. *Gastroenterology* 1990; 98:134-40.

[71] Garcia-Tsao G, Conn HO, Lerner E. The diagnosis of bacterial peritonitis: comparison of pH, lactate concentration and leukocyte count. *Hepatology* 1985; 5:91-6.

[72] Stassen WN, McCullough AJ, Bacon BR, Gutnik SH, Wadiwala IM, McLaren C, Kalhan SC, Tavill AS. Immediate diagnostic criteria for bacterial infection of ascitic fluid. Evaluation of ascitic fluid polymorphonuclear leukocyte count, pH, and lactate concentration, alone and in combination. *Gastroenterology* 1986; 90:1247-54.

[73] Yang CY, Liaw YF, Chu CM, Sheen IS. White count, pH and lactate in ascites in the diagnosis of spontaneous bacterial peritonitis. *Hepatology* 1985; 5:85-90.

[74] Campillo B, Richardet JP, Kheo T, Dupeyron C. Nosocomial spontaneous bacterial peritonitis and bacteremia in cirrhotic patients: impact of isolate type on prognosis and characteristics of infection. Clin. *Infect. Dis.* 2002; 35:1-10.

[75] González-Navajas JM, Bellot P, Francés R, Zapater P, Muñoz C, García-Pagán JC, Pascual S, Pérez-Mateo M, Bosch J, Such J. Presence of bacterial-DNA in cirrhosis identifies a subgroup of patients with marked inflammatory response not related to endotoxin. *J. Hepatol.* 2008; 48: 61-7.

[76] Runyon BA, Hoefs JC. Ascitic fluid analysis in the differentiation of spontaneous bacterial peritonitis from gastrointestinal tract perforation into ascitic fluid. *Hepatology* 1984; 4:447-50.

[77] Soriano G, Castellote J, Alvarez C, Girbau A, Gordillo J, Baliellas C, Casas M, Pons C, Román EM, Maisterra S, Xiol X, Guarner C. Secondary bacterial peritonitis in cirrhosis: a retrospective study of clinical and analytical characteristics, diagnosis and management. *J. Hepatol.* 2009; 52:39-44.

[78] Wu SS, Lin OS, Chen YY, Hwang KL, Soon MS, Keeffe EB. Ascitic fluid carcinoembryonic antigen and alkaline phosphatase levels for the differentiation of primary from secondary bacterial peritonitis with intestinal perforation. *J. Hepatol.* 2001; 34:215-21.

[79] Runyon BA. Ascitic fluid bilirubin concentration as a key to the diagnosis of choleperitoneum. *J. Clin. Gastroenterol.* 1987; 9:543-5.

[80] Angeloni S, Nicolini G, Merli M, Nicolao F, Pinto G, Aronne T, Attili AF, Riggio O. Validation of automated blood cell counter for the determination of polymorphonuclear cell count in the ascitic fluid of cirrhotic patients with or without spontaneous bacterial peritonitis. *Am. J. Gastroenterol.* 2003; 98:1844-8.

[81] Riggio O, Angeloni S, Parente A, Leboffe C, Pinto G, Aronne T, Merli M. Accuracy of the automated cell counters for management of spontaneous bacterial peritonitis. *World J. Gastroenterol.* 2008; 14:5689-94.

[82] Cereto F, Genesca J, Segura R. Validation of automated blood cell counters for the diagnosis of spontaneous bacterial peritonitis. *Am. J. Gastroenterol.* 2004; 99:14.

[83] Nousbaum JB, Cadranel JF, Nahon P, Khac EN, Moreau R, Thévenot T, Silvain C, Bureau C, Nouel O, Pilette C, Paupard T, Vanbiervliet G, Oberti F, Davion T, Jouannaud V, Roche B, Bernard PH, Beaulieu S, Danne O, Thabut D, Chagneau-Derrode C, de Lédinghen V, Mathurin P, Pauwels A, Bronowicki JP, Habersetzer F, Abergel A, Audigier JC, Sapey T, Grangé JD, Tran A; Club Francophone pour l'Etude de l'Hypertension Portale; Association Nationale des Hépato-Gastroentérologues des Hôpitaux Généraux de France. Diagnostic accuracy of the Multistix 8 SG reagent strip in diagnosis of spontaneous bacterial peritonitis. *Hepatology* 2007; 45:1275-81.

[84] Conn HO. Unusual presentations of SBP. In: Conn HO, Rodes J, Navasa M, eds. London: *Informa Healthcare*, 2000:47-74.

[85] Ortiz J, Soriano G, Coll P, Novella MT, Pericas R, Sàbat M, Sánchez F, Guarner C, Prats G, Vilardell F. Early microbiologic diagnosis of spontaneous bacterial peritonitis with BacT/ALERT. *J. Hepatol.* 1997; 26:839-44.

[86] Pelletier G, Salmon D, Ink O, Hannoun S, Attali P, Buffet C, Etienne JP. Culture-negative neutrocytic ascites: a less severe variant of spontaneous bacterial peritonitis. *J. Hepatol.* 1990; 10:327-31.

[87] Bruns T, Sachse S, Straube E, Assefa S, Herrmann A, Hagel S, Lehmann M, Stallmach A. Identification of bacterial DNA in neutrocytic and non-neutrocytic cirrhotic ascites by means of a multiplex polymerase chain reaction. *Liver Int.* 2009; 29:1206-14.

[88] Francés R, Benlloch S, Zapater P, González JM, Lozano B, Muñoz C, Pascual S, Casellas JA, Uceda F, Palazón JM, Carnicer F, Pérez-Mateo M, Such J. A sequential study of serum bacterial DNA in patients with advanced cirrhosis and ascites. *Hepatology* 2004; 39:484-91.

[89] Zapater P, Francés R, González-Navajas JM, de la Hoz MA, Moreu R, Pascual S, Monfort D, Montoliu S, Vila C, Escudero A, Torras X, Cirera I, Llanos L,Guarner-Argente C, Palazón JM, Carnicer F, Bellot P, Guarner C, Planas R, Solá R, Serra MA, Muñoz C, Pérez-Mateo M, Such J. Serum and ascitic fluid bacterial DNA: a new independent prognostic factor in noninfected patients with cirrhosis. *Hepatology* 2008; 48:1924-31.

[90] Wong CL, Holroyd-Leduc J, Thorpe KE, Straus SE. Does this patient have bacterial peritonitis or portal hypertension? How do I perform a paracentesis and analyze the results? *JAMA* 2008; 299: 1166-1178.

[91] Gerbes AL, Jüngst D, Xie YN, Permanetter W, Paumgartner G. Ascitic fluid analysis for the differentiation of malignancy-related and nonmalignant ascites. Proposal of a diagnostic sequence. *Cancer* 1991; 68:1808-14.

[92] Wang SS, Lu CW, Chao Y, Lee MY, Lin HC, Lee SD, Tsai YT, Chen CC, Lo KJ. Malignancy-related ascites: a diagnostic pitfall of spontaneous bacterial peritonitis by ascitic fluid polymorphonuclear cell count. *J. Hepatol.* 1994; 20:79-84.

[93] Viallon A, Zeni F, Pouzet V, Lambert C, Quenet S, Aubert G, Guyomarch S, Tardy B, Bertrand JC. Serum and ascitic procalcitonin levels in cirrhotic patients with spontaneous bacterial peritonitis: diagnostic value and relationship to proinflammatory cytokines. *Intensive Care Med.* 2000; 26: 1082-1088.

[94] Spahr L, Morard I, Hadengue A, Vadas L, Pugin J. Procalcitonin is not an accurate marker of spontaneous bacterial peritonitis in patients with cirrhosis. *Hepatogastroenterology* 2001; 48: 502-505.

[95] Parsi MA, Saadeh SN, Zein NN, Davis GL, Lopez R, Boone J, Lepe MR, Guo L, Ashfaq M, Klintmalm G, McCullough AJ. Ascitic fluid lactoferrin for diagnosis of spontaneous bacterial peritonitis. *Gastroenterology* 2008; 135: 803-807.

[96] França A, Giordano HM, Sevá-Pereira T, Soares EC. Five days of ceftriaxone to treat spontaneous bacterial peritonitis in cirrhotic patients. *J. Gastroenterol.* 2002; 37: 119-122.

[97] Ricart E, Soriano G, Novella MT, Ortiz J, Sàbat M, Kolle L, Sola-Vera J, Miñana J, Dedéu JM, Gómez C, Barrio JL, Guarner C. Amoxicillin-clavulanic acid versus cefotaxime in the therapy of bacterial infections in cirrhotic patients. *J. Hepatol.* 2000; 32: 596-602.

[98] Navasa M, Follo A, Llovet JM, Clemente G, Vargas V, Rimola A, Marco F, Guarner C, Forné M, Planas R, Bañares R, Castells L, Jimenez De Anta MT, Arroyo V, Rodés J. Randomized, comparative study of oral ofloxacin versus intravenous cefotaxime in spontaneous bacterial peritonitis. *Gastroenterology* 1996; 111: 1011-1017.

[99] Terg R, Cobas S, Fassio E, Landeira G, Rios B, Vasen W, Abecasis R, Rios H, Guevara M. Oral ciprofloxacin after a short course of intravenous ciprofloxacin in the treatment of spontaneous bacterial peritonitis: Results of a multicenter, randomized study. *J. Hepatol.* 2000; 33:564-9.

[100] Angeloni S, Leboffe C, Parente A, Venditti M, Giordano A, Merli M, Riggio O. Efficacy of current guidelines for the treatment of spontaneous bacterial peritonitis in the clinical practice. *World J. Gastroenterol.* 2008; 14:2757-62.

[101] Castellote J, Ariza X, Girbau A, et al. Antibiotic-resistant bacteria in spontanous bacterial peritonitis. Is it time to change? *J. Hepatol.* 2010; 52:S69.

[102] Pitout JD, Laupland KB. Extended-spectrum beta-lactamase producing Enterobacteriaceae: an emerging public-health concern. *Lancet Infect. Dis.* 2008; 8:159-66.

[103] Song KH, Jeon JH, Park WB, Park SW, Kim HB, Oh MD, Lee HS, Kim NJ, Choe KW. Clinical outcomes of spontaneous bacterial peritonitis due to extended-spectrum betalactamase-producing Escherichia coli and Klebsiella species: a retrospective matched case-control study. *BMC Infect. Dis.* 2009; 9:41.

[104] Park YH, Lee HC, Song HG, Jung S, Ryu SH, Shin JW, Chung YH, Lee YS, Suh DJ. Recent increase in antibioticresistant microorganisms in patients with spontaneous bacterial peritonitis adversely affects the clinical outcome in Korea. *J. Gastroenterol. Hepatol.* 2003; 18:927-33.

[105] Rodríguez-Baño J, Picón E, Gijón P, Hernández JR, Cisneros JM, Peña C, Almela M, Almirante B, Grill F, Colomina J, Molinos S, Oliver A, Fernández-Mazarrasa C, Navarro G, Coloma A, López-Cerero L, Pascual A. Risk factors and prognosis of nosocomial bloodstream infections caused by extended-spectrum-beta-lactamase-producing Escherichia coli. *J. Clin. Microbiol.* 2010; 48:1726-31.

[106] Rodríguez-Baño J, Picón E, Gijón P, Hernández JR, Ruíz M, Peña C, Almela M, Almirante B, Grill F, Colomina J, Giménez M, Oliver A, Horcajada JP, Navarro G, Coloma A, Pascual A; Spanish Network for Research in Infectious Diseases (REIPI). Community-onset bacteremia due to extended-spectrum beta-lactamase-producing Escherichia coli: risk factors and prognosis. *Clin. Infect. Dis.* 2010; 50:40-8.

[107] Such J, Hillebrand DJ, Guarner C, Berk L, Zapater P, Westengard J, Peralta C, Soriano G, Pappas J, Francés R, Muñoz C, Runyon BA. Nitric oxide in ascitic fluid is an independent predictor of renal impairment in patients with cirrhosis and spontaneous bacterial peritonitis. *Eur. J. Gastroenterol. Hepatol.* 2004; 16:1-7.

[108] Sort P, Navasa M, Arroyo V, Aldeguer X, Planas R, Ruiz-del-Arbol L, Castells L, Vargas V, Soriano G, Guevara M, Ginès P, Rodés J. Effect of intravenous albumin on renal impairment and mortality in patients with cirrhosis and spontaneous bacterial peritonitis. *N. Engl. J. Med.* 1999; 341: 403-409.

[109] Singh N, Wagener MM, Gayowski T. Changing epidemiology and predictors of mortality in patients with spontaneous bacterial peritonitis at a liver transplant unit. *Clin. Microbiol. Infect.* 2003; 9:531-7.

[110] Runyon BA: Monomicrobial non-neutrocytic bacterascites: A variant of spontaneous bacterial peritonitis. *Hepatology* 1990; 12:710-15.

[111] Garcia-Tsao G. Current management of the complications of cirrhosis and portal hypertension: variceal hemorrhage, ascites, and spontaneous bacterial peritonitis. *Gastroenterology* 2001; 120: 726-748.

[112] Ginés P, Rimola A, Planas R, Vargas V, Marco F, Almela M, Forné M, Miranda ML, Llach J, Salmerón JM. Norfloxacin prevents spontaneous bacterial peritonitis recurrence in cirrhosis: results of a double-blind, placebo-controlled trial. *Hepatology* 1990; 12: 716-724.

[113] Terg R, Llano K, Cobas SM, Brotto C, Barrios A, Levi D, Wasen W, Bartellini MA. Effects of oral ciprofloxacin on aerobic gram-negative fecal flora in patients with cirrhosis: results of short- and long-term administration, with daily and weekly dosages. *J. Hepatol.* 1998; 29: 437-42.

[114] Singh N, Gayowski T, Yu VL, Wagener MM. Trimethoprimsulfa-methoxazole for the prevention of spontaneous bacterial peritonitis in cirrhosis: a randomized trial. *Ann. Intern. Med.* 1995; 122:595-8.

[115] Fernández J, Ruiz del Arbol L, Gómez C, Durandez R, Serradilla R, Guarner C, Planas R, Arroyo V, Navasa M. Norfloxacin vs ceftriaxone in the prophylaxis of infections in patients with advanced cirrhosis and hemorrhage. *Gastroenterology* 2006; 131:1049-56.

[116] Runyon BA. A pill a day can improve survival in patients with advanced cirrhosis. *Gastroenterology* 2007; 133:1029-31.

[117] Kalambokis GN, Mouzaki A, Rodi M, Tsianos EV. Rifaximin for the prevention of spontaneous bacterial Peritonitis. *World J. Gastroenterol.* 2012 Apr 14; 18(14):1700-2.

In: Advances in Medicine and Biology. Volume 77   ISBN: 978-1-63117-444-5
Editor: Leon V. Berhardt   © 2014 Nova Science Publishers, Inc.

Chapter 5

Chronic Subdural Hematomas in Elderly Patients Treated by Burr Hole Craniostomy with One-Year Follow-Up: A Single Centre Experience

M. Luongo*, M.D., Michelangelo Grassi, M.D.
and Umberto Godano, M.D.
Department of Neurosurgery, "San Carlo" Hospital,
Potenza, Italy

Abstract

Chronic subdural hematoma (CSDH) is frequently seen in daily neurosurgical practice. It is becoming more and more a disease of the elderly, often following a trivial head trauma. Even if diagnosis and treatment are well established, there are still debated questions about recurrences, complications and outcome, especially in elderly patients. In this study we evaluated clinical characteristics, surgical results and long term follow-up in 142 consecutive patients (109 males and 33 females) surgically treated at our Department between 1th January 2009 and 31th December 2010, extracted by a total population of 257 patients (172 males and 84 females) harboring CSDH. Patients were followed up by neurological examinations and CT scan, one, three and twelve months after surgery. We obtained good results in 105 cases (73,9%) after one month, 103 cases (72,5%) after three months and 99 cases (69,7) after one year, with a recurrence rate of 9,1% and a mortality rate of 6,3%. Burr hole craniostomy is a good therapy for management of CSDHs, leading to a good outcome in a significant percentage, even in elderly people. The distinctive feature of this study is the remarkably large series of patients treated through the same surgical technique at the same Department and followed up for at least one year. At our knowledge, no previous study has examined the outcome

---

* Corresponding author: Marianna Luongo, M.D., Department of Neurosurgery, "San Carlo" Hospital, via Potito Petrone – 85100 Potenza (Italy), Postal Address: Via Palmanova, 1 – 85100 Potenza (Italy), Email: marianna.luongo@gmail.com, Mobile Phone: +393389754505; Fax number: +39971612535

of CSDHs such a long time after surgery in a relatively homogeneous population of elderly patients, who all underwent the same surgical technique, with a steady cure rate of almost 70% one year after surgery.

Keywords: Chronic subdural hematoma, burr hole, recurrence, outcome, follow-up, cure rate

Introduction

Chronic subdural hematoma (CSDH) is frequently encountered in neurosurgical practice, with a reported incidence of 1-5,3 cases per 100,000 per year, even if more recent studies have shown a higher incidence, probably because of better images techniques [1], and it tends to predominantly occur in elderly patients, in whom the incidence is estimated at 7,4/100,000. Several theories have been postulated about pathophysiologic mechanism, diagnosis and treatment are well recognized, but problems regarding recurrences, complications and cure rate are yet to be completely known especially in elderly patients.

Even the latest published literature, despite the important evaluations provided about peri-operative risks, complications and outcome in elderly people, are lacking of a long enough follow-up period [2-4].

We describe our results with 142 consecutive surgical cases, among a total population harboring CSDH of 257 patients over two years, with a follow-up of at least one year after surgery.

Materials and Methods

From 1th January 2009 and 31th December 2010, we observed at the Department of Neurosurgery of San Carlo Hospital, 257 patients (172 males and 84 females) affected by CSDH. The overall mean age was 77.3 (±11.5 years). Among them, in this report, we retrospectively reviewed medical records of 142 consecutive adult patients surgically treated by burr hole craniostomy, during the above mentioned period, focusing the attention on surgical results in such an old population, treated by using the same surgical technique.

There were 109 men and 33 women, the overall mean age was 78,1 (±10.6 years), with a range from 36 to 99 years. Factors conditioning the surgical treatment were clinical characteristics determined by the hematoma associated with a midline shift more than 5 mm. Patients not underwent to surgery were clinically and radiologically controlled, because their clinical conditions and the entity of midline shift didn't required surgery but only a conservative treatment, mainly based on hydration.

The diagnosis of CSDHs was confirmed by computer tomography (CT), also performed to control surgical results and during follow-up, respectively one month, three months and one year after surgery. From this point we'll refer only to surgical patients.

Clinical Characteristics

The most frequent clinical symptoms were hemiparesis (97 cases, 68,3%), followed by incontinence (59 cases, 41,5%) and motor aphasia (49 cases, 34,5%). (Table 1).

Patients characteristics are described in Table n. 4. Head trauma, often trivial, is well recognized to be probably the main risk factor for the development of CSDHs.

Nevertheless, a clear history of head injury is reported in 39 patients (27,4%) in our series. At the time of diagnosis of CSDHs, 32 patients received anticoagulant or antithrombotic therapy (22,5%). Most patients didn't have any definite cause of CSDHs or, most probably, couldn't remember any episode of head trauma. The distribution of clinical symptoms is described in Table 1. The main pathological conditions associated to CSDHs was arterial hypertension (66 patients, 46,4%), followed by diabetes mellitus (20 patients, 14,8%).(Table 4)

Table 1. Presenting Symptoms in 142 patients with CSDH

Symptoms	Number of patients	Male	Female
Hemiparesis	97 (68,3%)	73	24
Consciousness Disturbances	75 (52,8%)	57	18
Ideomotor slowdown	22 (15,5%)	21	1
Disorientation	36 (25,3%)	26	10
Drowsiness	16 (11,2%)	10	6
Coma	1 (0,7%)	0	1
Incontinence	59 (41,5%)	40	19
Motor Aphasia	49 (34,5%)	36	13
Gait Disturbances	20 (14,08%)	12	8
Headache	13 (9,1%)	12	1
Cranial nerves deficits	13 (9,1%)	12	1

Table 2. Results in 142 patients with CSDH

	Good Recovery	No Changes	Recurrence	Exitus	No Response
In-Hospital	127 (89,4%)	6 (4,2%)	7 (4,9%)	2 (1,4%)	-
Post-Discharge:	Good Recovery	No Changes	Recurrence	Exitus	No Response
One Month	105 (73,9%)	-	4 (2,8%)	-	28 (19,7%)
Three Months	103 (72,5%)	-	2 (1,4%)	1 (0,7%)	-
Long term Follow-up	Good Recovery	No Changes	Recurrence	Exitus	No Response
One Year	99 (69,7%)	-	-	6 (4,2%)	-
TOT	-	6 (4,2%)	13 (9,1%)	9 (6,3%)	28 (19,7%)

Table 3. Markwalder's grading system and summary of clinical results in 142 patients with CSDH

		Pre-op	1 month	3 months	1 year
		n. of patients	n. of patients	n. of patients	n. of patients
Grade 0	Patient neurologically normal	3	53	64	61
Grade 1	Patient alert and oriented; mild symptoms, such as headache; absent or mild symptoms or neurological deficits	60	50	38	36
Grade 2	Patient drowsy or disoriented with variable neurological deficit, such as hemiparesis	69	2	1	2
Grade 3	Patient stuporous but responding appropriately to noxious stimuli; severe focal signs, such as hemiparesis	7	-	-	-
Grade 4	Patient comatose with absent motor response to painful stimuli; decerebrate or decorticate posturing	3	-	-	-
TOT		142	105	103	99

Surgical Treatment

142 cases of CSDHs were treated (under general anesthesia or sedation, according to patient's condition and anesthesiologist's preference) through a single burr hole performed 2-3 cm in front of parietal eminence, enlarged through a ribbed cutter with a maximum diameter of 17 mm. The hematomas were spontaneously evacuated and repeatedly irrigated with warm saline by means of nelathon catheter, inserted in several directions through the enlarged hole. The enlargement degree (reaching a maximum diameter of 2 cm) was established, from time to time, by the neurosurgeon according to the characteristics of the hematoma, showed by preoperative CT scan. The nelathon catheter was also used as subdural drain, by connecting it to a sterile pocket, avoiding negative pressure. This closed system subdural dranaige was left in the hematoma cavity for 24-48 hours, and was removed according to clinical conditions of the patient and to the amount of the liquid drained.

Patients Assessment

Mobilization began, after removing the drainage, as soon as possible, compatibly with patients' conditions, with no precise early or delayed protocol of mobilization. Subcutaneous low weight molecular heparin admnistered until a completely mobilization had been reached. Patients with no complications were discharged on the 5th-8th day after surgery and followed up for one year, with a first clinical and radiological assessment one month later, to evaluate the postoperative state and to compare it with the preoperative one. Postoperative conditions were classified in four categories: good recovery, no change, recurrence and exitus (Table 2). The neurological performance of the patients was preoperatively and postoperatively evaluated with the "Markwalder's Neurological Grading System", the most commonly used grading system for CSDHs (Table 3) [5-6]. Clinical and radiological follow-up was performed by CT scan in all patients three months and one year after surgery.

Results

Outcome

Overall good outcome was achieved in most of cases (105 patients of 142): after surgery, in fact, the mean neurological status improved in most but 6 cases, which show no changes. The overall mortality rate was 6,3%, corresponding to 9 patients, 2 of which (1,4%) died during the hospitalization because of complications. The remaining 7 patients died, beyond discharge, due to other conditions, not related to evacuation of CSDH and, particularly: 2 respiratory arrests, 1 ischemic stroke, 1 pulmonary embolism, 1 pancreatic failure, 1 complication related to an abdominal operation and 1 not explained reason. Three months after surgery, the clinical and radiological assessment showed 103 patients (72,5%) with good recovery and this trend was confirmed at the assessment one year after surgery when 99 patients (69,7%) showed good results, especially if we consider the mean age of this series: 78,1 (±10.6 years). (Table 2)

Complications and Recurrence

As complications, we observed 7 cases of pneumocephalus, 4 acute subdural hematomas and 1 ponto-mesencephalic hemorrhage (Figure 1). Patients with acute subdural hematomas underwent to urgent surgical operation, while pneumocephalus spontaneously absorbed, helped by a postoperative hydration. Overall, 2 patients (1,4%) died, during hospitalization, because of complications (acute subdural hematoma and ponto-mesencephalic hemorrhage), while the other patients with complications had a good outcome, with no permanent deficits. The rate of recurrence was 4,9% during the hospitalization, when 7 patients underwent reoperation through the previous burr hole, and 4,2% post-discharge, within three months, with an overall recurrence rate of 9,1% (13 of 142 patients).

Table 4. Clinical characteristics of 142 patients with CSDHs

Clinical characteristics:	Male (%)	Female (%)	TOT (%)
Sex	109 (76,7)	33 (23,2)	142
Mean age	77,5	80,4	78,2
Left side hematoma	59 (41,5)	16 (11,2)	75 (52,8)
Right side hematoma	33 (23,2)	7 (4,9)	40 (28,1)
Anticoagulant therapy	19 (13,3)	13 (9,1)	32 (22,5)
History of head trauma	31 (21,8)	8 (5,63)	39 (27,4)
Coexisting disease:	Male (%)	Female (%)	TOT (%)
Arterial hypertension	51 (35,9)	15 (10,5)	66 (46,4)
Diabetes mellitus	17 (11,97)	3 (2,1)	20 (14,08)
Dyslipidemia	7 (4,9)	2 (1,4)	9 (6,3)
Hepatitis	3 (2,1)	0	3 (2,1)
Cardiac arrhythmia	1 (0,7)	0	1 (0,7)
Epilepsy	1 (0,7)	0	1 (0,7)

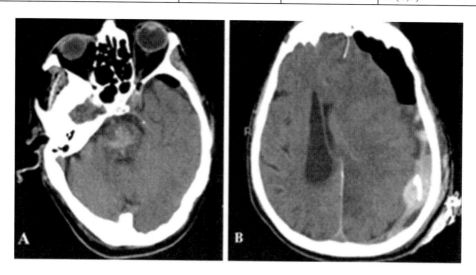

Figure 1. CT scan showing complications determining in-hospital mortality;
A: ponto-mesencephalic hemorrhage; B: left acute subdural hematoma.

Discussion

Chronic subdural hematoma is a common entity seen in neurosurgery and it is becoming more and more an elderly disease. It is an encapsulated collection of blood first described as "pachymenigitis haemorragica interna" by Virchow in 1857 and afterwards by Trotter, in 1914, as "chronic subdural hemorrhage of traumatic origin", introducing the theory of trauma to the bridging veins [7-8]. The clinical picture of CSDH varies widely. There are no pathognomonic signs or symptoms that allow one to make the diagnosis solely on the basis of clinical data and it is not even clear which pathophysiologic aspect causes the clinical symptoms that's why Potter, in 1977, described CSDH as "the great neurological imitator"

[9]. After the description of Virchow, first surgical attempts to treat "pachymeningitis haemorragica interna" failed, so leading to the assumption that it was an incurable disorder. Successful neurosurgical treatment was marked by the publication of Hulke in The Lancet, in 1883; a reported "cure rate" of 83%, after a large craniotomy with marsupialization of the membranes, was achieved with Horrax and Poppen in 1937 [10]. During the following year, surgical techniques improved and the same good results were achieved by less invasive methods in largest series. Markwalder's review on CSDHs of 1981 was an important step in minimizing the invasiveness of surgical treatment, confirming that twist drill or burr hole craniostomy with closed system drainage, described by Tabaddor and Shulman, should have been the initial procedure of choice for patients affected by CSDHs. [11] Before then, in fact, neurosurgical point of view on treatment was influenced by the idea that CSDHs was a possibly lethal disorder so, the option of a large craniotomy with capsulectomy was currently considered for surgical treatment [12]. Nowadays, the development of mini-invasive techniques is aimed to achieve sufficient drainage, especially in elderly people, in a minimally invasive manner as possible, and to prevent early and late recurrence and to avoid complications related to surgery or anesthesiology. Sometimes they were referred to as "bedside techniques", to underline the character of low invasiveness. These strategies vary from replacement of hematoma by injecting oxygen, to puncture of the hematoma with a butterfly needle ("trans-marrow puncture") and drainage to the exterior, or to facilitate the spontaneous outflow of the CSDHs after positioning the hollow screw, followed by irrigation with Ringer to dilute the hematoma, or by using a stainless evacuating port, radiolucent silicone tubing and a bulb suction device [13-16]. The necessity to identify the most effective surgical approach lead to a well-designed meta-analysis based on the existing data published, which confirmed burr hole craniostomy as superior to twist drill craniostomy and craniotomy, as regards a lower incidence of recurrence and of highly morbid complications [17]. Even if the goal of surgical treatment is removing the hematoma, it has been established that removal of hematoma's membrane doesn't reduce the risk of recurrence. The risk is in fact increased by the concentration of inflammatory mediators and fibrinolytic factors contained in the hematoma fluid so its removal, simply achievable by burr hole craniostomy, enables to reach the primary goal of surgery. The breaking up of the hematoma and the dilution of its inflammatory and fibrinolytic content represent the rationale behind the use of irrigation in conjunction with burr hole craniostomy (or with any of the other surgical techniques used); it has been demonstrated to determine a decrease in recurrence rate [18]. Since the variation in outcome in the literature likely reflects differences in surgical evacuation techniques, we chose to investigate the outcome of CSDH one year after surgery in a relatively homogeneous cohort of patients, treated exclusively by a single technique, at the same institution. The most frequent early symptoms in our series (hemiparesis, incontinence and motor aphasia) were consistent with other reported in literature. (Table 1) Anticoagulant or antiaggregant therapy were used in 32 patients (22,5%) at time of diagnosis. A history of head injury, often trivial, has been reported in 39 cases (27,4%). Epilepsy is traditionally considered a rare presentation; in our series there was just one case (0,7%), even though it has been reported in up to 6% of cases as an initial symptom. All of our patients were surgically treated with a single enlarged burr hole performed 2-3 cm in front of the parietal eminence. It really took short operation time, avoiding in elderly people respiratory and anesthesiologic complications, and leading to an overall recurrence rate of 9,1%. Recurrence, as the occurrence of signs and symptoms due to an increase in hematoma volume in the ipsilateral

space documented by CT scan, happened in 9,1% of our patients; all of them underwent surgery in the previous operation site. After a patient has successfully undergone surgery, a major concern is prevention of recurrence so many authors, in different studies, focused the attention on the role of several aspects (i.e. localization of drainage, patient's position after surgery, coagulopathy, anticoagulant/antiaggregant therapy, timing of mobilization etc.), in determining CSDH's recurrence. It has been accepted that the use of drain reduces recurrences and, according to Nagakuchi, its placement over the frontal convexity was ideal to reduce them [19].

As regards positioning, Abouzari et coworkers asserted that assuming an upright position soon after surgery was not recommended for elderly because significantly associated with increased incidence of recurrence; on the contrary, Nakajima had previously affirmed that elderly should assume an upright position as soon as possible [20-21]. Coagulopathy and postoperative low molecular weight heparin thromboprophylaxis may be a contributing risk factor for recurrence, so that a delayed protocol of mobilization [24, 25, 26]. The rate of anticoagulant/antiaggregant drugs reported by Gelabert-Gonzàlez and coworkers in a population older than 70 years was 11,3%, with a low recurrence rate found (6,1%) [22]. Similar studies by Mori or Baechli respectively reported 18,5% and 13,6%, in this subpopulation of elderly patients. [23-24] In our series, patients assumed a supine position for 24-48 hours, until removal of drainage; the subdural drainage didn't systematically follow a specific direction, although preferring an "opposite to the vertex" position; subcutaneously bemiparin thromboprophylaxis was administrated by the day after surgery and mobilization began, after removing drainage, as soon as possible, (compatibly with their clinical conditions) and received anticoagulant drugs in a percentage of 22,5%. This surgical and clinical behavior led to an overall recurrence rate of 9,1%, all within three months after surgery, but we couldn't demonstrate a cause and effect relationship with this result. CSDHs is known to have a significant recurrence rate reported by different authors, with ranges from 5% to 30%, as underlined by Oh and colleagues, according to which this is due to a lack of working criteria of the recurrence of CSDHs. Since more than half of recurrent CSDHs recurred within one month and 70% of them within 3 months, the authors suggested that follow-up for 2 months after surgery is not enough and proposed to set the term of 3 months as cut off, classifying recurrence in "*early recurrence*" within 3 months from surgery and "*late recurrence*" beyond 3 months [24-25].

We classified recurrences considering three months as a cut off, but depending on they occur during the hospitalization or post discharge. We observed recurrence in 13 cases, so our recurrence rate (9,1%) is quite low compared with literature data, but we distinguished in-hospital recurrence (7 patients, 4,9%) from post-discharge recurrence, within three months too, (6 patients, 4,2%) [26]. We also debated about long term results, referring to this literature data according to which there is a worsening of remote recovery [4]. Our results let us be fairly optimistic on the long term follow-up because, one year after surgery, the trend towards good recovery is quite firm, especially considering the mean age of patients (78,1 ±10.6 years) and the fact that the mortality was determined by causes not related to CSDHs. (Table 2)

We have found little data focusing the attention on elderly people harboring CSDHs published. In 2011, Miranda et al. reported the first review of the long term outcome following treatment of CSDHs in the elderly, retrospectively analyzing 209 patients admitted to their institution between September 2000 and February 2008, with a mean age of 80,6 years; they undertook an examination of the long term mortality rate in patients affected by CSDHs. They found that whereas the in-hospital mortality rate was 16,7%, modestly exceeding the average reported rate they referred to of 0-15,6%, 6 months and 1 year later rates continue to increase to 26,3 and 32%, respectively. These results compared with lifetable matched actuarial survival underlined that CSDH confers significant excess mortality for up to 1 year post discharge [4]. Furthermore, they assumed that CSDHs unmask and exacerbate some associated pathological conditions that lead to that progressive increasing in post-discharge mortality. Authors referred to Weigel's review article which summarized the data from 48 publications, focusing on a cure rate of 80% and mortality rate of 2,8%, but not indicating the follow-up duration [27]. According to Miranda, a short follow-up could lead to underestimate a condition that progressively gets worse, becoming not a so "benign disease" for elderly people [4]. Their population was the oldest cohort to be reported in literature with a mean of about 26 cases per year. No other series of patients affected by CSDHs has examined the long term outcome after surgery in such old group, but we must emphasized, according to Burchiel, that 35% of 209 cases have been conservatively treated so there wasn't a direct correlation between surgical treatment and mortality rate [28]. The latest reported study regarding CSDHs in elderly patients, by Borger et al., evaluated the outcome and peri-operative risks and complications in these patients. They reported on 322 patients treated, during seven years, by a single burr hole, irrigation and positioning of subdural drain. The mean age was 76. Results in this series are encouraging, with an overall rate of peri-operative complications of 6% and a mortality rate of 2,75%. Despite a different distribution of patients, our results were similar, but the great difference between the studies regards the follow-up that was performed in very short period (14 days post discharge or until the resolution of the subdural fluid, in case of its persistence documented by CT scan) while, in our series, is at least of one year [2].

In a recent study, Han and colleagues compared the postoperative recurrence rates between one and two burr hole craniostomy, with closed system drainage, concluding that CSDH can be sufficiently evacuated through one burr hole craniostomy and this technique has two additional advantages, especially for elderly people: is less invasive and takes short operation time, even with lower recurrence rate, compared with reported ones, ranging from 9,2 to 26,5%, they analyzed [26]. The necessity in elderly patients to obtain mini-invasivity and shorter operation time led to the development of some "bedside techniques". The great limitation of the studies reporting about these techniques is represented by not clear interpretation of results: the authors sometimes don't consider as recurrence the failure of the first treatment and the necessity to repeat it, or don't indicate the follow-up period, so it is difficult to really evaluate the efficacy of mini-invasive techniques in elderly people [28, 16]. We can say that burr hole craniostomy has a good cure to complication ratio and a low recurrence rates: we obtained a cure rate of 72,5% one month after surgery and an overall percentage of recurrence of 9,1%, considering that recurrences all occurred within three months. All our 142 surgical patients were treated with the same procedures and recurrences underwent surgery through the previous burr hole: this enables to really evaluate the outcome, so allowing a correlation between surgical results and a single surgical technique. Although during last decades different important on surgical treatment of CSDHs have been published, analyzing different aspects from surgical techniques to outcome and recurrence, this study on surgical treatment on 142 consecutive cases of CSDHs is "unusual" for different aspects: the remarkable number of elderly patients treated at a single Institute (71/year), the same surgical technique used to treat all patients, one of the longest follow-up [2, 4, 24-26, 29].

Comparing ours with the other studies, we analyzed clinical findings, surgical results and long term outcome of 142 consecutive cases, extracted by a population of 257 patients affected by CSDH, observed over two years at our Department. This remarkable series could be justified by the fact that our Neurosurgical Unit is the only one in a region populated by about 587.000 inhabitants.

We think that some other studies are necessary to better understand the trend forwards an increasing incidence of this condition, if it should be related to some unrecognized predisposing factor or to an increased indication to anticoagulant or antithrombotic therapy, even if it was present in 32 cases in our series (22,5%), a lower rate compared to literature data [23]. Another aspect to be analyzed is the correlation between increased incidence and quite good results.

We think that surgical technique could play a role: the enlargement of the burr hole, in fact, though being less invasive, lead the surgeon better to aid the spontaneous evacuation of hematoma and consent an optimal irrigation with warm saline, thus removing factors determining rebleeding and leading to a modest recurrence rate. The single surgical technique, in our opinion, consents to really evaluate the recurrence rate, which is not influenced by several surgical options. The "innovation" of this study, compared to the vast majority of the previous ones, is represented by a longer follow-up: our population has been evaluated also one year after surgery and, unlike Miranda et al. and their worsening of clinical conditions and increasing of mortality, we could have observed an overall mortality of 6,3% with a satisfying cure rate (69,7%), especially considering the mean age and the percentage of patients lost to follow-up (19,7%) [4].

Limitations

Our study present several limitations. The data analysis was performed retrospectively (although the quality and completeness of data are satisfying) and our results come from a single center experience, because our Department is the only one in the Region. Another limitation is the observational nature of the data and the absence of a control group so conclusions on cause and effect relationship should be carefully drawn.

Conclusion

To our knowledge, no previous study has examined the outcome of CSDHs such a long time after surgery in a relatively homogeneous population of elderly patients, who all underwent the same surgical technique. In our experience, burr hole craniostomy is a an effective way to manage CSDHs, leading to a good outcome in a significant percentage. Further study are necessary to better manage prognosis and life expectancy in such a selected subgroup of older patients.

Acknowledgments

We are grateful to Dr. Paolo Severino, Director of the Department of Neurosurgery - "San Carlo" Hospital - from March 2003 to September 2010, and to Carmela Pietrafesa for helping us in collecting patients' data.

References

[1]   Senturk S, Guzel A, Bilici A, Takmaz I, Guzel E, Aluclu MU, et al. CT and MR imaging of chronic subdural hematomas: a comparative study. *Swiss Med Wkly*. 2010;140:335-340.

[2]   Borger V, Vatter H, Oszvald A, Marquardt G, Seifert V, Guresir E. Chronic subdural haematoma in elderly patients: a retrospective analysis of 322 patients between the ages of 65-94 years. *Acta. Neurochir (Wien)*. 2012;154:1549-1554.

[3]   Dumont TM, Rughani AI, Goeckes T, Tranmer BI. Chronic Subdural Hematoma: A Sentinel Health Event. *World Neurosurg*. 2012.

[4]   Miranda LB, Braxton E, Hobbs J, Quigley MR. Chronic subdural hematoma in the elderly: not a benign disease. *J. Neurosurg*. 2011;114:72-76.

[5]   Lee JK, Choi JH, Kim CH, Lee HK, Moon JG. Chronic subdural hematomas: a comparative study of three types of operative procedures. *J. Korean Neurosurg. Soc*. 2009;46:210-214.

[6]   Markwalder TM, Steinsiepe KF, Rohner M, Reichenbach W, Markwalder H. The course of chronic subdural hematomas after burr-hole craniostomy and closed-system drainage. *J. Neurosurg*. 1981;55:390-396.

[7]   Virchow. Das Heamotom der dura mater. *Verhandlungender Phys Med Gesellesh*. 1857;24:134-142.

[8]   Trotter W. Chronic subdural hemorrage of traumatic origin and its relation to pachymeningitis haemorragica interna. *Br. J. Surg*. 1914;2:271.

[9]   Potter JF, Fruin AH. Chronic subdural hematoma--the "great imitator". *Geriatrics*. 1977;32:61-66.

[10]   Hulke. Severe blow on the right temple, followed by right hemiplegia and coma, and then by spastic rigidity of the left arm; trephining; evacuation of inflammatory fluid by incision through dura mater; quick disappearance of cerebral symptoms; complete recovery. *Lancet*. 1883;2:814.

[11]   Tabaddor K, Shulmon K. Definitive treatment of chronic subdural hematoma by twist-drill craniostomy and closed-system drainage. *J. Neurosurg*. 1977;46:220-226.

[12]   Markwalder TM. Chronic subdural hematomas: a review. *J. Neurosurg*. 1981;54:637-645.

[13]   Singla A, Jacobsen WP, Yusupov IR, Carter DA. Subdural evacuating port system (SEPS)—minimally invasive approach to the management of chronic/subacute subdural hematomas. *Clin. Neurol. Neurosurg*. 2013;115:425-431.

[14]   Krieg SM, Aldinger F, Stoffel M, Meyer B, Kreutzer J. Minimally invasive decompression of chronic subdural haematomas using hollow screws: efficacy and safety in a consecutive series of 320 cases. *Acta. Neurochir (Wien)*. 2012;154:699-705.

[15] Latini MF, Fiore CA, Romano LM, Spadaro E, Zorrilla JP, Gonorazky SE, et al. [Minimally invasive treatment of chronic subdural hematoma in adults. Results in 116 patients]. *Neurologia.* 2012;27:22-27.

[16] Takeda N, Sasaki K, Oikawa A, Aoki N, Hori T. A new simple therapeutic method for chronic subdural hematoma without irrigation and drainage. *Acta. Neurochir (Wien).* 2006;148:541-546.

[17] Lega BC, Danish SF, Malhotra NR, Sonnad SS, Stein SC. Choosing the best operation for chronic subdural hematoma: a decision analysis. *J. Neurosurg.* 2010;113:615-621.

[18] Goldstein H, Sonabend AM, Connolly ES, Jr. Chronic subdural hematomas: perspective on current treatment paradigms. *World Neurosurg.* 2012;78:66-68.

[19] Nakaguchi H, Tanishima T, Yoshimasu N. Relationship between drainage catheter location and postoperative recurrence of chronic subdural hematoma after burr-hole irrigation and closed-system drainage. *J. Neurosurg.* 2000;93:791-795.

[20] Abouzari M, Rashidi A, Rezaii J, Esfandiari K, Asadollahi M, Aleali H, et al. The role of postoperative patient posture in the recurrence of traumatic chronic subdural hematoma after burr-hole surgery. *Neurosurgery.* 2007;61:794-797; discussion 797.

[21] Nakajima H, Yasui T, Nishikawa M, Kishi H, Kan M. The role of postoperative patient posture in the recurrence of chronic subdural hematoma: a prospective randomized trial. *Surg. Neurol.* 2002;58:385-387; discussion 387.

[22] Gelabert-Gonzalez M, Iglesias-Pais M, Garcia-Allut A, Martinez-Rumbo R. Chronic subdural haematoma: surgical treatment and outcome in 1000 cases. *Clin. Neurol. Neurosurg.* 2005;107:223-229. 16.

[23] Baechli H, Nordmann A, Bucher HC, Gratzl O. Demographics and prevalent risk factors of chronic subdural haematoma: results of a large single-center cohort study. *Neurosurg. Rev.* 2004;27:263-266.

[24] Mori K, Maeda M. Surgical treatment of chronic subdural hematoma in 500 consecutive cases: clinical characteristics, surgical outcome, complications, and recurrence rate. *Neurol. Med. Chir. (Tokyo).* 2001;41:371-381.

[25] Oh HJ, Lee KS, Shim JJ, Yoon SM, Yun IG, Bae HG. Postoperative course and recurrence of chronic subdural hematoma. *J. Korean Neurosurg. Soc.* 2010;48:518-523.

[26] Han HJ, Park CW, Kim EY, Yoo CJ, Kim YB, Kim WK. One vs. Two Burr Hole Craniostomy in Surgical Treatment of Chronic Subdural Hematoma. *J. Korean Neurosurg. Soc.* 2009;46:87-92.

[27] Weigel R, Schmiedek P, Krauss JK. Outcome of contemporary surgery for chronic subdural haematoma: evidence based review. *J. Neurol. Neurosurg Psychiatry.* 2003;74:937-943.

[28] Burchiel KJ. Outcome in chronic subdural hematoma. *J. Neurosurg.* 2011;114:71; discussion 71.

[29] Kwon TH, Park YK, Lim DJ, Cho TH, Chung YG, Chung HS, et al. Chronic subdural hematoma: evaluation of the clinical significance of postoperative drainage volume. *J. Neurosurg.* 2000;93:796-799.

In: Advances in Medicine and Biology. Volume 77   ISBN: 978-1-63117-444-5
Editor: Leon V. Berhardt   © 2014 Nova Science Publishers, Inc.

Chapter 6

Basic Approach to Metabolic Acidosis

Consolación Rosado, PhMD, Rosario Manzanedo,
Carmen Felipe, PhMD, Begoña Alaguero, Amelia Fidalgo,
Carlos Chacón and Jesús Martín, PhMD
Service of Nephrology of the Care Complex of Ávila, Spain

Abstract

Metabolic acidosis is a disorder of the acid-base balance due to excessive acid production, kidney maladjustment to such production or excessive loss of base. The consequence is the reduction of serum bicarbonate (when combined with excess acid or lost by the kidney or gastrointestinal tract), the secondary decrease in partial carbon dioxide blood pressure and the reduction in blood pH.

It is a symptom of various diseases and its severity can range from mild discomfort to the possibility of imminent death.

Depending on the anion gap [Na+ - (Cl - + HCO3-)], metabolic acidosis are classified into two types: hyperchloremic (normal anion gap), which are caused by bicarbonate losses through the digestive or urinary tract and normocloremic (anion gap increased), caused by acid gain, which can be endogenous or exogenous. The latter group includes lactic acidosis, ketoacidosis, renal failure acidosis, and intoxication by ethanol, methanol, ethylene glycol, aldehydes and acetyl salicylic acid.

Any type of metabolic acidosis significantly alters both hydroelectrolytic balance and extracellular volume. Thus, in acute stages hyperkalemia, distal reuptake inhibition of sodium, volume depletion and hypercalcemia (protein bound calcium displacement) occur. At this stage the cardiovascular system is affected in a very obvious way, as both contractility and cardiac output are reduced and arterial vasodilation occurs, which contributes to the development of hypotension. Other signs include tachypnea, diaphoresis, gastrointestinal discomfort and depression of the central nervous system.

In chronic stages hypokalemia, increased natriuresis (as sodium gets out of the bone, this acting as acid buffer) and increased renal loss of calcium, phosphorus and magnesium occur. At this stage the musculoskeletal system is most affected, since metabolic acidosis can cause or exacerbate pre-existing bone disease, accelerate muscle breakdown to produce muscle loss and cause growth deficiency in children.

The diagnosis of metabolic acidosis is based on four points: confirmation of the state of acidosis, respiratory compensation assessment, quantification of the anion gap and comparison of the anion gap increase with decreasing plasma bicarbonate. This requires having a blood gas test, which can be venous, arterial or capillary and quantifying the plasma sodium, potassium and chlorine.

Regarding the treatment it is essential to assess the magnitude and speed of the onset of acidosis, determine the cause, apply a specific treatment and ensure advanced life support for severe cases. The general treatment is to stop the production of acid, increase endogenous bicarbonate production, apply exogenous bicarbonate and maintain homeostasis of the internal environment.

Definition

Metabolic acidosis is characterized by a primary reduction in serum bicarbonate (HCO_3^-) concentration, a secondary decrease in arterial partial pressure of carbon dioxide ($PaCO_2$) and a reduction in blood pH [1,2].

If we consider the reaction of the proton (H^+) with HCO_3^-, the main extracellular buffer:

$$H^+ + HCO_3^- \Leftrightarrow H_2CO_3 \Leftrightarrow CO_2 + H_2O$$

It is clear that metabolic acidosis is due to an increase in H^+ or a decrease in the HCO_3^-. Thus, this condition is caused by the inability of the kidney to excrete the H^+ charge obtained in the diet, the increase in the generation of H^+ or intestinal or renal loss of HCO_3^-.

It can be acute, lasting from minutes to several days and is relatively common among severely ill patients or chronic, that can last from weeks to years, is rare and usually occurs in patients with impaired renal function [3].

Both forms can produce significant adverse effects on cell function and may contribute to increased morbidity and mortality.

Pathophysiology

Maintaining the arterial pH between 7.35 and 7.45 is essential for normal cell function, since even small fluctuations in the concentration of H^+ significantly affect the activity of various enzymatic systems [4]. The optimum pH is achieved through the extracellular and intracellular buffers, along with respiratory and renal regulatory mechanisms. Thus, the response to the elevation of the concentration of H^+ involves four processes: extracellular buffering by HCO_3^-, intracellular and bone buffering, respiratory compensation and renal excretion of acid load. The first three mechanisms are the first to act, although the renal excretion of excess H^+ achieves the final restoration of acid-base balance.

In the acid-base balance, the production of acid and the renal handling of HCO_3^- play a key role.

With a normal diet, 50-100 mEq/day of H^+ are generated, as sulfuric acid from the catabolism of the amino acids, organic acids not metabolized, phosphoric acid and other acids. However, the metabolic alterations, as the ones that occur in the synthesis of lactic acid or ketogenesis and ingestion of substances that are metabolized to organic acids, such as methanol or ethylene glycol, can increase the production of acid [3,4].

These H^+ are buffered at early stages by HCO_3^- and other cell and bone buffers to minimize intracellular pH drop. However, the acid-base balance is restored by the excretion of H^+ in the urine, which regenerates the HCO_3^- lost in the buffer reaction [5].

The kidney is the key organ for the maintenance of acid-base balance, as it is the only one that excretes daily non-volatile acid load resulting from the daily protein intake and endogenous catabolism by the proximal reabsorption of HCO_3^- filtered, the total excretion of H^+ and regeneration of HCO_3^- in the distal nephron, a third combined with urinary phosphate and sulfate (titratable acidity) buffers, and the remaining two thirds with ammonia forming ammonium anion.

When the glomerular filtration rate falls below 20 ml/min these mechanisms are altered, so that metabolic acidosis occurs [6].

Classification

To make an etiological classification of metabolic acidosis we must know the anion GAP, since it is affected differently by the various conditions that cause metabolic acidosis.

This anion is defined as $[Na^+] - ([Cl^-] + [HCO_3^-])$ and its normal range is relatively large (6-10 mmol/L), due to biological variability of their components [1].

It can be affected by different factors. It is reduced approximately 2.3 mmol/L per 10 g/L of reduced serum albumin concentration. It may also be decreased or become negative due to the serum accumulation of cationic paraprotein, bromide or iodide. Oppositely, a serum increase of anionic paraprotein or hyperphosphatemia can elevate it. Thus, the most significant increases in anion GAP (figures greater than 45 mmol/L) are associated with severe hyperphosphatemia. However, the most common cause of increased anion GAP is the accumulation of organic or inorganic anions in metabolic acidosis [2].

Given the involvement of the anion GAP, the acidosis can be classified into:

– *Hyperchloremic*: occur with normal anion GAP and are produced by bicarbonate loss. In this type of acidosis, anion GAP does not increase because, as the acid accumulated in blood is HCl, the Cl^- retained is equal to HCO_3^- entitled for protons. Serum anion GAP may drop slightly due to the acid titration of circulating proteins.

– *Normocloremic*: anion GAP is increased. They are caused by the gain of acid that, since it contains a different anion to the Cl^-, the drop in the concentration of seric HCO_3^- is associated with an elevation in the anion GAP.

We conclude that, in metabolic acidosis with increased anion GAP, the HCO_3^- is "used" in the buffer of the accumulation of endogenous or exogenous acids, whereas the metabolic acidosis that occur with normal anion GAP is the HCO_3^- buffer that is lost primarily.

Metabolic Acidosis with Normal Anion GAP (Hyperchloremic)

They may be caused by digestive and urinary loss of HCO_3^- or the net gain of Cl^-, situation known as cloroacidosis [7].

Intestinal Loss of HCO $_3^-$

Biliopancreatic secretions contain 200 mEq/day of HCO_3^-, of which 150 mEq are neutralized by stomach acid. Thus, the remaining 50 mEq must be reabsorbed in the gastrointestinal tract. When this is altered by derivation or disease, metabolic acidosis is caused by loss of HCO_3^-.

The most common causes are diarrohea, biliary drainage, ostomy (duodenostomy, ileostomy, jejunostomy), paralytic ileus, intestinal fistulas or villous adenomas [2].

This type of metabolic acidosis has two particular characteristics: hypokalemic, as the loss of HCO_3^- is accompanied by loss of K^+ and the hypovolemia that is produced activates the renin-angiotensin II-aldosterone axis, which may contribute to increased disposal of K^+ and the subsequent generation of a metabolic alkalosis (typical of chronic diarrohea and laxative abuse) [8].

Urinary Loss of HCO₃⁻ Filtering (Proximal Tubular Acidosis)

Most filtered bicarbonate (80-85%) is reabsorbed in the proximal convoluted tubule by the Na^+/H^+ pump and H^+-ATPase. At this level, carbonic anhydrase facilitates the division of cytosolic H_2CO_3 in HCO_3^- and H^+, thus generating H^+ to be secreted. The HCO_3^- formed escapes out of the cell through the basolateral cotransporter Na^+/HCO_3^-.

In the proximal renal tubular acidosis (type II) the role of carbonic anhydrase or secretion of H^+ can not reabsorb all the HCO_3^- filtrated, so that this reaches the collecting duct that is impermeable. Na^+ reuptake attracts K^+ and H^+, which are lost in the urine together with the Na^+, so hypokalaemia occurs.

The proximal renal tubular acidosis is an inherited or acquired alteration in the proximal transport of HCO_3^-. Although this condition may be present as an isolated defect in the reabsorption of HCO_3^- (hereditary defects on the function of the S1C4A4 gene and deficiency of carbonic anhydrase), is more frequent the coexistence of defects in other carriers of the proximal tubule, which generate fosfaturia, aminoaciduria and glucosuria, which is known as the Fanconi syndrome [3]. Hereditary disorders that occur with this syndrome include Wilson's disease, cystinosis and fructose intolerance. Diseases such as multiple myeloma, renal transplant rejection or the administration of carbonic anhydrase inhibitors may cause acquired Fanconi syndrome [9].

Defect in Synthesis of Renal HCO₃⁻ (Distal Tubular Acidosis I and IV)

The type A intercalated cells of the collecting duct, stimulated by aldosterone, synthesize daily the HCO_3^- lost during metabolism. To be able to do this, H_2O and CO_2 are extracted from the capillary side and, in the presence of carbonic anhydrase, HCO_3^- and H^+ are obtained. The main cells send the HCO_3^- with Na^+ into the capillary lumen and the H^+ through a pump of H^+ and the pump K^+-H^+-ATPase into the tubular lumen.

To remove a sufficient amount of H^+ is required to have elements to neutralize it and prevent the accumulation of H^+ in the urine, such as NH_3, which is excreted along with the H^+ as NH_4 or HPO_4^{2-}, in which the H^+ forms H_2PO_4.

For the HCO_3^- to be synthesized and the H^+ to be eliminated, the integrity of certain elements is necessary, since the absence or alteration of any will generate distal renal tubular acidosis [10].

These elements are: the presence of aldosterone, an electronegative luminal gradient allowing correct exchange of ions, intercalated cell integrity, availability of items combining with H^+ and urinary tract to be covered with endothelium, to avoid back diffusion of H^+ [2].

- *Aldosterone:* primary or secondary deficit of aldosterone or the receptors, cause distal renal tubular acidosis.
- *Primary deficit:* Mineralocorticoid deficiency, adrenogenital syndrome with deficit in C-21 hydroxylase, Addison's disease.
- *Secondary deficit:* Hyporeninemic hypoaldosteronism, renin synthesis inhibition by nonsteroidal antiinflammatories or beta-blockers, inhibition of synthesis of angiotensin II by inhibitors of the converting enzyme or its receptors.

The causes of hyporeninemic hypoaldosteronism are detailed in the following table:

Table 1. Causes of hyporeninemic hypoaldosteronism

CAUSES OF HYPORENINEMIC HYPOALDOSTERONISM	
Diabetes mellitus	Interstitial nephritis
Arterial Hypertension	Gout
Glomerulonephritis	Analgesic induced nephropathy
Obstructive uropathy	Mixed cryoglobulinemia
Lead nephropathy	Sickle-cell disease
Amyloidosis	Systemic lupus erythematosus
Renal transplantation	

Deficiency of aldosterone receptors: Pseudohypoaldosteronism type I (due to mutations in the epithelial sodium channel or the mineralocorticoid receptor), and spironolactone.

- *Defect in the formation of an electronegative gradient in the distal tubule lumen:* that may be caused by an increase in permeability to Cl^- or decreased permeability to Na^+.

The causes responsible for the increased permeability to Cl^- are type II pseuhypoaldosteronism or Gordon syndrome which is associated with increased distal transport of Na^+ and Cl^- and the use of cyclosporine.

The permeability to Na^+ is reduced by the consumption of various drugs such as triamterene, amiloride, and atrial natriuretic peptide.

- *Defective H^+ pump:* This may be caused by distal tubular acidosis type I, in which only the interleaved cell is affected, and may result from congenital forms, the use of inhaled glue or amphotericin B or distal tubular acidosis type IV, in which both intercalated and principal (responsible for the exchange of Na^+ by K^+) cells are affected, and that generates a salt-losing nephropathy with hyperkalaemia and entities such as chronic interstitial nephritis or chronic pyelonephritis can occur.

−   *Availability of items combining with H^+:*

Defect in proximal synthesis of NH_3: Hyperkalaemia inhibits the synthesis of NH_3 and medullary cystic disease and obstructive uropathy prevent its arrival to the distal tubule.

Defect in the availability of titratable acidity: Reduced glomerular filtration makes difficult the removal of H^+ and HCO_3^- synthesis by the distal tubule.

−   *Integrity of the urothelium:* In patients with an ureterosigmoidostomy, colecistoplasty or ileocystoplasty, acidic urine contacts the intestinal epithelium and H^+ go back to the capillaries, so that HCO_3^- cannot be generated.

Cloroacidosis

This type of metabolic acidosis with Cl^- occurs when the body comes into contact with large amounts of HCl [3]:

$$HCl \rightarrow Cl^- + H^+ \rightarrow H^+ + HCO_3^- \rightarrow CO_2 + H_2O$$

In these cases a net gain of Cl^- occurs and HCO_3^- is lost to neutralize the H^+.

Table 2. Hyperchloremic metabolic acidosis as potassium levels

METABOLIC ACIDOSIS WITH NORMAL ANION GAP (HYPERCHLOREMIC)		
serum K^+ increased or normal		low serum K^+
Administration of HCl or precursors		Diarrohea
Administration of cationic amino acids		Intestinal, pancreatic or biliary fistula
Chronic kidney disease		Proximal renal tubular acidosis
Primary or secondary adrenal insufficiency		Distal renal tubular acidosis
Hyporeninemic hypoaldosteronism		Ureterosigmoidostomy / Ureteroileostomy
Hyperkalemic distal renal tubular acidosis		Diabetic ketoacidosis
Pseudoaldosteronism type I		Toluene poisoning
Pseudoaldosteronism type II (Gordon syndrome)		D-Lactic acidosis
Medication	Spironolactone Prostaglandin inhibitors Triamterene Amiloride Trimethoprim Pentamidine Ciclosporin	

The most frequent causes of acidosis are using derived clorohidrated lysine or arginine, parenteral nutrition, hypertonic saline, ammonium chloride or sevelamer.

Metabolic acidosis with normal anion GAP may be associated with hyperkalemia or hypokalemia [7]. A classification of these entities in relation to serum potassium is detailed next.

Metabolic Acidosis with Elevated Anion GAP (Normocloremic)

This type of acidosis is caused by the accumulation of endogenous or exogenous acids.

Accumulation of Endogenous Acids

Occurs when there is an imbalance between the synthesis of endogenous acids and their use or disposal, which is typical for situations such as:

− *Renal impairment:* Both acute and chronic renal failure can cause this type of metabolic acidosis, the latter being the most common cause of chronic metabolic acidosis.

Kidney failure is the cause of metabolic acidosis for two reasons: the distal acidification does not work, which is necessary for regenerating HCO_3^- and the reduction in glomerular filtration causes retention of inorganic anions, increasing the anion GAP [1,2].

− *Lactic acidosis:* Different types of lactic acidosis may occur [8]:
  1 Type A lactic acidosis: It is generated by a sudden decrease of oxygen supply to the tissues which prevents the aerobic metabolism of carbohydrates, causing pyruvate to be transformed into lactate. For each lactate that appears, HCO_3^- is destroyed, so metabolic acidosis occurs with increased anion GAP:

$$\text{lactic acid} \rightarrow \text{lactate}^- + H^+ \rightarrow H^+ + HCO_3^- \rightarrow CO_2 + H_2O$$

  2 Type B lactic acidosis: It is due to the inability of the liver to metabolize lactic acid which is normally produced, because of liver failure, which may be due to different causes, such as myocardial infarction or extensive ischemia, severe hypoperfusion due to shock, defects in the transport or use of oxygen (CO or cyanide poisoning), or defects in pO_2.
  3 It can also be observed when the hepatic metabolism of lactic acid is interfered with by substances such as ethanol or metformin.
  4 D-lactic acidosis: It is a rare disorder, occurring when intestinal flora is disturbed, so that the organic acids in the D system, such as D-lactic acid, cannot be metabolized. This acidosis is often found in episodes of bacterial translocation or short bowel syndrome. The process is not a very severe acidosis with neurological signs and symptoms such as ataxia and dysarthria.
− *Ketoacidosis:* This occurs when there is a deficit of oxaloacetate, which is necessary for the acetyl-CoA to be integrated into the Krebs cycle to generate energy.

Oxaloacetate deficiency exists when this is used for gluconeogenesis because the liver cannot dispose of glucose. Thus, the ketone bodies formed by the acetyl-CoA that has accumulated are used by muscle and brain for energy after long periods of fasting. When liver cells spend long time unable to import glucose, the maintained gluconeogenesis generates lots of ketones, as in situations like: great aerobic exercise, insulin deficiency, prolonged fasting, gluconeogenesis type I, sustained alcohol intake without consuming carbohydrates or salicylate poisoning. The latter occurs most commonly in suicide attempts or in the elderly who take medication for the treatment of rheumatic diseases. In the absence of a history of ingestion of salicylates, the presence of respiratory alkalosis is an important clue to the diagnosis of this entity [3].

$$\text{Ketoacids} \rightarrow \text{acetoacetate}^- \text{ or } \beta\text{-Hydroxybutyrate}^- + H^+ \rightarrow HCO_3^- + H^+$$

These anions accumulate as the bicarbonate is consumed, so that a metabolic acidosis occurs with increased anion GAP.

Diabetic ketoacidosis and lactic acidosis are the most common causes of acute metabolic acidosis, and together account for 85% of cases when metabolic acidosis (blood pH <7.1) is severe.

Accumulation of Exogenous Acids

These may be alcohols or aldehydes [2].

- *Alcohols* The toxic alcohols, including methanol, ethylene glycol, diethylene glycol and propylene glycol can produce a metabolic acidosis with increased risk of mortality.

This metabolic acidosis is unusual in that causes an increase in blood osmolality. This is because, as those alcohols have a low molecular weight (32-106 kDa), their accumulation raises serum osmolality and causes a mismatch between the estimated and measured serum osmolality called osmolal gap. Serum osmolality can be estimated using the following formula:

Serum osmolality (mOsm/L) = 2x [Na$^+$] (mmol/L) [BUN] (mg/dL) / 2.8 [Glucose] (mg/dL) /18

Typically, the difference between the estimated and measured serum osmolality is ≤ 10 mOsm/L (<10 mmol/kg). Osmolal anion GAP > 20 mOsm/L (> 20 mmol/kg) consistently indicates the accumulation of one of the toxic alcohol or ethanol, although no increase of the serum osmolality will not preclude the ingestion of toxic alcohols. If enough time has passed for most of the alcohol to have been metabolized to organic acids, serum osmolality is altered minimally [1].

The determination of ethanol, methanol, ethylene glycol, diethylene glycol, and in some cases, propylene, is indicated in the presence of a osmolal gap or when intoxication by toxic alcohols is suspected based on clinical findings.

- *Aldehydes*: Paraldehyde, which was used as a hypnotic produces severe metabolic acidosis with increased anion GAP but does not raise the osmolality by its high molecular weight. It was used as a sedative and hypnotic, but has been displaced by barbiturates, neuroleptics and benzodiazepines.

Clinical Effects

The clinical effects are different in the case of an acute or chronic acidosis.

Acute Metabolic Acidosis

The most significant effect is produced in the cardiovascular system because contractility and cardiac output are reduced and arterial vasodilation and hypotension develop. These phenomena depend on the figures of blood pH: when it drops from 7.4 to 7.2, the cardiac output increases due to increased catecholamine levels, but when the pH falls below 7.1-7.2 cardiac output falls, in part due to resistance development to inotropic and vasoconstrictor effects of catecholamines infused. With these levels of acidosis, the predisposition to the development of ventricular arrhythmias increases [1,11].

Even with very slight changes in the cerebrospinal pH, mental confusion and lethargy can be observed.

The affinity of hemoglobin for oxygen is also affected. Thus, already in the first 8 hours, the production of 2,3-diphosphoglycerate (which increases the affinity of hemoglobin for oxygen) decreases.

Acute metabolic acidosis alters the immune response in various ways: the chemotactic properties and bactericidal capacity of leukocytes are weakened, production of interleukins by macrophages are stimulated and lymphocyte function is suppressed [2].

Cellular energy production and cellular responses to insulin are dependent on pH figures, so are also altered.

Finally, there is an increased susceptibility to cell death, since the acute metabolic acidosis stimulates apoptosis phenomena.

Chronic Metabolic Acidosis

The target of chronic acidosis is the musculoskeletal system, as it causes or exacerbates bone disease and muscle breakdown is accelerated, which generates muscle wasting and stunting. These abnormalities are more frequent and severe with greater degrees of metabolic acidosis, but even mild acidosis may contribute to the development of bone disease and muscle breakdown [1].

Secretion and action of different hormones is also altered, such as corticosteroids, the thyroid and parathyroid hormone and insulin.

Albumin synthesis is reduced, while increasing the production of β2-microglobulin, which predisposes patients to amyloidosis.

This type of acidosis has no direct effect on cardiovascular function, although mortality by this cause is increased in patients with chronic kidney disease, when serum bicarbonate concentration falls to 22 mmol/L.

A generalized stimulation of inflammation also appears to contribute to the adverse effects of chronic metabolic acidosis.

Table 3. Clinical manifestations of metabolic acidosis

ACUTE	Impaired leukocyte function and suppression of lymphocyte function
	Predisposition to ventricular arrhythmias
	Arterial vasodilation with hypotension
	Resistance to catecholamines and insulin
	Altered cellular energy production
	Stimulation of apoptosis and the production of interleukins
	Changes in mental status
	Alterations in the binding of oxygen to haemoglobin
	Venoconstriction
	Decreased contractility and cardiac output
CHRONIC	Generation or worsening of bone disease
	Stunting
	Impaired glucose tolerance.
	Accelerated progression of chronic kidney disease
	Muscle spending increased
	Albumin synthesis reduction
	Increased production of β 2microglobulina

Diagnosis

The diagnosis of acid-base disorders requires a systematic approach, in which a complete medical history and the thorough physical examination are very useful because they determine whether the acidosis is acute or chronic.

In addition to an arterial or venous blood gas test, plasma and urinary ionograms are essential, since the former allows us to calculate the anion GAP and thus classify the type of metabolic acidosis and the second helps differentiate the loss of HCO_3^+ from defect in urine acidification in metabolic hyperchloremic acidosis [12,13].

Below is a detailed diagnosis algorithm to determine the cause of the metabolic acidosis:

Treatment

Metabolic acidosis is caused by a loss of HCO_3^- or by the net addition of strong acids. The elimination or control of the underlying cause, if feasible, is obviously a high priority in the treatment of all forms of metabolic acidosis [3].

Decisions about the type of therapy depend on the duration and severity of the disorder.

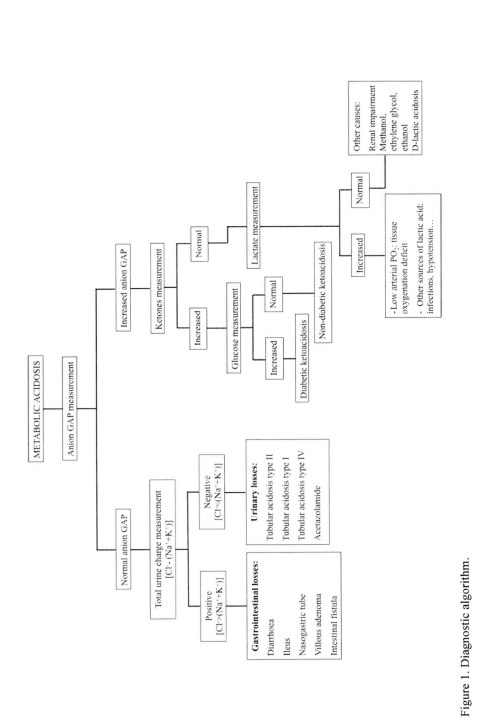

Figure 1. Diagnostic algorithm.

Acute Metabolic Acidosis

Changes in the intracellular and extracellular pH are responsible for the adverse effects of metabolic acidosis. This is the reason why, traditionally, base management (especially $NaCO_3^-$ compounds) has been the therapy of choice. However, this treatment does not result in a reduction in morbidity or mortality or a improvement in cardiovascular dysfunction.

Consequently, there is disagreement among clinicians about the value of the administration of HCO_3^- in these acid-base disorders and the criteria for administration [3].

The failure of the administration of $NaCO_3^-$ to improve cardiovascular function, morbidity and mortality could be partly ascribed to the adverse affects of the therapy, including exacerbation of intracellular acidosis caused by the generation of CO_2 in the process buffering, hypertonicity of the extracellular fluid when HCO_3^- is given as a hypertonic solution, volume overload, reflect metabolic alkalosis, enhancing the synthesis of organic acids and acceleration of cellular Na^+, K^+, causing a deleterious rise in cellular Na^+ and Ca^{2+} [2,3].

This is the reason why the therapy must be individualized in these cases, with the use of HCO_3^- solutions only in the cases when they are actually needed.

It is necessary to assess the severity and the presence of other electrolyte and acid-base disorders associated.

Acidosis severity depends on:

- HCO_3^- in arterial blood, an indicator of the remaining buffer capacity. When lower than 5 mmol/l, acidosis is very severe.
- Adequate compensation of pCO_2: arterial pCO_2 higher than expected indicates a disorder in alveolar ventilation and will have a big impact on the final figure of pH. A pCO_2 <15 mmHg indicates that respiratory compensation is reaching its limit. The venous pCO_2 is an index of tissue perfusion, which will be compromised if it exceeds the arterial pCO_2 by 10 mmHg.
- Etiology of acidosis: lactic acidosis caused by hypoxia is the most serious, since their rate of production of H^+ is far superior to other acidosis. The acidosis caused by alcohol intoxication are severe for their rapid development [4].

The serum potassium is the main parameter to be evaluated to establish the treatment. Each 0.1 units that the pH decreases, the K^+ increases by 0.6 mmol/l. In severe acidosis, normal values of K^+ indicate that there is an underlying hypokalaemia that may go unnoticed and worsen during the correction of acidosis, favouring respiratory muscle fatigue. In these cases, the hypokalaemia correction must be done simultaneously to the acidosis [2].

Metabolic acidosis with increased anion GAP: treatment is based on slowing the source of acid production. The addition of bicarbonate should be limited only to certain specific circumstances (extreme hyperkalaemia or life-threatening decreases in pH), always assessing risks and benefits. It is useful in extreme acidosis to gain time while what caused the acidosis is corrected, preferably as non-hyperosmolar preparations (bicarbonate 1/6 M) [15].

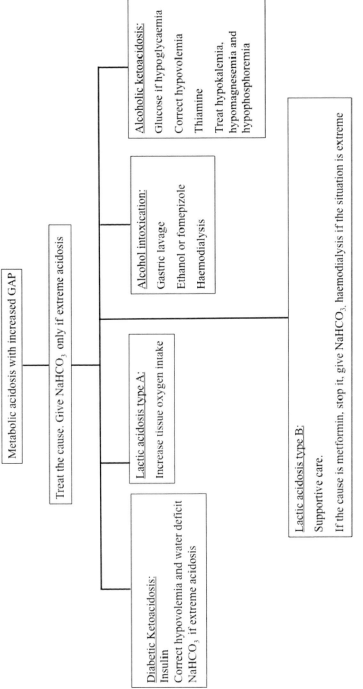

Figure 2. Scheme of treatment of metabolic acidosis with increased anion GAP.

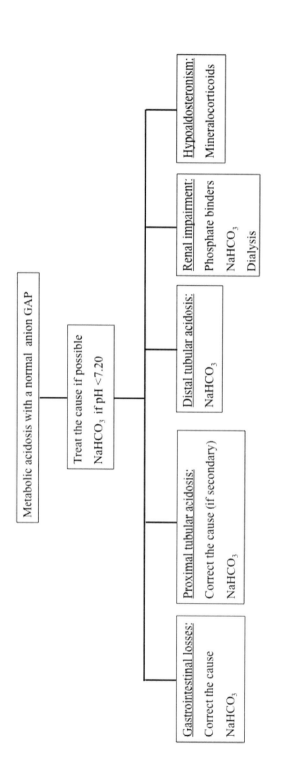

Figure 3. Scheme of treatment of metabolic acidosis with normal anion GAP.

The target serum bicarbonate in the replacement calculations shall not exceed 10 to 12 mEq/l.

Bicarbonate deficit = Δ HCO$_3^-$ x 0.5* x body weight

Δ HCO$_3^-$ = target HCO$_3^-$ - plasma HCO$_3^-$

* In extreme acidosis ([HCO3] $\leq$ 5 mEq/l) replace the value of 0.5 with 0.8.

Metabolic acidosis with normal anion GAP: treatment with NaHCO$_3$ is less restrictive, because in the origin of acidosis there is a primary loss of bicarbonate, which is typically used if the pH is <7.20 [14,15].

Chronic Metabolic Acidosis

The administration of bases improves or slows the progression of bone disease, normalizes growth and albumin synthesis, reduces muscle breakdown and delays the progression of chronic renal disease. Serum HCO$_3^-$ should be raised at least to 22-23 mmol/L.

Patients with normal renal function or chronic renal disease without dialysis can be treated with HCO$_3^-$ oral salts. These drugs can cause abdominal discomfort and, if so, should be replaced by sodium citrate [2].

Base therapy may exacerbate pre-existing hypertension and volume overload occurs, so it is necessary to maintain the balance of neutral sodium.

Mineralocorticoid treatment is indicated in chronic metabolic acidosis of individuals with hiporeninemic states, but should be used with caution in patients with pre-existing hypertension. In these patients, the acidosis and hyperkalaemia can be controlled with diuretics or sodium polystyrene sulfonate [15].

In haemodialysis patients, the use of dialysate with high bicarbonate concentration (approximately 40 mmol/L) is sufficient to correct metabolic acidosis. In peritoneal dialysis a dialysate with high concentration of base is enough.

References

[1]   Palmer BF. Approach to fluid and electrolyte disorders and acid-base problems. *Prim Care* 2008;35(2):195-213.
[2]   Kraut JA, Madias NE. Metabolic acidosis: pathophysiology, diagnosis and management. *Nat Rev Nephrol.* 2010 May;6(5):274-85.
[3]   Ayers P, Dixon C. Simple acid-base tutorial. *JPEN J Parenter Enteral Nutr.* 2012 Jan;36(1):18-23.
[4]   Liamis G, Milionis HJ, Elisaf M. Pharmacologically-induced metabolic acidosis: a review. *Drug Saf.* 2010 May 1;33(5):371-91.

[5]   Bruno CM, Valenti M. Acid-base disorders in patients with chronic obstructive pulmonary disease: a pathophysiological review. *J Biomed Biotechnol.* 2012;2012:915150.

[6]   Halperin ML, Kamel KS: Some observations on the clinical approach to metabolic acidosis. *J Am Soc Nephrol* 21: 894–897,2010.

[7]   DuBose TD Jr: Hyperkalemic hyperchloremic metabolic acidosis: Pathophysiologic insights. *Kidney Int* 51: 591–602,1997.

[8]   Andersen LW, Mackenhauer J, Roberts JC, Berg KM, Cocchi MN et al. Etiology and therapeutic approach to elevated lactate levels. *Mayo Clin Proc.* 2013 Oct;88(10):1127-40.

[9]   Haque SK, Ariceta G, Batlle D. Proximal renal tubular acidosis: a not so rare disorder of multiple etiologies. *Nephrol Dial Transplant.* 2012 Dec;27(12):4273-87.

[10] Batlle D, Haque SK. Genetic causes and mechanisms of distal renal tubular acidosis. *Nephrol Dial Transplant.* 2012 Oct;27(10):3691-704.

[11] Renda F, Mura P, Finco G, Ferrazin F, Pani L et al. Metformin-associated lactic acidosis requiring hospitalization. A national 10 year survey and a systematic literature review. *Eur Rev Med Pharmacol Sci.* 2013 Feb;17 Suppl 1:45-9.

[12] Kraut JA, Madias NE. Differential diagnosis of nongap metabolic acidosis: value of a systematic approach. *Clin J Am Soc Nephrol.* 2012 Apr;7(4):671-9.

[13] Ayers P, Warrington L. Diagnosis and treatment of simple acidbase disorders. *Nutr Clin Pract.* 2008;23:122-128.

[14] Adrogue HJ, Madias NE. Medical progress: management of lifethreatening acid-base disorders: first of two parts. *N Engl J Med.*1998;338(1): 26-34.

[15] Kraut JA, Madias NE. Treatment of acute metabolic acidosis: a pathophysiologic approach. *Nat Rev Nephrol.* 2012 Oct;8(10):589-601.

In: Advances in Medicine and Biology. Volume 77
Editor: Leon V. Berhardt

ISBN: 978-1-63117-444-5
© 2014 Nova Science Publishers, Inc.

Chapter 7

The Biomechanics of the Ankle Joint

M. R. Nannaparaju, W. S. Khan and K. Vemulapall
UCL Institute of Orthopaedics and Musculoskeletal Sciences,
Royal National Orthopaedic Hospital, Stanmore, London, UK

Abstract

Ankle joint is one of the most complex joints in the human body. Anatomists, biomechanical engineers, and clinicians have studied the foot and ankle complex for centuries.

Each discipline has provided its unique insight into the structure and function of this unit. The differences of approaches have also led to varying interpretations, resulting in considerable confusion regarding the operation of this complex.

The purpose of this article is to discuss the basic biomechanical characteristics and forces acting on the ankle under static conditions and their influences on artificial total ankle replacement designs.

Introduction

The ankle joint has been an area of study for centuries. It is a complex joint form by the articulation of many bones and helps in transforming body load onto the foot. It is one of the most important joints of the body as pain, discomfort and other pathology may have significant impact on the functional life of an individual. Due to its structure, the biomechanical forces acting on the ankle are very different and complicated to those acting on the hip or knee.

Having a clear understanding of these is very important for a clinician to diagnose the ankle pathology and choose the appropriate means of treatment. This article discusses the anatomy, biomechanical aspects of the ankle and their implications in designing total ankle replacement prosthesis.

Anatomy of the Ankle Joint

The ankle joint complex consists of three joints namely the ankle joint (or talocrural), the subtalar joint and the midtarsal joints. The ankle joint consists of three bones namely, the tibia, fibula, and talus (figure 1). The average thickness of the ankle cartilage is approximately 1.6mmwhereas the thickness of thc knee cartilage is 6–8mm (Shepherd and Seedhom, 1999).

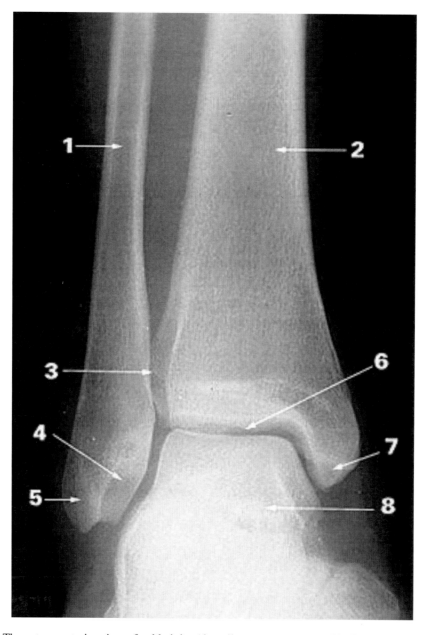

Figure 1. The anteroposterior view of ankle joint (http://www.szote.u-szeged.hu/Radiology/ Anatomy/skeleton) 1. Fibula; 2. Tibia; 3. Distal tibiofibular joint; 4. Malleolar fossa; 5. Lateral malleolus; 6. Ankle joint; 7. Medial malleolus; 8. Talus.

The ankle joint experiences higher forces than any other articulation. During the stance phase, the ankle joint experiences forces of magnitude 5 to 7 times the body weight (BW) whereas it is 3 to 4BW in the knee joint and 2 to 3BW in the hip joint (Stauffer et al., 1977). Although the surface area of the ankle joint is similar to that of the hip and knee joints,the contact area during loading is only one-third of these. (Kimizuka et al., 1980; Brown and Shaw, 1983; Ihn et al., 1993).

The ankle joint gains its stability from bony congruence, the joint capsule as well as ligamentous support.Medial ankle stability comes from the medial malleolus and the deltoid ligament, which is by far the strongest stabilizer of the ankle with a tensile strength of 714N. CFL is the strongest ligament on the lateral side with a tensile strength of 346N (Attarian et al, 1985).

Gait Cycle

The proper concept of gait cycle is very important to understand the biomechanics of ankle. Gait cycle has two different phases, the stance phase and the swing phase. The stance phase constitutes about 60% of the gait cycle in order of occurrence it is divided into these divisions: heel strike, foot flat, heel rise, pushoff and toeoff. The swing phase takes up the other 40% of the gait cycle and is divided into acceleration, toe clearance, and deceleration. Muscular activity during gait affords control of the foot such that the centre of gravity of the body progresses smoothly forward without excessive frontal plane motion.

Gait may also be specifically considered in relation to foot motion in the sagittal plane using the rocker theory (Perry,1992). During the first rocker the ankle plantarflexes after heel-strike bringing the forefoot into contact with the ground. Ankle plantarflexion is brought under control by eccentric (lengthening) contraction of the extrinsic anterior compartment. Next during the second rocker the ankle dorsiflexes as the centre-of-gravity of the body moves over the joint muscles. The final third rocker occurs as the metatarsophalangeal joints dorsiflex in preparation for toe-off. Here the windlass mechanism is activated, tensioning the plantar fascia under the metatarsophalangeal joints and transforms into a rigid lever which can transmit a propulsive force to the ground.

Biomechanics of the Static Ankle

Patil et al. (1993) developed a 2D finite element (FE) model of a normal foot and simulated the joint forces acting on it to determine the ground reaction forces in different stages of the gait cycle. In their study the foot bone material was assumed to be isotropic, homogenous and linearly elastic with a young's modulus of 7.3Gpa and poisson's ratio of 0.3. Table 1 shows the ankle joint forces, ground reaction forces, highest principal tensile stresses, highest principal compressive stress, and highest vonMises stress contour during various phases of gait cycle. (Patil et al,1993).This data reveals that the ankle joint exerts almost twice the magnitude of ground reaction forces to maintain stability during each phase of gait cycle. Although a 2D model gives us a good understanding of the distribution of forces(ankle joint force, ground reaction force) and stresses (highest principal tensile, compressive stresses and vonMises stress contour) it cannot effectively depict the inticacies of the ankle joint complex. Gefen et al. (2000) designed a 3D foot model using MRIs from the feet of a 27 year old male, a 25 year old female and a cryosection from a 39 year ols male. They used a young's modulus of 7.3Gpa for the foot bones and 1Mpa for cartilage. The finite element method was selected for numerical analysis of the model. The results are shown in table 2 and 3 which show the areas experiencing increased vonMises stresses and the loads acting on the ankle joint during various subphases of gait cycle respectively.

Cheung et al. (2005) also used a 3D finite element model to study the peak vonMises stresses, during balanced standing, in the talus and calcaneum. They used the MRI of right foot from a normal male aged 26, height 174cm and weight 70 kg.Young's modulus of 7.3Gpa and poisson's ratio of 0.3 for foot bones, 1Mpa and 0.4 for cartilage, 260Mpa and 0 for ligaments were used respectively. The nominal stress values were multiplied by a factor of 2, 3, and 5 to investigate the biomechanical effect of soft tissue stiffening in different stages.

Table 1. Ankle Joint stresses during various subphases of gait

Model phase	Ankle joint force,N	Ground reaction force,N	Highest principal tensile stress,%[a]	Highest principal compressive stress,%[a]	Highest vonMises stress contour,%[a]
Midstance	2.0W	600	52.0	38	32.5
Heel phase	2.25W	961(0.77W)	--	24	22.0
Push-off	3.5W	904.8(1.51W)	82.5	61	60.0

W-Body weight of a person weighing 600N.
a-Percentage of yield stress of the bone material.

Table 2. Areas experiencing increased vonMises stresses during gait

Sub-stage	Location of stress	Maximum stress value(Mpa)	Location of stress	Maximum stress value(Mpa)	Location of stress	Maximum stress value(Mpa)
Initial contact	Plantar calcaneus	0.45	Posteriorand medial calceneus	1.21	Dorsal talus	1.07
Heel strike	Medial Calcaneus	1.24	--	--	-	-
Midstance	Posterior calcaneus	3.48	Dorsal talus	2.72	Lateral talus	2.61
Forefoot-contact	Posterior calcaneus	3.18	Dorsal talus	3.37	-	-
Push-off	Posterior calcaneus	3.80	Dorsal talus	3.55	-	-
Toe-off	Posterior calcaneus	0.61	Dorsal talus	1.04	-	-

Table 3. Loads acting on ankle joint during various subphases of gait cycle

Region	Initial contact	Heel strike,N	Midstance,N	Forefoot contact,N	Push-off,N	Toe-off,N
Ankle joint load	675	1350	2100	2550	3000	300

Table 4. vonMises stress of the foot during standing

Bone	Normal	F2	F3	F5
Talus	2.89	2.47	2.33	2.11
Calcaneum	3.94	3.50	3.27	2.99

F2,F3 and F5 correspond to simulations of 2,3and 5 times the stiffness of normal tissue.

The results are summarized in table 4 which show that with a 5% increase in tissue stiffness there is a reduction in the peak vonMises stress of 0.78Mpa at the talus and 0.95Mpa at the calcaneum.

As ligaments play a vital role in various motions of the ankle joint, the relationship between the changes in ligament strain during these motions is very important. Renstrom et al. (1988) used Hall effect transducers to determine the strain in the anterior talofibular and calcaneofibular ligaments. Measurements of 5 cadaveric ankles were made in neutral position and during the motion from 10deg dorsiflexion to 40deg plantar flexion. It was found that the strain increased in the anterior talo fibular ligament when the ankle motion ranged from 10deg dorsiflexion through 40deg plantarflexion to 3.3% as well as in the calcaneofibular ligament with supination and eversion. The strain was found to decrease in the calcaneofibular ligament with increased plantarflexion and in the anterior talofibular ligament with eversion to 1.9%. In conclusion, these two ligaments were found to be synergistic, that is when one of the ligaments is strained the other one is relaxed and vice versa.

Another important parameter which has been widely studied is the stress change in the articulating surface of the tibio-talar (TT) interface during various motions of the joint. To study the relationship between the stress changes in the TT interface, geometry of the articulating surface of the TT interface was modelled through an experiment conducted with six normal cadaveric ankles with a material testing system, Bionix MTS (Tochigi et al., 2006).The contact stress at the TT articulation was monitored by realtime contact stress sensor (Tekscan 5033). The ankles were loaded with the normal body weight (primary axial force). Also, the anterior/posterior shear forces, the inversion/ eversion torques and the internal/external rotation torque were applied independently while the other two were constrained. From the experiment it was found that the anterior/posterior shear forces produce reproducible positive changes (elevation in the values) in the anterior/posterior regions respectively. Similarly, the version torques produce corresponding reproducible positive changes in the medial/lateral regions while internal/external rotation torques produce reproducible positive changes in two diagonal locations namely anterolateral and posteromedial or anteromedial, and posterolateral. With these forces and torques as input, a model of the articulating surface was generated using MATLAB, version 7.0. The talus consists of two domes adjacent to each other on its upper surface in the frontal plane

(Saltzman et al., 2005). Hence the surface was modelled as two adjacent spheres with radii of 25 mm and the distance between the centres of the spheres was 20 mm. The radius of the sphere is taken to be 25 mm since the radius of the talar dome is 21.3 ± 1.8 mm. The analysis of the articulating surface revealed that the changes were seen with respect to altered external load to retain stability. The contribution of the articulating surface to the joint stability was 70% of the anterior/posterior stability, 50% of inversion/eversion stability and 30% of internal/external rotation stability.

Application of Biomechanics in Designing Total Ankle Replacements

TAR's were first developed in early 1970's (Alvine, 2000).They are broadly discussed as the first and second generation prostheses.

First Generation TAR's

The first generation TARs were of two types namely constrained and unconstrained. Constrained prostheses limit motion to the sagittal plane. They were typically spherical, spheroidal, conical, cylindrical or sliding cylindrical in shape (Lewis, 1994). They provided greater stability (Waugh et al., 1976), minimized impingement of the malleoli against the talus (Conti and Wong, 2001), and decreased wear of the polyethylene insert due to larger contacting surfaces. The only disadvantage of the prostheses was increased stresses at the bone cement implant interfaces leading to early failure due to aseptic loosening. Examples of this prostheses type are Imperial College London Hospital (ICLH), Conaxial, St.Georg/ Buchholz. Unconstrained prostheses were typically trochlear, bispherical, concaveconvex, and, convexconvex in shape (Lewis, 1994). They provided improved range of motion but stability was greatly reduced.The results of unconstrained prostheses proved to be a total failure (Evanski and Waugh, 1977). Though the constrained prostheses produced comparatively better initial results they also proved to be discouraging.

Second Generation TAR's

The second generation prostheses were developed to overcome the disadvantages and complications associated with the first generation prostheses (Thomas and Timothy, 2003). These implants were intended to reproduce the anatomical characteristics of the ankle joint, joint kinematics, ligament stability and mechanical alignment. The sliding and rotational motions of the ankle joint were achieved by the two or three component designs. Agility ankle is the prototype of the two component semiconstrained design. The incongruency between the talar and tibial articulations in this design allows sliding as well as the rotational motions that mimic ankle kinematics (Saltzman et al., 2000). Examples of threecomponent TARs are Scandinavian total ankle replacements (STAR), Mobility, Ankle evolutive system (AES), Bologna Oxford (BOX) TAR and Eclipse Total Ankle Implant.

Michael et al. (2008) compared the long term outcomes of the second generation prostheses and concluded that the survivability rate of TAR models is influenced by various factors such as component loosening, component migration, deep or superficial infection, delayed wound healing, nonunion of bones, intraoperative fractures of malleoli, tibia, or talus. Out of these, the major reason for TAR failure is the loosening of components, the cause being either malposition of the components during initial procedure or wear debris of the cement (polymethyl methacrylate, PMMA) particles that leads to abrasive wear in the polyethylene liner. Though the clinical outcomes of TARs are reported extensively, the reasons behind the failure are not explained. A broad comparison of their outcomes revealed that the results of most of the existing TAR models are unsatisfactory. (Leardini et al., 1999a,b; Leardini, 2001) developed A computer based geometrical model, fourbar linkage (4BL), to describe the ankle motion in passive conditions in the sagittal plane. They concluded that the shape of the articulation surface compatible with the ligament rotation during various ankle motions was an arc of a circle which is polycentric and polyradial in nature. Michael et al(2008) developed three models of TAR's based on the above model but further analysis is to be carried out to review the biomechanics of the ankle after replacement with these designs.

Conclusion

Understanding the complex anatomy and the effects of the different biomechanical forces acting on the ankle joint is very important for orthopaedic practice. A clear knowledge of these aids the correct decision making in treating ankle pathology. The unique bony structure and multi ligamentous configuration render the stability needed in ankle which exerts almost twice the magnitude of ground reaction forces during each gait cycle phase. As it is very difficult to mimic this natural configuration with an artificial joint, research is ongoing to design a total ankle replacement system with satisfactory long term results.

References

Alvine, F. G., 2000. In: Myerson, M.S. (Ed.), Total Ankle Arthroplasty. In: Foot and Ankle Disorders, vol. 2. Saunders, Philadelphia, p. 1087.

Attarian D. E., McCrackin H. J., Devito D. P., McElhaney J. H., Garrett Jr W. E. Biomechanical characteristics of human ankle ligaments. *Foot Ankle*, 1985 Oct; 6: 54e8.

Brown, T. D., Shaw, D. T., 1983. In vitro contact stress distributions in the natural human hip. *Journal of Biomechanics*, 16, 373–384.

Cheung, J. T. M., Zhang, M., Leung, A. K. L., Fan, Y. B., 2005. Threedimensional finite element analysis of the foot during standing — a material sensitivity study. *Journal of Biomechanics*, 38, 1045–1054.

Conti, S. F., Wong, Y. S., 2001. Complications of total ankle replacement. *Clinical Orthopaedics and Related Research,* 391, 105–114.

Evanski, P. M., Waugh, T. R., 1977. Management of arthrodesis of the ankle: An alternative to arthrodesis. *Clinical Orthopaedics and Related Research*, 122, 110–115.

Gefen, A., Ravid, M. M., Itzchak, Y., Arcan, M., 2000. Biomechanical analysis of the three dimensional foot structure during gait: A basic tool for clinical applications. *Journal of Biomechanical Engineering,* 122 (6), 630–639.

Ihn, J. C., Kim, S. J., Park, I. H., 1993. In vitro study of contact area and pressure distribution in the human knee after partial and total meniscectomy. *International Orthopaedics,* 17 (4), 214–218.

Kimizuka, M., Kurosawa, H., Fukubayashi, 1980. Load bearing pattern of the ankle joint: Contact area and pressure distribution. *Archives of Orthopaedic and Trauma Surgery,* 96, 45–49.

Leardini, A., O'Connor, J. J., Catani, F., Giannini, S., 1999a. A geometric model of the human ankle joint. *Journal of Biomechanics,* 32, 585–591.

Leardini, A., O'Connor, J. J., Catani, F., Stagni, R., Giannini, S., 1999b. Lever arm lengths of the flexor and extensor muscles at the ankle joint complex. In: Proceedings of the 45th Annual Meeting of the orthopaedic Research Society, Anaheim, CA. p. 216.

Leardini, A., 2001. Geometry and mechanics of the human ankle complex and ankle prosthesis design. *Clinical Biomechanics,* 16 (8), 706–709.

Lewis, G., 1994. The ankle joint prosthetic replacement: Clinical performance and research challenges. *Foot and Ankle International,* 15 (9), 471–476.

Michael, J.,Golshani, A.,Gargac,s.,Goswani, T., 2008. Biomechanics of the ankle joint and clinical outcomes of total ankle replacement. *Journal of the mechanical behaviour of biomedical materials,* 276-294.

Patil, K. M., Braak, L. H., Huson, A., 1993. Stresses in a simplified two dimensional model of a normal foot — A preliminary analysis. *Mechanics Research Communications,* 20 (1), 1–7.

Perry J. Gait analysis: normal and pathological function. Thorofare, NJ: SLACK Inc, 1992.

Renstrom, P.,Wertz, M., Incavo, S., Pope, M., Ostgaard, H. C., Arms, S., Haugh, L., 1988. Strain in the lateral ligaments of the ankle. *Foot Ankle,* 9 (2), 59–63.

Saltzman, C. L., Salamon, M. L., Blanchard, G. M., Huff, T., Hayes, A., Buckwalter, J. A., Amendola, A., 2005. Epidemiology of ankle arthritis: Report of a consecutive series of 639 patients from a tertiary Orthopaedic center. *Iowa Orthopaedic Journal,* 25, 44–46.

Saltzman, C. L., McIff, T. E., Buckwalter, J. A., Brown, T. D., 2000. Total ankle replacement revisited. *Journal of Orthopaedic and Sports Physical Therapy,* 30 (2), 56–67.

Shepherd, D. E., Seedhom, B. B., 1999. Thickness of human articular cartilage in joints of the lower limb. *Annals of the Rheumatic Diseases,* 58 (1), 27–34.

Stauffer, R. N., Chao, E. Y. S., Brewster, R. C., 1977. Force and motion analysis of the normal, diseased, and prosthetic ankle joint. *Clinical Orthopedics,* 127, 189–196.

Thomas, R. H., Timothy, R. D., 2003. Ankle arthritis. *Journal of Bone and Joint Surgery,* 85, 923–936. American Volume.

Tochigi, Y., Rudert, M. J., Saltzman, C. L., Amendola, A., Brown, T. D., 2006. Contribution of articular surface geometry to ankle stabilization. *Journal of Bone and Joint Surgery,* 88, 2704–2713. American Volume.

Waugh, T. R., Evanski, P. M., McMaster, W. C., 1976. Irvine ankle arthroplasty. Prosthetic design and surgical technique. *Clinical Orthopaedics,* 114, 180–184.

In: Advances in Medicine and Biology. Volume 77
Editor: Leon V. Berhardt

ISBN: 978-1-63117-444-5
© 2014 Nova Science Publishers, Inc.

Chapter 8

Mitochondrial Dysfunction in Severe Hemorrhagic Shock

Ke-seng Zhao, Rui Song and Xingmin Wang

Dept of Pathophysiology, Guangdong Key Lab of Shock and Microcirculation Research,
Southern Medical University, Guangzhou, China

Abstract

Severe or irreversible shock is the late stage of shock with persistent or refractory hypotension and often is a life-threatening situation, in which the therapeutic anti-shock measures including infusion, transfusion, and vasoactive agent are generally ineffective, indicating that besides microcirculatory disturbance, other events may be involved in the genesis. It was shown by us and others that the depletion of ATP in arteriolar smooth muscle cells (ASMCs) in severe shock led to activate ATP-sensitive potassium channels (K_{ATP}) with hyperpolarization of ASMCs, which inhibited L-type calcium channels in norepinephrine-stimulated ASMCs. The consequently reduced influx Ca^{2+} resulted in depression of contractile vasoresponsiveness and persistent hypotension. The depressed ASMCs ATP levels, with ensuing activation of K_{ATP} channels, existed even after improvement of microcirculation, which indicated that lower ATP level might not only result from insufficient delivery of nutrient and oxygen, but also from damage of ATP factory. Mitochondrion is the power plant with 90% ATP production in cell. Mitochondrial injury may lead to energy exhaustion with ROS production, release of apoptosis enzymes, and calcium overload, which finally results in cell damage or death. Therefore, an acute severe hemorrhagic shock rat model (the duration of 4 h in the experiment including 2 h for hemorrhage and 2 h after reinfusion of shed blood) was reproduced in our lab, then the arteriolar smooth muscle cells were isolated and the mitochondrial function including 5 indices was measured. In the shock group, the mitochondria appeared apparently swollen with poor defined cristae under electron microscope; the mitochondrial permeability transition pore often opened with the calcein-Co^{2+} technique; the inner mitochondrial membrane potential (ψm) was reduced with JC_1 method; the lysosomal stability was decreased with acridine orange base method and LPO content was increased using LPO assay kit, which led to injury mitochondria through the lysosomal-mitochondria axis; and the intracellular ATP level apparently decreased to 17.6 ± 7.9% of normal condition, although treatment of reinfusion was taken. The above change of morphology (ultrastructure), metabolic (ψm, mPTP), and function (ATP content) indicated the presence of ASMCs mitochondrial damage or mitochondrial dysfunction. Administration of mitochondrial protector (cyclosporine A, resveratrol, and polydatin) could partially recover the variables mentioned above. Among them the best one was polydatin, which could return intracellular ATP level to 90.7±7.5% with prolonged survival time. With ATP level recovery in ASMCs, PD also suppressed the activation of K_{ATP} channels, ASMCs hyperpolarization, and reduced vasoresponsiveness, which led recover the MAP and significantly prolong the survival time. Besides ASMCs and brain neurons, hepatocytes and platelets were also studied in rat with severe shock, which showed similar alterations of mitochondrial dysfunction including ultrastructure alterations, ψm, mPTP, activation of lysosomal-mitochondrial axis, and ATP content. The study demonstrated that mitochondrial dysfunction was a common phenomenon among diverse organs, which involved in the genesis of severe shock, and administration of mitochondrial protector might be a new approach to treatment of severe shock.

Introduction

The course of shock can be devided into 4 stages: initial stage, compensated stage, decompensated, and irreversible stage [1]. The irreversible stage is the final stage of shock with refractory hypotension, which is a life-threatening situation, since the therapeutic measures are ineffective. Therefore, the research concentration is focused on the mechanism and treatment of severe or irreversible shock (IS). In the literature there are some reports about mitochondrial dysfunction in sepsis or sepsis-induced MODS, in which a long term (≥24 h) model was usually used for the research that rarely involved in the acute severe shock including the acute irreversible shock [2-7].

It was shown by us and others that the ATP depletion of arteriolar smooth muscle cells (ASMCs) in a short term (≤6h) hemorrhagic shock model led to activate ATP-sensitive potassium channels (K_{ATP}) with hyperpolarization of ASMCs, which inhibited L-type calcium channels in norepinephrine-stimulated ASMCs. The consequently reduced influx Ca^{2+} resulted in depression of contractile vasoresponsiveness and persistent hypotension [8-16]. Blockages of ASMCs K_{ATP} channels could restitute the vasoreactivity and improve the outcome in severe shock [17-19]. The depressed ATP levels, with ensuing activation of K_{ATP} channels of ASMCs, existed even after administration of infusion, transfusion, and vasoactive agent with improvement of microcirculation, which indicated that lower ATP level might not only result from insufficient delivery of nutrient and oxygen, but also from the damage of ATP factory. Mitochondrion is the power plant with 90% ATP production in cell. It is reasonable to consider mitochondrial dysfunction involving in the genesis of irreversible shock [15].

1. Mitochondrial Dysfunction

The first case of mitochondrial dysfunction was described by Luftin in 1962 [20]. A euthyroid femal patient presented with myopathy, excessive perspiration, heat intolerance, polydipsia and increased basal metabolic rate. The patient suffered from an uncoupling of oxidative phosphorylation in mitochondria of skeletal muscle, which led to the production of heat in muscle cells without generation ATP. Since then, 50 years have passed through and the mitochondrial dysfunction has been implicated in nearly all pathologic genesis of diseases, such as cardiovascular disease, diabetes mellitus, Alzheimer disease, Parkinson disease, nonalcoholic steatohepatitis, cancer, obesity, etc. It has also been demonstrate that the functions of mitochondria involved in many processes essential for cell alive, including energy production, redox control, calcium homeostasis, reactive oxygen species (ROS) generation, physiologic cell death, and certain metabolic and biosynthetic pathway, etc. Mitochondrial dysfunction may be involved in all the functions mentioned above. However, mitochondrial dysfunction usually indicates the inability of the mitochondria to make ATP appropriately in response to energy demands, since most of ATP is produced by mitochondria and calcium homeostasis, ROS generation, and apoptosis, etc. can be caused not only by mitochondria but also by other organelles or events [21,20].

2. Assessing Mitochondrial Dysfunction

Mitochondrial dysfunction can be assessed by measurement of following variables in intact cells [23].

(1) Intracellular ATP level

Production of ATP is the main function of mitochondria. The reduced intracellular ATP content is an important variable for determination of mitochondrial dysfunction [17]. However, the decrease of ATP may also come from the insufficient delivery of oxygen and nutrient in shock. Therefore, the assessment of mitochondrial dysfunction should combine the intracellular ATP level with other pathological morphologic and metabolic indices. The ATP level of isolated cells is usually measured by a luciferase–based assay and the luminescence is tested with an automatic microplate reader (Spectra Max Ms) [24,29].

(2) The Mitochondrial Permeability Transition Pore

The mitochondrial permeability transition pore (mPTP) is a multi-component protein aggregate in mitochondria that comprises proteins in the inner membrane and outer membranes located at contact sites. The exact molecular composition of mPTP remains uncertain. PT pore is redox, Ca^{2+}, voltage adenine nucleotide, Pi, and pH sensitive. The mPTP of the inner mitochondrial membranes normally remain closed, but can open under a pathological condition, such as ischemia-reperfusion injury. Ischemia-reperfusion injury is associated with increase in mPT pore activators (Ca^{2+}, ROS, Pi) and reductions in mPT pore inhibitors (ATP/ADP). The open state of mPTP possesses a channel~3nm wide in diameter thus allowing diffusion of all molecules with molecular masses less than 1.5 kDa. This causes equilibration of H^+ across the inner membrane, which dissipates $\Delta\psi$m with the inhibition of

ATP synthesis by the $F_1 F_0$-ATPase. A concomitant influx of water causes swelling of the mitochondria, which stretches the membranes to the point where the outer membrane fails. The permeabilization of the outer membrane to an extent allows the release of pro-apoptotic proteins (cytoehrome C, etc) from the inter-membrane space into cytosol, resulting in apopotosis [18, 19, 20]. Therefore, the mPTP is a critical determinant for the genesis of mitochondrial dysfunction and apoptosis. The assessment of mPTP opening can be measured by ^{3}H-DOG entrapment technique [32]. However, Calcein-AM and $CoCl_2$ technique recently replaces the DOG technique [27, 28], since ^{3}H-DOG is a radioactive molecule. Calcein is a fluorescent molecule. Upon its esterification to generate calcein-AM, it turns non-fluorescent. Once inside the cell, the probe is deesterified and trapped in its free, fluorophoric form. Co^{2+} causes quenching of cytosolic and nuclear calcein, but it does not easily permeate the mitochondrial inner membrane. However, if the pores open, Co^{2+} can distribute itself inside mitochondria, resulting in quenched mitochondrial fluorescence. The density of mitochondrial fluorescence can be analyzed by flow cytometry [29].

(3) Mitochondrial Morphology

Mitochondrial swelling is a prominent phenomenon in mitochondrial dysfunction which can be semiquantitatively assessed with a scoring system that is based on the swelling level (scale of 0-5). Disruption of mitochondrial membranes and a loss of defined crystal take place with the increase of swelling. Mitochondrial swelling can occur through two distinct mechanisms: energy-dependent swelling and colloid osmotic swelling. Energy-dependent swelling is a consequence of solute accumulation (monovalent cations and anions), which is driven by the proton motive force or by simple concentration gradients. This kind of swelling appears without a loss of respiratory function. It is reversible and is not associated with "membrane damage". Colloid osmotic swelling occurs when mPTP opens, which is driven by the colloid osmotic pressure differential that exists across the inner mitochondrial membrane because proteins remain trapped within the matrix space. Swelling of this kind can be difficult to reverse, and is accompanied by a loss of mitochondrial function [23, 24]. Therefore, large swelling, disrupted mitochondrial membrane, and a loss of defined crystae are important morphological signs for assessment of mitochondrial dysfunction, which can be seen under transmission electron microscope [34, 35].

(4) Mitochondrial Membrane Potential

The reduced mitochondrial membrane potential ($\Delta\psi m$) is another index for assessment of mitochondrial dysfunction. The decrease of $\Delta\psi m$ is caused by two events. One is deficiency of oxidization or blockage of respiration, especially in hypoxia and shock state, which leads to the reduction of H^+ pumping into the intermembrane space. Another one is mPTP opening, which leads the H^+ from the intermembrane space, where exits high proton gradient, through the opened mPT pore into the matrix, resulting in low $\Delta\psi m$. ATP synthase is a reversible coupling device that interconverts the energies of the electrochemical proton gradient and chemical bonds. Lower $\Delta\psi m$ causes the uncoupling of oxidative phosphorylation which in turn causes the reverse mode activation of APTase leading to ATP hydrolysis rather than ATP synthesis. Mitochondrial membrane potential can be measured by fluorescent probe, such as JC_1, rhodamine 123, TMRM. JC_1 monomers in mitochondrial matrix (the presence of which indicates low $\Delta\psi m$) emit at 527 nm (green fluorescence), and JC-1 mitochondrial aggregates (indicating normal $\Delta\psi m$) at 590 nm (red fluorescence). A shift in fluorescence mission from red to green indicates depolarization. The percentage of cells with abnormally low $\Delta\psi m$ (green fluorescence) can be measured by flow cytometer [36, 37].

(5) Lysosomal Membrane Permeabilization and Intracellular LPO Content

Lysosome rupture with release of chelatable ferrous iron, ROS, and cathepsins has been demonstrated to induce mitochondrial damage including mPTP opening. Ischemia-reperfusion is well known to induce severe oxidative stress that induces iron-mediated intra lysosomal production of hydroxyl radicals (Fento-type reactions) with ensuing lysosomal membrane permeabilization (LMP). Under the condition of LMP, relocated lysosomal enzymes may attack mitochondria through so-called "Lysosomal-Mitochondrial Axis"[38, 39]. Therefore, measuring LMP and intracellular LPO level are indirect variables for assessment of mitochondrial dysfunction. The lysosomal membrane stability is usually measurand with AO uptake test. Acridine orange(AO) is a classic lysosomotropic fluorochrome exhibiting red flurescence when highly concentrated (as is in intact lysosomes). The percentage of "Pale" cells (i.e., cells with fewer than normal intact, red lysosomes) may be used to identify the lysosomal membrane permeabilization [28].

(6) Efficiency of Mitochondrial Protector

Treatment with mitochondrial protector, can be attenuated the reduced intracellular ATP content with other pathological variables mentioned above in severe shock, which leads to the reduction of K_{ATP} channel activation and ASMCs hyperpolarization with the recovery of vasohyporeactivity and MAP. These gives a counterevidence of mitochondrial dysfunction in vivo during severe shock. Therefore, the efficiency of mitochondrial protector also is a assessment index of mitochondrial dysfunction. According to the mechanism, the mitochondrial protectors can be divided into different groups [30, 40, 41]. One is inhibition of mPTP opening, such as cyclosporine A (CsA), which is assumed to bind to CyP-D with nanomolar affinity and prevents the interaction of this protein with the adenine nucleotide translocator, thus inhibiting mPTP opening. The second one is inhibition the generation of ROS in mitochondrial, such as trans-resveratrol(Res), which can decrease complex III activation with less ROS generation. Polydatin(PD) is a glucoside of Res, a natural polyphenolic compound [42, 43]. Both PD and Res belong to stilbene-type of compounds and share same pharmacological effects. The third one is inhibition of inner membrane Ca^{2+} regulated channels, such as ruthenium red, which can chelate Ca^{2+} or inhibit mitochondrial uniporter, preventing mPTP opening. The forth one is activation of $MitoK_{ATP}$ channel, such as diazoxide, which shows protective effect against ischemia- reperfusion injury in heart and neuron, but the exact mechanism remains to explore. The beneficial effect of diazoxide could be the consequence of the partial dissipation of the membrane potential caused by the net influx of K^+. This would reduce Ca^{2+} entry or release an excess of Ca^{2+}, preventing Ca^{2+} overload.

3. Existing Mitochondrial Dysfunction in SevereShock

An acute severe hemorrhagic shock model in rat was reproduced with 4 h duration (2 h hemorrhage to keep MAP 30 mmHg and 2 h observation after reinfusion of shed blood), then isolated the investigating cell (Arterial smooth muscle cells ASMCs; Brain Neurons, BN) to make following assessment experiments. The experiments were performed on 5 groups: control (sham) group, shock + NS group, shock + CsA group, shock + Res group, shock + PD group, in which the rats were subjected to hemorrhage 2 h followed by administration NS, CsA(6mg/kg), Res (15mg/kg), PD(30mg/kg respectively), then reinfusion of shed blood.

Mitochondrial Damage

Mitochondria of ASMCs in severe shock group appeared spherical or irregularly shaped, apparently swollen with electron-lucent matrix, and poorly defined crystae. The mean area of mitochondria (μm^2) was increased to 2.9 times more than normal (Figure 1).

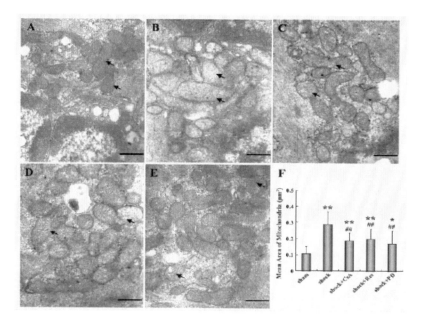

Figure 1. Ultrastructural alterations of arteriolar smooth muscle cells (ASMC) mitochondria following shock. A: Mitochondria are normal (some arrowed) in the control (sham) group. B: mitochondria (some arrowed) are swelled with poorly efined cristae in the shock group. These alterations are partially prevented in the shock + CsA (C), shock + Res (D), and shock + PD groups (E), respectively (some mitochondria arrowed). Scale bars: 1.0 μm. The column graphs (F) show results of morphologic assessments of ASMC total mitochondria areas from the five groups.*$P<0.05$, **$P<0.01$ vs. sham group; ##$P<0.01$ vs. shock group.

The similar alterations occur in the mitochondria of BN. The ultrastructure damage of mitochondria in the shock were partially protected by CsA, Res, and PD, especially PD heas the best protective effect. The morphological damage of mitochondria made a crucial bases for the assessment of mitochondrial dysfunction in irreversible shock (IS).

Mitochondrial Transition Pore Opening

The mean fluorescence intensity (MFI) of ASMCs calcein was 156.6±11.8 in the control group and 48.9±7.1 in the shock group, which meant that the calcein MIF value was decreased by 68.8% in ASMCs of shock group, indicating substantial mPTP opening.

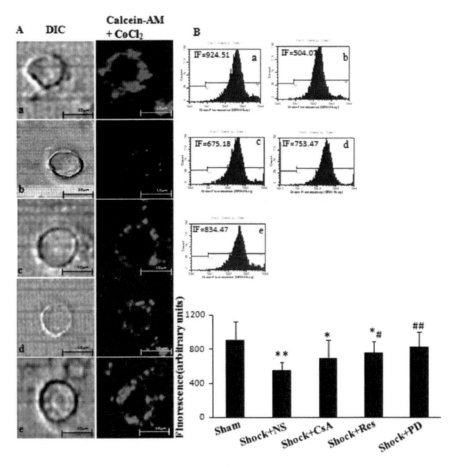

Figure 2. Changes in neuronal mPTP in neurons during severe shock. (A) Neurons are showed at left, and neuronal mitochondria exposed to calcein-AM and CoCl2 are showed at right. Normal mitochondrial fluorescence in the sham group (A right), obviously decreased in the shock + NS group (A right), and partially preserved in the shock + CsA group (A right) and in the shock + NS group (A right) the best preserved effect is found in the shock + PD group (A right). (B) Neurons stained with calcein-AM and CoCl2 were analyzed by FACS for green fluorescence. The result shows that normal mitochondrial fluorescence in the sham group (Ba) significantly reduce in the shock + NS group (Bb). This alteration was partially inhibited by the three protectors, PD showing the best effect (Be). *p < 0.05. zp < 0.01 versus sham group. §p < 0.05. {p < 0.01 versus shock + NS group. (DIC: differential interference contrast).

The MIF values were preserved to 59.7±13.4, 62.3±24.8 and 79.6±8.6 in CsA+shock, Res+shock, and PD+shock group respectively, which showed that the protective effect of PD was much better than both CsA and Res. The similar results occurred in mitochondria of brain neuron (BN) following severe shock, which showed that the MFI decreased to 60.77±10.06% of normal condition in the shock + NS group and returned to 91.32±18.57% in the PD-treated group (Figure 2).

Reduced Mitochondrial Membrane Potential

Mitochondrial depolarization (low Δψm) of ASMCs results in increased group contained 80.34±9.01% of green cells, which was substantially higher than the value of 13.44±7.73% in the control group (p<0.01).

The percentage of cells with low Δψm was 75.38±18.33%, 53.69±17.10%, and 31.57±6.12% in shock+CsA, shock+Res, shock+PD group respectively, indicating a better protective effect of PD than CsA or Res on ASMCs mitochondrial depolarization in shock. (Table 1). A similar phenomenon occurred in BN, which showed mitochondrial depolarization in severe shock.

Lysosomal Destabilization and Increased Intracellular LPO

The "pale" cell (lysosomal membrane permeabilization cell) of ASMCs was 51.6±5.2% in the shock group, which was much higher than value of 28.5±5.2% in the control group (p<0.01). The percentage of pale cells was 42.0±2.8%, 47.5±3.1% and 36.8±3.8% in shock+CsA, shock+Res, and shock+PD group respectively. The LPO level in ASMCs was increased from 10.01±1.56 nmol in the sham group to 15.00±2.23 nmol in the shock group (p<0.01), while the LPO content was reduced to 10.41±0.99 nmol in the shock+PD group, which was significantly lower than that in shock group (p<0.01). The PD antioxidative effect was apparently better than that of CsA and Res group. (Table 2).

Table 1. Changes of ASMCs mitochondrial membrane potential in shock (Δψm) ($\bar{\chi}$ ±s)

Group	n	Percentage of Cells with JC-1 Monomer (%)
Sham	5	13.44 ± 7.73
Shock	5	80.34 ± 9.01**
Shock + CsA	5	75.38 ± 18.33*ΔΔ
Shock + Res	5	53.69 ± 17.10*Δ
Shock + PD	5	31.57 ± 6.12*##

Quantification of mitochondrial depolarization expressed as JC-1 monomer (green fluorescence) in different treatments. ASMC, arteriolar smooth muscle cells; CsA, cyclosporin A; Res, resveratrol; PD, polydatin. * $P<0.05$, ** $P<0.01$ vs. sham group; ## $P<0.01$ vs. shock group; Δ$P< 0.05$, ΔΔ$P < 0.01$ vs. shock+PD group.

Table 2. Changes of ASMC intracellular LPO content in shock (($\bar{\chi}\pm$s)

Group	n	LPO Content, nmol
Sham	5	10.01 ± 1.56
Shock	5	$15.00 \pm 2.23**$
Shock + CsA	5	$14.10 \pm 1.42**\Delta\Delta$
Shock + Res	5	$14.18 \pm 1.59**\Delta\Delta$
Shock + PD	5	$10.41 \pm 0.99\#\#$

LPO, lipid hydroperoxide. ** $P<0.01$ vs. sham group; ## $P<0.01$ vs. shock group; $\Delta\Delta$ $P<0.01$ vs. shock+PD group.

Reduced Intracellular ATP Content

Severe shock caused significant decrease in the ATP level of ASMCs to 17.6±7.9% of the control value (p<0.01). Treatment with CsA, or Res increased ATP level to 32.7±5.4% or 62.1±11.5% of normal value, respectively (p<0.05), while exposure to PD was almost fully protective and resulted in 90.7±7.5% of the control value, which was no difference from the control group (p>0.05) Figure 3.

The similar results was got in brain neuron in severe shock, which demonstrated that intracellular ATP level changed from 44.14±13.81% of normal value in shock group to 89.57±9.21% in PD treated group

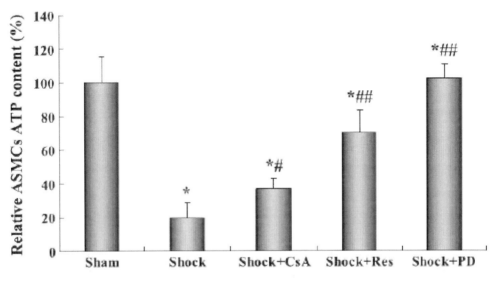

Figure 3. Changes in ASMC ATP levels following shock. Intracellular ATP levels of the shock group decreased to 17.6 ± 7.9% of that of the sham group. The ATP content was significantly better preserved in the shock + PD group than in the shock + CsA and shock + Res groups (n = 6 for each group). * P < 0.01 vs. sham group; # P < 0.05, ## P < 0.01 vs. shock group.

4. MD Involving in the Genesis of Severe Shock

Protection of MD Inhibits K_{ATP} Activation and ASMCs Membranes Hyperpolarization in IS

The K_{ATP} current densities of ASMCs increased remarkably during shock with ASMCs membrane hyperpolarization (membrane potential increasing from -31.7 ± 5.7 mV in control group to -49.7 ± 5.3 mV in shock group). Exposure to PD before reperfusion led to the K_{ATP} current density decreased by 40% (from 15.7 ± 7.3 pA/pF in shock group to 9.4 ± 4.2 pA/pF in shock+PD group) and suppression of the ASMCs membrane potential (from -49.7 ± 5.3 mV in shock group to -36.9 ± 7.2 mV **in** shock + PD group) Table 3.

Protection of MD Recovers Low Vasoreactivity and MAP in IS

The NE threshold concentration, that is an index for assaying vasoreactivity, increased to 29.3 times of the prehemorrhage level at the end of a period (2 h of hemorrhage and 2 h of treatment) and MAP had then decreased to 47.23 ± 11.28 mmHg in shock group. In the shock+CsA and shock+Res group the NE threshold concentration increased to half of the shock group (10.4 and 11.8 times of the prehemorrhage level, respectively), while MAP increased to 55.23 ± 9.92 and 57.10 ± 15.74 mmHg, respectively, at the same time points. Meanwhile, in the shock+PD group, the NE threshold concentration increased 1/4 of the shock group (4.8 times of the prehemorrhage level) during the same period, while MAP returned to 89.38 ± 16.31 mmHg, which was significantly higher than that of the shock group ($p<0.01$).

Atractyloside (ATR) can induce mPTP opening and mitochondrial damage in vitro. ATR was used to produce a cell model, in which ATR was added to normal ASMCs. It was demonstated that ATR treatment in vitro can induce morphological damage of ASMCs mitochondria with the reduction of $\Delta\psi m$ and ATP level, which finally led ASMC hyperpolarization and low vasoreactivity. This experiment gave a collateral evidence that ASMCs mitochondrial damage even caused by toxicant drug might also result in ASMC ATP depletion and low vasoreactivity.

Table 3. Changes of ASMC membrane potential in shock ($\bar{x}\pm s$)

Group	n	Membrane Potential, mV
Sham	25	-31.7 ± 5.3
Shock	29	-49.7 ± 9.3**
Shock + CsA	27	-42.0 ± 9.5*#
Shock + Res	24	-41.5 ± 10.3**#
Shock + PD	27	-36.9 ± 7.2*##

* $P <0.05$, ** $P < 0.01$ vs. sham group; # $P < 0.05$, ## $P < 0.01$ vs. shock group.

Protection of MD Prolongs the Survival Time in IS

The mean survival time was 5.4±2.6 h and an 100% animal death within 24 h. after reinfusion of shed blood in the shock group, since it was a severe hemorrhagic shock model with MAP reduced to 30 mmHg and lasted for 120 min.

However, the survival time in shock+CsA and shock+Res group was prolonged 2.05 and 1.9 times that of the shock group, respectively, which was significantly longer than that of shock group (p<0.01).

In the shock+PD group, the survival time was significant prolonged to 4.35 times that of shock group, and the 24 h survival rate was 5/8, which was significantly higher than the value of the shock group (p<0.01, Table 4). Therefore, administration of mitochondrial protector, especially PD could significantly enhance the survival time even in a severe hypotension (MAP 30 mmHg for 120 h) condition.

Table 4. Rat survival time following hemorrhagic shock ($\bar{x}\pm s$)

Group	n	Body Weight, g	Blood Loss, ml/100 g body wt	Survival Time, h	24-h Survival Rate
Sham	8	207.1±6.2	0	>72.0	8/8
Shock	8	208.9±5.4	2.9±0.1	5.4±2.6	0/8
Shock + CsA	8	210.4±10.0	3.0±0.1	9.0±4.8	0/8
Shock + Res	8	215.4±5.2	2.9±0.1	10.6±6.7	0/8
Shock + PD	8	211.6±5.6	2.9±0.1	23.7±3.7 [##]	5/8 [##]

P< 0.01 vs. shock group.

Conclusion

The study demonstrated that based on the functional (ATP), morphologic (ultrastructure damage), and metabolic (mPTP, $\Delta\psi m$, LMP, LPO) assessment, mitochondrial dysfunction existed in ASMCs and BN of IS, which involved in the genesis of refractory hypotension during severe or irreversible shock, and maybe the reason for usual antishock measures (infusion, transfusion, vasoactive agent) ineffective in irreversible shock. Besides ASMCs and BN, similar alterations were also demonstrated in hepatocytes and platelets similar alterations of MD, which implied that mitochondrial dysfunction might be a common phenomenon among divers' organs.

Therefore, mitochondrial dysfunction is an important therapeutic target in shock treatment (Figure 4) and mitochondrial protector, especially Polydatin which has been got the permission of SFDF for clinical trial and entered stage II now, may be a new approach to treatment of irreversible shock.

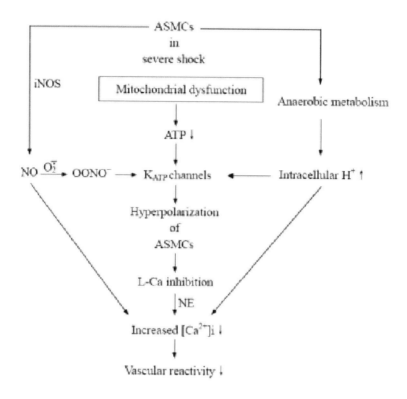

Figure 4. A tentative scheme on the role of ASMC mitochondrial dysfunction in the genesis of low vasoreactivity in hemorrhagic shock.

References

[1]   Porth CA. Circulatory Failure (Shock)-stages. In Porth CA eds, *Pathophysiology - Concepts of Altered Health States*. 7th ed, Linppincott Williams & Wilkins: Philadelphia, 2005, p617-625.

[2]   Dare AJ, Phillips AR, Hickey AJ, Mittal A, Loveday B, Thompson N, Windsor JA. A systematic review of experimental treatments for mitochondrial dysfunction in sepsis and multiple organ dysfunction syndrome. *Free Radic. Biol. Med.,* 2009, 1; 47(11): 1517-1525.

[3]   Víctor VM, Espulgues JV, Hernández-Mijares A, Rocha M. Oxidative stress and mitochondrial dysfunction in sepsis: a potential therapy with mitochondria-targeted antioxidants. *Infect. Disord. Drug Targets.,* 2009, 9(4): 376- 389.

[4]   Harrois A, Huet O, Duranteau J. Alterations of mitochondrial function in sepsis and critical illness. *Curr. Opin. Anaesthesiol.,* 2009, 22(2): 143-149.

[5]   Brealey D, Karyampudi S, Jacques TS, Novelli M, Stidwill R, Taylor V, Smolenski RT, Singer M. Mitochondrial dysfunction in a long-term rodent model of sepsis and organ failure. *Am. J. Physiol. Regul. Integr. Comp. Physiol.,* 2004, 286 (3): R491-R497.

[6]   Singer M. Mitochondrial function in sepsis: acute phase versus multiple organ failure. *Crit. Care Med.,* 2007, 35(9 Suppl): S441-S448.

[7]   Sayeed MM. Mitochondrial dysfunction in sepsis: a familiar song with new lyrics. *Crit. Care Med.,* 2002, 30(12):2780-2781.

[8]   Zhao KS, Liu J, Jin C. The role of membrane potential and calcium kinetic changes in the pathogenesis of vascular hyporeactivity during severe shock. *Chin. Med. J.,* 2000, 113: 59-64.

[9]   Chen SJ, Wu CC, Yang SN, Lin CI, Yen MH. Hyperpolarization contributes to vascular hyporeactivity in rats with lipopolysaccharide -induced endotoxic shock. *Life Sci.,* 2000, 68: 659-668.

[10]   Zhao Q, Zhao KS. Inhibition of l-type calcium channels in arteriolar smooth muscle cells is involved in the pathogenesis of vascular hyporeactivity in severe shock. *Shock.,* 2007, 28:717-721.

[11]   Zhao KS, Liu J, Yang GY, Jin C, Huang Q, Huang X. Peroxynitrite leads to arteriolar smooth muscle cell membrane hyperpolarization and low vasoreactivity in severe shock. *Clin. Hemorhe. Microc.,* 2000, 23: 259-267.

[12]   Zhao G, Zhao Y, Pan B, Liu J, Huang X, Zhang X, Cao C, Hou N, Wu C, Zhao KS, Cheng H. Hypersensitivity of BKCa to Ca^{2+} sparks underlies hyporeactivity of arterial smooth muscle in shock. *Circ. Res.,* 2007, 101:493-502.

[13]   Pan BX, Zhao GL, Huang XL, Jin JQ, Zhao KS. Peroxynitrite induces arteriolar smooth muscle cells membrane hyperpolarization with arteriolar hyporeactivity in rats *Life Sciences.,* 2004, 74:1199-1210.

[14]   Pan BX, Zhao GL, Huang XL, Zhao KS. Calcium mobilization is required for peroxynitrite-mediated enhancement of spontaneous transient outward currents in arteriolar smooth muscle cells. *Free Rad. Biol. Med.,* 2004, 37:823-838.

[15]   Landry DW, Oliver JA. The ATP-sensitive K^+ channel mediates hypotension in endotoxemia and hypoxic lactic acidosis in dog. *J. Clin. Invest.,* 1992, 89: 2071 – 2074.

[16]   Zhao KS. Ion channels and low vasoreactivity in severe shock. In Zhao KS and Xu Q eds < *Molecular Mechanism of Severe Shock* >, Research Signpost: Kerala (India), 2009, p107-129.

[17]   Zhao KS, Huang X, Liu J, Huang Q, Jin C, Jiang Y, Jin J, Zhao G. New approach to treatment of shock-restitution of vasoreactivity. *Shock.,* 2002, 18:189-192.

[18]   Szabó C, Salzman AL. Inhibition of ATP-activated potassium channels exerts pressor effects and improves survival in a rat model of severe hemorrhagic shock. *Shock.,* 1996, 5:391-394.

[19]   Maybauer DM, Salsbury JR, Westphal M, Maybauer MO, Salzman AL, Szabó C, Westphal-Varghese BB, Traber LD, Traber DL. The ATP-sensitive potassium channel inhibitor glibenclamide improves outcome in an ovine model of hemorrhagic shock. *Shock.,* 2004, 22:387-391.

[20]   Luft R, Ikkos D, Palmieri G, Ernster L, Afzelius B. A case of severe hypermetabolism of nonthyroid origin with a defect in the maintenance of mitochondrial respiratory control: a correlated clinical, biochemical, and morphological study. *J. Clin. Invest.,* 1962, 41(9): 1776-1804.

[21]   Pieczenik SR, Neustadt J. Mitochondrial dysfunction and molecular pathways of disease. *Exp. Mol. Pathol.,* 2007, 83(1):84-92.

[22]   Sivitz WI, Yorek MA. Mitochondrial dysfunction in diabetes: from molecular mechanisms to functional significance and therapeutic opportunities. *Antioxid. Redox. Signal.*, 2010,12(4):537-577.

[23]   Brand M D, Nicholls D G. Assessing mitochondrial dysfunction in cells. *Biochem. J.*, 2011, 15; 435(2):297-312.

[24]   Levy RJ. Mitochondrial dysfunction, bioenergetic impairment, and metabolic down-regulation in sepsis. *Shock.*, 2007, 28(1):24-28.

[25]   Grimm S, Brdiczka D. The permeability transition pore in cell death. *Apoptosis.*, 2007, 12(5): 841-855.

[26]   Baines CP. The mitochondrial permeability transition pore and ischemia- reperfusion injury. *Basic Res. Cardiol.*, 2009, 104(2):181-188.

[27]   Petronilli V, Miotto G, Canton M, Brini M, Colonna R, Bernardi P, Di Lisa F. Transient and long-lasting openings of the mitochondrial permeability transition pore can be monitored directly in intact cells by changes in mitochondrial calcein fluorescence. *Biophys. J.*, 1999, 76(2): 725-734.

[28]   Jones RA, Smail A, Wilson MR. Detecting mitochondrial permeability transition by confocal imaging of intact cells pinocytically loaded with calcein. *Eur. J. Biochem.*, 2002, 269(16): 3990-3997.

[29]   Song R, Bian H, Wang X, Huang X, Zhao KS. Mitochondrial injury underlies hyporeactivity of arterial smooth muscle in severe shock. *Am. J. Hypertens.*, 2011, 24(1): 45-51.

[30]   Javadov S, Karmazyn M. Mitochondrial permeability transition pore opening as an endpoint to initiate cell death and as a putative target for cardioprotection. *Cell Physiol. Biochem.*, 2007, 20(1-4):1-22.

[31]   Song R, Bian H, Huang X, Zhao KS. Atractyloside induces low contractile reaction of arteriolar smooth muscle through mitochondrial damage. *J. Appl. Toxicol.*, 2012, 32(6): 402-408.

[32]   Halestrap AP, Clarke SJ, Javadov SA. Mitochondrial permeability transition pore opening during myocardia.l reperfusion – a target for cardioprotection. *Cardiovasc. Res.*, 2004, 1:372-385.

[33]   Petronnilli V, Miotto G, Canton M, Colonna R, Bernardi P, Lisa D. Imaging the mitochondrial permeability transition pore in intact cells. *BioFactors.*, 1998, 8:263-272.

[34]   Crouser ED. Mitochondrial dysfunction in septic shock and multiple organ dysfunction syndrome. *Mitochondrion.*, 2004, 4(5-6):729-741.

[35]   Crouser ED, Julian MW, Blaho DV, Pfeiffer DR. Endotoxin-induced mitochondrial damage correlates with impaired respiratory activity. *Crit. Care Med.*, 2002, 30(2): 276-284.

[36]   Salvioli S, Ardizzoni A, Franceschi C, Cossarizza A. JC-1, but not DiOC6(3) or rhodamine 123, is a reliable fluorescent probe to assess delta psi changes in intact cells: implications for studies on mitochondrial functionality during apoptosis. *FEBS Lett.*, 1997, 7; 411(1):77-82.

[37]   Adrie C, Bachelet M, Vayssier-Taussat M, Russo-Marie F, Bouchaert I, Adib-Conquy M, Cavaillon JM, Pinsky MR, Dhainaut JF, Polla BS. Mitochondrial membrane potential and apoptosis peripheral blood monocytes in severe human sepsis. *Am. J. Respir. Crit. Care Med.*, 2001, 1;164(3): 389-395.

[38] Kon K, Kim JS, Uchiyama A, Jaeschke H, Lemasters JJ. Lysosomal iron mobilization and induction of the mitochondrial permeability transition in acetaminophen-induced toxicity to mouse hepatocytes. *Toxicol. Sci.,* 2010, 117(1): 101-108.

[39] Zhao M, Antunes F, Eaton JW, Brunk UT. Lysosomal enzymes promote mitochondrial oxidant production, cytochrome c release and apoptosis. *Eur. J. Biochem.,* 2003, 270(18): 3778-3786.

[40] Szewczyk A, Wojtczak L. Mitochondria as a pharmacological target. *Pharmacol. Rev.,* 2002, 54(1): 101-27.

[41] Morin D, Papadopoulos V, Tillement J P. Prevention of cell damage in ischaemia: novel molecular targets in mitochondria. *Expert. Opin. on Ther. Targets.,* 2002, 6(3): 315-334.

[42] Wang X, Song R, Bian HN, Brunk UT, Zhao M, Zhao KS. Polydatin, a natural polyphenol, protects arterial smooth muscle cells against mitochondrial dysfunction and lysosomal destabilization following hemorrhagic shock. *Am. J. Physiol. Regul. Integr. Comp. Physiol.,* 2012, 302(7): R805-R814.

[43] Wang X, Song R, Chen Y, Zhao M, Zhao KS. Polydatin--a new mitochondria protector for acute severe hemorrhagic shock treatment. *Expert Opin. Investig. Drugs.,* 2013, 22(2): 169-179.

In: Advances in Medicine and Biology. Volume 77
Editor: Leon V. Berhardt

ISBN: 978-1-63117-444-5
© 2014 Nova Science Publishers, Inc.

Chapter 9

Early Hematoma Enlargement after ICH: Current Diagnosis and Treatment

Qi Li[1], Bernard Yan[2], Xinyu Zhou[1] and Peng Xie[1,]*
[1]Department of Neurology, The First Affiliated Hospital of Chongqing Medical University, Chongqing, China
[2]Department of Neurology, The Royal Melbourne Hospital, University of Melbourne, Melbourne, Australia

Abstract

Hematoma enlargement is reported in a significant proportion of patients with intracerebral hemorrhage (ICH). Early hematoma enlargement is associated with poor clinical outcome after ICH. Imaging studies play an important role in prompt identification of high risk patients for hematoma enlargement. Selection of patients at high risk for hematoma enlargement is crucial for treatment. Current knowledge of the clinical and imaging predictors for hematoma enlargement is discussed in detail. The contrast extravasation on CT angiography (CTA) is a well-established imaging predictor for subsequent hematoma expansion. The presence of contrast extravasation may be used as a useful imaging marker to guide therapies. The CTA spot sign is also associated with early hematoma enlargement. Hemostatic treatment may limit hematoma expansion, but fail to change clinical outcome. Rapid intensive lowering of blood pressure reduces hematoma growth, but fails to result in a significant reduction in death or major disability. However, intensive lowering of blood pressure may improve functional outcomes in selected patients. The safety and possible benefit of intensive blood pressure lowering in treatment of patients with intracerebral hemorrhage needs further validation.

---

* Corresponding author: Prof. Peng Xie, Department of Neurology, The First Affiliated Hospital of Chongqing Medical University, Chongqing, China.

Introduction

Spontaneous intracerebral hemorrhage (ICH) is a medical emergency that is associated with high morbidity and mortality [1]. It is one of the least treatable form of stroke and a major public health burden worldwide. Early hematoma enlargement has been reported in a significant proportion of patients [2]. The early hematoma enlargement is associated with poor functional outcome in patients with ICH. CT scan of the head is the preferred method for evaluation of patients with ICH and should be performed as early as possible. CTA spot sign is a reliable imaging marker for prediction of early hematoma expansion [3]. Blood pressure modulation may theoretically limit hematoma growth and reduction of blood pressure is probably safe and feasible. The benefit of surgical evacuation of hematoma is still controversial.

Definition of Early Hematoma Enlargement

Early hematoma enlargement was reported in approximately 28% to 38% of patients scanned within 3 hours of ICH onset [4]. In a study of 103 patients with ICH, Brott et al defined early hematoma expansion as an increase in the volume of hematoma of >33% as measured by follow-up CT scan as compared with the baseline CT scan [5]. The number of 33% was chosen because the volume corresponds to a 10% increase in diameter which is readily identifiable by the naked eye of a physician. The authors found that 38% of ICH patients had >33% hematoma growth during the first 24 hours after symptom onset. In a study of 204 patients with spontaneous intracerebral hemorrhage, Kazui and colleagues have defined early hematoma enlargement as an increase in hematoma volume by ≥ 12.5 cm^3 or by ≥ 1.4 times based on the follow-up CT scan [6]. They found 20% of the cohort had hematoma expansion based on their judging criteria. Hematoma enlargement was common among those who underwent the initial CT scan early. The definition of hematoma expansion proposed by Brott and Kazui has gained worldwide acceptance. The large randomized controlled trials including INTERACT and ATTACH have defined hematoma enlargement as increase of the hematoma volume >33% or >12.5 ml [7].

Diagnosis of Hematoma Expansion

ICH is a medical emergency that requires prompt diagnosis and management. Although the clinical signs and symptoms may give a clue to the diagnosis, it is difficult and inaccurate for physicians to distinguish intracerebral hemorrhage from acute ischemic stroke and stroke mimics. Rapid imaging is crucial to differentiate between ischemic and hemorrhagic strokes. Computed tomography (CT) is considered the first line imaging method for evaluation of patients with ICH [8]. The non-contrast CT is fast, cost-effective and readily available worldwide. It is thus commonly used in emergency departments for detection of clinically relevant acute hemorrhages. Magnetic resonance imaging (MRI) is also reasonable for initial evaluation. T2* weighted, gradient-echo and sensitivity weighted MR imaging sequences are more sensitive than CT for detection of cerebral microbleed [9]. MR sequences are also useful for identification of prior hemorrhage. Brain MRI is also more sensitive than CT for identification of secondary causes of ICH, including arteriovenous malformation, cerebral amyloid angiopathy and stroke from tumor [10, 11]. However, the cost, time and availability of MRI have limited its use in the emergency setting for ICH.

Assessment of Hematoma Volume

CT is widely used to assess the volume of hematoma. To date, several volumetric methods are used to measure hematoma. The most commonly used method for bedside assessment of hematoma volume is the ABC/2 method [12]. Briefly, the largest area of hemorrhage on the CT slice was identified. Then, the largest diameter (A) of the hematoma on this slice was measured. The largest diameter (B) perpendicular to A was measured on the same slice. Multiply the number in which the ICH is visible by the slice thickness in centimeters (C).

Recently, semi-automated planimetry methods have been used to assess the hematoma volume. The semi-automated techniques are more accurate than the ABC/2 method [13]. Assessment of hematoma size is important for predicting 30-day mortality.

CTA and Contrast Enhanced CT

Although the location of hemorrhage may give a clue to a particular underlying etiology of ICH, this approach is inaccurate and may miss a significant proportion of secondary causes [14]. Therefore, angiographic studies are necessary to identify secondary vascular causes in patients with ICH.

CT angiography (CTA) has been widely used for evaluation of the underlying cause of ICH, such as arteriovenous malformations, aneurysms and moyamoya disease. Recently, CTA is increasingly used for visualizing the CTA spot sign [15]. The sign was defined as small (1 to 2 mm) foci of contrast enhancement within the hematoma identified on CTA source images. The CTA spot sign is associated with the presence of hematoma expansion [16]. The presence of the spot sign is a reliable indicator of active bleeding and has been associated with increased mortality in patients with ICH [17].

Extravasation of contrast material on contrast enhanced CT scan may also identify patients at risk for hematoma expansion [18, 19]. The spot sign has a high sensitivity and specificity for determining hematoma expansion.

Recently, a spot sign score has been developed to assess the risk of hematoma expansion [20]. The spot sign could be better visualized using a "spot windows" with window width of 200. The CTA spot sign appears as a focus of contrast within the hematoma with an attenuation of approximately 120-180 Hounsfield units. The spot sign score is based on the number of spot signs, maximum axial dimension and maximum attenuation.

Risk Factors of Early Hematoma Expansion

Several predictors for hematoma enlargement have been identified. The size of the baseline hematoma volume is a reliable predictor for hematoma expansion. Large hematomas are more likely to enlarge than small hematomas [21]. The time of presentation after symptom onset to CT scan may also influence the rate of hematoma expansion [22]. It is well-established that earlier time from symptom onset to initial neuroimaging scan is associated with increased likelihood of hematoma expansion on follow-up scan. The density and shape of the hematoma on initial CT scan is also a novel predictor for early hematoma enlargement [23]. Regular shaped hematomas with smooth margins are less likely to have hematoma expansion than irregular shaped hematoma with multinodular margins. Hematoma heterogeneity is also an independent predictor for early hematoma enlargement. Patients with APOE ε2 allele also increases the risk of hematoma expansion in patients with lobar ICH [24]. The CTA spot sign is a reliable imaging marker of active bleeding [16]. The CTA spot sign is strongly associated with hematoma expansion and poor functional outcome. However, a significant number of patients with negative spot CTA sign will have hematoma expansion.

Treatment Options for Hematoma Expansion

Medical and surgical approaches are the major therapeutic strategies to restrict hematoma expansion.

Blood Pressure Modulation

Hypertension has thought to be one of the most important causes of intracerebral hemorrhage. In patients with ICH, the systolic blood pressure is frequently elevated [25]. Increased blood pressure in the acute phase of ICH may lead to hydrostatic expansion of hematoma and increased intracranial pressure. Several large randomized controlled trials have assessed the effect of intensive blood pressure lowering in ICH. The INTensive Blood Pressure Reduction in Acute Cerebral Hemorrhage Trial (INTERACT), published in 2008, was a large randomized, controlled pilot study to compare intensive with guideline-recommended blood pressure reduction in patients with ICH [26]. The INTERACT trial has included 404 patients with elevated systolic BP (150-220 mm Hg) within 6 hours of the onset of ICH. The primary endpoint of the INTERACT trial was the proportional change in hematoma volume assessed at 24 hours. The authors found that relative risk of hematoma growth was significantly lower in the intensive blood pressure reduction group (target systolic BP <140 mm Hg) than the guideline group (target systolic BP <180 mm Hg). However, intensive blood pressure reduction treatment did not alter the risks of adverse events. The recently published INTERACT 2 trial randomly assigned 2839 patients with ICH who had elevated systolic blood pressure to intensive blood pressure reduction treatment and guideline-recommended treatment [27]. The authors reported that intensive lowering of blood pressure failed to result in a significant reduction in the rate of the primary outcome of death or severe disability. However, ordinal analysis of modified Rankin scores suggested improved functional outcomes in patients receiving intensive blood pressure reduction. The results of the INTERACT 2 trial have further reinforced the safety and efficacy of rapid blood pressure lowering for treatment of ICH. Therefore, acute lowering of systolic BP to 140 mm Hg is probably safe and may benefit patients with ICH. The Antihypertensive Treatment of Acute Cerebral Hemorrhage (ATACH) trial is another randomized trial assessing reduction of blood pressure in ICH [28]. A total of 60 patients with lobar ICH were included in the ATACH trial and received intravenous nicardipine within 6 hours to achieve the blood pressure at three different target tiers. The results of the ATTACH trial also confirmed safety and feasibility of systolic blood pressure reduction in patients with ICH. Based on these findings, the ASA guideline recommended acute blood pressure reduction of systolic BP to 140mmHg in ICH patients with elevated systolic BP.

Hemostasis

Patients taking oral anticoagulants (OACs) constitute an important proportion of patients with ICH. Anticoagulants have been increasingly used in clinical practice, leading to a growing number of ICH. For ICH patients with the use of OACs, rapid reversal of warfarin anticoagulation should be done as quickly as possible [29]. Anticoagulants should be discontinued to stop further hematoma expansion. Traditionally, intravenous vitamin K, fresh frozen plasma and activated recombinant factor VIIa (rFVIIa) are frequently used [30, 31]. More recently, prothrombin complex concentrates has emerged as a new therapeutic option to reversal the coagulopathy [32]. The risk of hematoma expansion may be lower in patients receiving prothrombin complex concentrates than those treated with fresh frozen plasma.

The rFVIIa is considered to be a promising drug that may limit hematoma expansion in large randomized controlled trials. In a large randomized controlled trial, the authors evaluated the effect of rFVIIa on hematoma expansion in patients with ICH [33]. The authors randomly assigned 399 patients to receive placebo or 40µg per kilogram, 80µg per kilogram, or 160µg per kilogram of rFVIIa. The authors report that rFVIIa limits hematoma expansion and improves functional outcomes at 90 days. The phase III Factor Seven for Acute Hemorrhagic Stroke (FAST) trial confirmed the effect on hematoma expansion, but did not report benefit in functional outcome [34]. The use of rFVIIa has been disappointing in large randomized trials and it is not routinely recommended in patients with ICH.

Surgical Treatment of ICH

The benefit of surgical removal of the clot is uncertain in patients with ICH. Theoretically, surgical removal of the clot may alleviate the mechanical mass effects of the growing hematoma as well as the toxic effects of blood degradations on the surrounding brain tissue [35]. However, open craniotomy may damage normal brain tissues resulting in surgery induced brain damage.

To date, several large randomized trials have been published to assess the effect of surgery versus medical treatment in patients with ICH. The surgical trial in intracerebral hemorrhage (STICH) is a large randomized trial assessing early surgery with hematoma evacuation with medical treatment [36]. The Glasgow outcome scale at 6 months follow-up was used as the primary outcome measurement. The authors found that no statistical significant benefit in patients receiving early neurosurgical intervention than those receiving initial conservative treatment. However, the STICH trial authors found that patients may have a trend to benefit from surgical intervention if the lobar hematoma extending to within 1 cm of the cortical surface. In 2013, the recently published STICH II trial compared early surgical hematoma evacuation plus medical treatment with medical treatment alone in patients with ICH [37]. In the STICH II trial, the authors randomly assigned 307 patients were to early surgery and 294 to conservative treatment. The outcome at 6 months did not differ significantly between the surgical treatment group and the medical treatment group. The STICH II results also showed that early surgery might have a small benefit for patients with spontaneous superficial intracerebral hemorrhage. Based on these results, surgical evacuation of supratentorial ICH might be beneficial for patients presenting with lobar hemorrhage >30 mL and within 1 cm of the surface.

Minimally invasive surgery has been used for treatment of patients with ICH. Endoscopic surgery and stereotactic aspiration are two minimally invasive surgical techniques that are alternatively used approach for ICH in some hospitals [38]. Minimally invasive surgery is less time-consuming than open craniotomy and could be performed under local anesthesia. However, the technique employs fibrinolytics and may lead to potential risk of rebleeding. In addition, the use of indwelling catheters may also increase the chance of infection. A recently published Meta-analysis involved 12 high-quality randomized controlled trials. The authors reported that supratentorial intracerebral hemorrhage patients with Glasgow Coma Scale score of ≥9 and hematoma volume between 25 and 40 mL might benefit from minimally invasive surgery [39]. Although several studies have showed the benefit of minimally invasive surgery in patients with ICH, the role of minimally invasive surgery are not well established.

Future Directions

Given the high morbidity and mortality of ICH, early recognition and treatment of ICH is important. Despite recent technical advancements in diagnosis and treatment of intracerebral hemorrhage, the etiology of hematoma expansion is still not clear. Non-enhanced CT and MRI may give a clue to the etiology of ICH, angiographic examinations are needed to identify the cause of ICH. The CTA spot sign is a reliable imaging marker for hematoma expansion. Contrast extravasation is a sign for active bleeding, new imaging techniques are needed to identify the pathogenesis of hematoma expansion. To date, surgery has not proved to be effective for patents with ICH. Minimally invasive surgical techniques that may remove hematoma's toxic and pressure effects while avoiding the damage caused by other invasive surgical procedures have been emerged as promising method for treatment of ICH.

To date, no established effective targeted therapy exists for intracerebral hemorrhage. Blood pressure modulation is a safe and effective approach that may limit hematoma expansion. Surgical evacuation of hematoma may benefit a small number of patients with lobar hemorrhage. Future researches are needed to further clarify the pathogenesis of hematoma expansion and develop novel therapeutic intervention that improves functional outcome in patients with ICH.

References

[1]   Broderick J, Connolly S, Feldmann E., et al. Guidelines for the management of spontaneous intracerebral hemorrhage in adults: 2007 update: a guideline from the American Heart Association/American Stroke Association Stroke Council, High Blood Pressure Research Council, and the Quality of Care and Outcomes in Research Interdisciplinary Working group. *Stroke*, 2007; 38: 2001-23.

[2]   Dowlatshahi D, Demchuk AM, Flaherty ML, et al. Defining hematoma expansion in intracerebral hemorrhage: relationship with patient outcomes. *Neurology*, 2011; 76: 1238–1244.

[3]   Wada R, Aviv RI, Fox AJ, et al. CT angiography "spot sign" predicts hematoma expansion in acute intracerebral hemorrhage. *Stroke*, 2007;38:1257–1262.

[4]   Dowlatshahi D, Smith EE, Flaherty ML, et al. Small intracerebral haemorrhages are associated with less haematoma expansion and better outcomes. *Int. J. Stroke*, 2011; 6: 201–206.

[5]   Brott T, Broderick J, Kothari R, et al. Early hemorrhage growth in patients with intracerebral hemorrhage. *Stroke*, 1997;28:1–5.

[6]   Kazui S, Naritomi H, Yamamoto H, et al. Enlargement of spontaneous intracerebral hemorrhage: incidence and time course. *Stroke*, 1996;27: 1783-7.

[7]   Qureshi AI, Mendelow AD, Hanley DF. Intracerebral haemorrhage. *Lancet*, 2009; 373: 1632–1644.

[8]   Chalela JA, Kidwell CS, Nentwich LM, et al. Magnetic resonance imaging and computed tomography in emergency assessment of patients with suspected acute stroke: a prospective comparison. *Lancet*, 2007; 369: 293–298.

[9]   Fiebach JB, Schellinger PD, Gass A, et al. Stroke magnetic resonance imaging is accurate in hyperacute intracerebral hemorrhage: a multicenter study on the validity of stroke imaging. *Stroke*, 2004;35: 502–506.

[10]   Nussel F, Wegmuller H, Huber P. Comparison of magnetic resonance angiography, magnetic resonance imaging and conventional angiography in cerebral arteriovenous malformation. *Neuroradiology*, 1991;33:56–61.

[11]   Yoon HK, Shin HJ, Lee M, Byun HS, Na DG, Han BK. MR angiography of moyamoya disease before and after encephaloduroarteriosynangiosis. *AJR Am. J. Roentgenol.*, 2000;174: 195–200.

[12]   Ginde AA, Foianini A, Renner DM, Valley M, Camargo CA Jr. Availability and quality of computed tomography and magnetic resonance imaging equipment in US emergency departments. *Acad. Emerg. Med.*, 2008; 15: 780–783.

[13]   Divani AA, Majidi S, Luo X, et al. The ABCs of accurate volumetric measurement of cerebral hematoma. *Stroke*, 2011; 42: 1569–1574.

[14]   Delgado Almandoz JE, Romero JM. Advanced CT imaging in the evaluation of hemorrhagic stroke. *Neuroimaging Clin. N Am.*, 2011; 21: 197–213, ix.

[15]   Brouwers HB, Falcone GJ, McNamara KA, et al. CTA spot sign predicts hematoma expansion in patients with delayed presentation after intracerebral hemorrhage. *Neurocrit Care*, 2012; 17:421–428.

[16]   Wada R, Aviv RI, Fox AJ, et al. CT angiography "spot sign" predicts hematoma expansion in acute intracerebral hemorrhage. *Stroke*, 2007;38:1257–1262.

[17] Gazzola S, Aviv RI, Gladstone DJ, Mallia G, Li V, Fox AJ, Symons SP. Vascular and nonvascular mimics of the CT angiography "spot sign" in patients with secondary intracerebral hemorrhage. *Stroke,* 2008;39: 1177–1183.

[18] Kim J, Smith A, Hemphill JC III, et al. Contrast extravasation on CT predicts mortality in primary intracerebral hemorrhage. *Am. J. Neuroradiol., 2008*;29:520–525.

[19] Goldstein JN, Fazen LE, Snider R, et al. Contrast extravasation on CT angiography predicts hematoma expansion in intracerebral hemorrhage. *Neurology,* 2007;68: 889–894.

[20] Delgado Almandoz JE, Yoo AJ, Stone MJ, et al. The spot sign score in primary intracerebral hemorrhage identifies patients at highest risk of in-hospital mortality and poor outcome among survivors. *Stroke,* 2010;41: 54-60.

[21] Kazui S, Naritomi H, Yamamoto H, Sawada T, Yamaguchi T. Enlargement of spontaneous intracerebral hemorrhage. Incidence and time course. *Stroke,* 1996;27:1783–1787.

[22] Fujii Y, Takeuchi S, Sasaki O, Minakawa T, Tanaka R. Multivariate analysis of predictors of hematoma enlargement in spontaneous intracerebral hemorrhage. *Stroke,* 1998;29:1160 –1166.

[23] Barras CD, Tress BM, Christensen S, et al. Density and shape as CT predictors of intracerebral hemorrhage growth. *Stroke,* 2009;40:1325-31.

[24] Tzourio C, Arima H, Harrap S, et al. APOE genotype, ethnicity, and the risk of cerebral hemorrhage. *Neurology,* 2008;70:1322–1328.

[25] Willmot M, Leonardi-Bee J, Bath PM. High blood pressure in acute stroke and subsequent outcome: a systematic review. *Hypertension,* 2004;43:18 –24.

[26] Anderson CS, Huang Y, Wang JG, et al. INTERACT Investigators. Intensive blood pressure reduction in acute cerebral haemorrhage trial (INTERACT): a randomised pilot trial. *Lancet Neurol,* 2008;7:391–399.

[27] Anderson CS, Heeley E, Huang Y, et al. Rapid blood-pressure lowering in patients with acute intracerebral hemorrhage. *N. Engl. J. Med.,* 2013; 368: 2355-65.

[28] Qureshi AI. Antihypertensive Treatment of Acute Cerebral Hemorrhage (ATACH): rationale and design. *Neurocritical Care,* 2007;6:56–66.

[29] Hanley JP. Warfarin reversal. *J. Clin. Pathol.,* 2004;57:1132–1139.

[30] Hung A, Singh S, Tait RC. A prospective randomized study to determine the optimal dose of intravenous vitamin K in reversal of overwarfarinization. *Br. J. Haematol.,* 2000;109:537–539.

[31] Goldstein JN, Thomas SH, Frontiero V, et al. Timing of fresh frozen plasma administration and rapid correction of coagulopathy in warfarin-related intracerebral hemorrhage. *Stroke,* 2006;37:151–155.

[32] Leissinger CA, Blatt PM, Hoots WK, Ewenstein B. Role of prothrombin complex concentrates in reversing warfarin anticoagulation: a review of the literature. *Am. J. Hematol.,* 2008;83:137–143.

[33] Mayer SA, Brun NC, Begtrup K, et al. Recombinant Activated Factor VII Intracerebral Hemorrhage Trial Investigators. Recombinant activated factor VII for acute intracerebral hemorrhage. *N. Engl. J. Med.,* 2005;352:777–785.

[34] Mayer SA, Brun NC, Begtrup K, et al. FAST Trial Investigators. Efficacy and safety of recombinant activated factor VII for acute intracerebral hemorrhage. *N. Engl. J. Med.,* 2008;358:2127–2137.

[35] Mendelow AD, Unterberg A. Surgical treatment of intracerebral haemorrhage. *Curr. Opin. Crit. Care,* 2007;13:169 –174.

[36] Mendelow AD, Gregson BA, Fernandes HM, et al. STICH investigators. Early surgery versus initial conservative treatment in patients with spontaneous supratentorial intracerebral haematomas in the International Surgical Trial in Intracerebral Haemorrhage (STICH): a randomized trial. *Lancet,* 2005;365:387–397.

[37] Mendelow AD, Gregson BA, Rowan EN, Murray GD, Gholkar A, Mitchell PM. STICH II Investigators. Early surgery versus initial conservative treatment in patients with spontaneous supratentorial lobar intracerebral haematomas (STICH II): a randomised trial. *Lancet,* 2013;382:397-408.

[38] Wang WZ, Jiang B, Liu HM, et al. Minimally invasive craniopuncture therapy vs. conservative treatment for spontaneous intracerebral hemorrhage: results from a randomized clinical trial in China. *Int. J. Stroke,* 2009;4:11–16.

[39] Zhou X, Chen J, Li Q, et al. Minimally invasive surgery for spontaneous supratentorial intracerebral hemorrhage: a meta-analysis of randomized controlled trials. *Stroke,* 2012;43:2923-30.

In: Advances in Medicine and Biology. Volume 77
Editor: Leon V. Berhardt
ISBN: 978-1-63117-444-5
© 2014 Nova Science Publishers, Inc.

Chapter 10

Thoracic Hematomas

Walid Leonardo Dajer-Fadel
General Hospital of Mexico, Mexico

Abstract

Many are the causes of hematomas within the boundaries of the chest, these span from a natural origin such as vascular malformations or tumors; traumatic such as rib fractures, intra-parenchymal bleeding or vascular rupture; infectious such as chronic tuberculous lesions; post-operative complications, anticoagulation and idiopathic are also other type of associated etiologies. In this chapter a thorough review is made of each, emphasizing the mechanisms that led to a thoracic hematoma, weather it occurred in the chest wall, the mediastinum, cardiac tissue, lung parenchyma, diaphragm or pericardium, a conscious analysis is made with each case towards what produced it and how it is approached and managed with the best evidence based treatment available. This rare entity which usually transcends with a benign course, left unattended or undermined could lead to fatal consequences, hence the importance of understanding and applying today's technological tools and knowledge for the accurate diagnosis and treatment of these patients.

Introduction

Hematomas of the thorax are a relatively rare entity and the array of causes comprise many origins, due to these facts a high clinical suspicion should be maintained at all times with prompt management weather a surgical or medical treatment is indicated, knowledge of the mechanisms that produce these complications are essential for the physician to achieve success. In this chapter we will review the most common causes that lead to a hematoma, with individual evaluation of the available literature, with subsequent conclusions based on the best evidence, awareness should be made regarding the rarity of some hematomas and the poor amount of available information on the subject. In table 1 we provide a list of the reported causes of hematomas, which we will review one by one.

Vascular Malformations

Thoracic vasculature when in stress is known to cause aneurysms which will be described ahead, a very rare entity is spontaneous rupture of the vessels. The common denominator always associated originating these lesions are pressure variances within the their walls. Bageacu [1] and Hoetzencker [2] recently reported a Valsalva manouvre related rupture of the inferior thyroid arteries, the first in the right and the latter in the left, also Stenner et al. [3] reported a superior thyroid artery rupture, regardless of the affected side, when rapidly progressing cervical enlargement, dyspnea, tachycardia and hypertension ensue, airway management becomes prioritary to avoid a tracheotomy. A contrast enhanced computed tomography (CT) should be performed if the patient is stable enough where a retropharygeal hematoma will be evident, if possible, embolization of the bleeding vessel could be performed, if not, surgical exploration is indicated. Also if stable without progression a conservative conduct could be entertained.

Blunt Thoracic Trauma

Thoracic trauma accounts for 25% of the deaths occurred by trauma, [4] evidently, the penetrating lesions cause more deaths and are more obvious at the moment of diagnosis, on the other hand blunt trauma could have "discrete" fatal consequences that should be taken in to account when assessing a patient. The incidence of extrapleural hematomas is 7.1%. [5] Equimoses are much more common than hematomas in this scenario, however the mechanisms that produce blood accumulation in the third space large enough to call it hematoma due to trauma have been reported few times in the literature and almost always associated with fractures of the thoracic wall and/or other injuries. Nan and colleagues [6] reported a 40-year-old man with sternal fracture and dissection of the left main coronary artery, as a consequence of the fracture a mediastinal hematoma formed retro-sternally due to oozing of the fractured site; in special situations where drainage is left conservatively, it will resolve spontaneously in 2-9 weeks depending on the volume accumulated. [7] They could also present as extra-thoracic hematomas that can be resolved by a small incision for adequate drainage and quicker time for resolution. [8] Also an interesting mode of presentation is with the accumulation of blood within the parietal pleura and the thoracic wall, pushing the lung parenchyma with the potential to shift the mediastinum towards the not injured side mimicking a pleural effusion when it is very large. [9] A radiographical sign that could be present during a chest X-ray is a D-shape appearance in the wall with its base towards the contour of the chest, also the costo-phrenic angle remains intact and the pleural reflection formed by the accumulating blood could also be seen. [5,9] Attention has to be made to radiographic details so that the physician could discard the differential diagnoses; this presentation usually takes place when ribs fracture but the parietal pleura remains intact, this limits the growth of the hematoma (depending on the size of the lesion) forming its extra-pleural variance (Figure 1). [10] When in doubt a CT scan is indicated either to clarify diagnosis or to make a surgical plan if circulatory and respiratory disturbances are present. [11] A conservative approach could also be done depending on the clinical status of the patient and the progression of the lesion. Due to the nature and mode of presentation of these lesions, a video-assisted thoracoscopic surgery (VATS) approach is not recommended; rather a limited thoracotomy is most suitable. [12] Another type of tissue affected by trauma is the thymus, this was diagnosed in a 19-month-old-girl who sustained a 7m fall to the ground with a mandible fracture and widened mediastinum diagnosed on CT, during surgery the enlarged tissue demonstrated to be the cause of the mediastinal image, histology demonstrated intra-parenchymal hemorrhage, she was discharged uneventfully afterwards. [13] Finally, another cause after blunt trauma is injury of the internal thoracic vein due to the decelerating forces; this was described in a patient that underwent a sternotomy for evacuation of a retrosternal hematoma. [14]

Table 1. Causes of hematomas according to literature review

Causes of hematomas
Vascular malformations
Blunt thoracic trauma (thoracic wall and mediastinum)
Neoplastic
Post-operative complications
Myocardial infarct
Aneurysms (aorta, bronchial artery, lung parenchymal arteries)
Anticoagulation therapy
Spontaneous

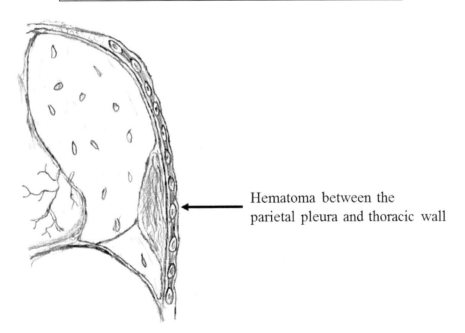

Hematoma between the parietal pleura and thoracic wall

Figure 1. Schematic representation of accumulated blood within the pleural cavity and thoracic wall.

Neoplastic Hematomas

Although rare, thoracic hematomas due to tumoral masses, are scarcely described. Type 1 neurofibromatosis (NF1), previously known as Von Recklinghausen disease, is a genetic disorder characterized by neurofibromas and hyperpigmented skin lesions [15], within various of its manifestations, hemorrhage is well known, with an incidence of 3.6% [16] Zhang et al. presented a case of a 20-year-old man with NF1 who had a left chest wall hematoma secondary to a 20 x 20 x 15-cm neurofibroma, bleeding was controlled by embolization so further surgery in a non emergent situation could be performed. [17] In NF1 patients vasculopathy is of great concern since it could present with fatal outcomes being one of the most important causes. Only three reports of such cases have been published, with different approaches each but all successful, wheather embolizing first followed by surgery or straight to surgery without embolization, all the authors agree that these patients must all be operated since embolization is just a temporary measure so that a more controlled scenario could be reached for the surgical phase of treatment. [17-19]

Postoperative Hematomas

Rarely hematomas are formed after a thoracic surgery was performed, Nanjaiah et al. reported a case that aroused after an aortic valve replacement in an octogenarian, [20] attributing it to a possible lesion of the perforating branches of the left internal thoracic artery, he also discusses the possibility of sarcopenia leading to physical frailty, [21] attention to detail should be always entertained since it could easily be confused for a pleural effusion on a simple radiography; once diagnosis is reached, surgical drainage with placement of a water seal system for the postoperative period and close follow-up are warranted, it is rare to find in the literature cases of this nature, but it is this author´s belief that this is an under reported complication, because of potential lesions to perforating intercostals (e.g. chest tube placement), hence the importance to carefully execute all the appropriate surgical steps. Agrifoglio et al. also described a variance secondary to rib fractures in a 79-year-old man after cardiac surgery who underwent a median sternotomy and coronary artery bypass grafting with an aortic graft replacement for an aneurysm. [22] At least from the two referred cases, octagenarians seem to be of increased risk, although more reports are needed to clarify this fact.

Cardiac Hematomas and Hemopericardium

Left ventricular free wall rupture after a myocardial infarction is the most common cause of death after arrhythmias and cardiogenic shock. [23] Almost invariably fatal when present, with survival very rarely reported. [23-26] Some authors suggest as a means of palliation previous to surgery, judicious pericardial aspiration and blood transfusion until definitive repair can be undertaken in the operating room. [24] Other forms of etiology are during percutaneous interventions of the coronary vessels with a reported incidence of 0.2-0.6% [27], graded from 1-3, the first two could be handled by reversal of anticoagulation and percutaneous techniques, grade 3 are associated with >1 mm ruptures with consequent bleeding, tamponade and death if not operated, with the evolution of percutaneous techniques, more aggressive interventions have been described, however these carry the burden of an increased rate of complications [28], Shekar et al. described a dilatation of an in-stent restenosis of a saphenous vein graft to the diagonal artery followed by a perforation of the anastomosis that lead to a large sub-epicardial hematoma shearing all epicardial vessels from the underlying myocardium eventually dying from the episode. [29] Decision has to follow echocardiographic and angiographic studies in order to determine the best and safest approach for the patient, of which could be direct repair of the vessel, revascularization or just decompression of the hematoma; that may or may not require ventricular assisting devices to reduce myocardial work and improve end organ perfusion.

Hematomas after cardiac surgery are also another cause worthy of attention, these occur within the myocardial fibers that form a neo-cavitation due to traumatic atrioventricular disruption of the perforating vessels, resulting in extravasation of blood into the muscles that could evolve into opening to the pericardial sac or self-limit to the muscle, this has been reported to happen in mitral valve surgery, coronary artery bypass grafting or even spontaneously. [30] Usually the site of lesion is the free left ventricular wall or interventricular septum, but also right ventricular free wall has been described. [30-33] When this occurs the result could be expansion, rupture or spontaneously resolve. It depends on the patient´s condition weather a surgical repair is in order or strict follow-up without intervention up until one year. [34] When a case presents with doubtful diagnosis of hemopericardium due to free wall rupture or after a traumatic event, many times it is advisable to perform a subxiphoid pericardial exploration, if the diagnosis is confirmed through a translucency of the blood in the pericardial sac, a complete median sternotomy should be done to explore and control the cause that is originating the hemorrhage.

Temporal pacing wires are used routinely during cardiac surgery, weather on the right free wall ventricle or ipsilateral auricle, they are attached at final stages of the surgery to serve both, diagnosing and treating brady- or tachyarrythmias following surgery. Very rarely complications have been reported, some groups withdraw the wires once they have completed their function, and others just cut them from the site where they emerge from the skin leaving the proximal section in the cavity. Few cases have been reported of bleeding, vascular perforation, atrial or ventricular laceration during wire removal with consequent tamponade, or in retained pacing wires, hematomas within the myocardium and extracardiac compression of cavities. [35-38] The main player in this physiopathologic process is believed to be the required anticoagulation therapy necessary for most of these patients, deeming them prone to events such as this. Based on these reports it is common practice to withdraw the pacing cables before initiating anticoagulation therapy and before retrieving drainage tubes, so if any bleeding is present it could be diagnosed immediately and treated accordingly, fortunately we have never experienced such complication.

Hematomas of the Aorta

Acute intramural hematoma (IMH) is defined as a result of injury to the aortic media with consequent hematoma within this space, triggered by rupture of the vasa vasorum and weakness of the wall, this entity could progress to rupture, aortic dissection, aneurysm, pseudoaneurysm or complete resolution. [39-40] This has to be differentiated from true aortic dissection due to their management and prognosis. Siriapisith et al. studied the tomographic differences between both pathologies, concluding that wall thickness less than a quarter of the aortic diameter, lesion extending around the entire aortic circumference, and ulcer like projections were the most useful indicators for distinguishing an IMH from a thrombosed false lumen of aortic dissection. [41] Treatment could be surgical or medical only, Moriyama and colleagues analyzed 51 patients and their therapeutic indications; candidates for surgery were patients with an enlarged ulcer, co-existing aneurysm, persistent pain with aneurysm, cardiac tamponade, superimposed dissection or recurrent pain with massive pleural effusion. The majority of patients with ascending IMH would require surgery with a 94% 2-year survival rate and a 25% operation-free rate. Twenty seven percent of descending aortic IMH required surgery with a 5-year survival rate of 63% and operation-free survival rate of 66%, Concluding that operation, in accordance with other authors, is recommended for almost all patients with ascending aortic IMH due to a high risk for serious complications; and medical therapy, primarily with anti-hypertensive drugs for those with descending aortic involvement unless a complication develops usually associated with ulcers of varying sizes, where the presence of these correlate to a significant risk for operation-free survival rates. [42-46]

Acute aortic rupture has a high mortality, approximately one third of patients don´t make it to the operating room, [47] these could present with the usual symptoms of aortic dissection mostly related to the left heart arterial system, such as symptoms or signs of aortic valve insufficiency, occlusion of major arterial vessels and cardiac tamponade, however in rare occasions, signs of pulmonary artery and superior vena cava stenosis could occur due to a mediastinal hematoma. [48] Survival of these patients depend on the physician's prompt diagnostic abilities and surgeon´s skills to achieve optimal results.

Anticoagulation Therapy Related Hematomas

Regarding the complications of anticoagulation, bleeding into the thoracic spaces have been published, Bapat et al. [49] reported a case of a retropharyngeal hematoma due to the use of warfarin, incidence varies between 0.3 and 0.7 per patient year, the risk rises when INR levels are above 4.5, although the retropharyngeal space isn´t considered thorax, but its direct relation with the retroesophageal space makes it a potential path for entry in the posterior mediastinum, Correction of INR is essential as it prevents further bleeding; for large or rapidly expanding hematomas surgical drainage is indicated.

Spontaneous Hematoma

Although rare these type of hematomas do scarcely occur as Sersar et al. [50] reported a pulmonary parenchymal aneurysm that warranted a right upper lobectomy to control the bleeding and hemoptysis. Usually found when a diferential diagnosis is in process and incidentally encountered on X-ray studies. Arterio-venous malformations have also been entertained in playing a "spontaneous" role, for which also surgical resolution is deemed. [51]

Also a possible cause is its relation to infectious diseases such as tuberculosis, where medical treatment is also added to the regimen, with good outcomes in any of the varying cases. [52]

Conclusion

As we have witnessed, thoracic hematomas have various origins with a wide array of severity at the time of diagnosis, physicians should always keep a keen eye to reach plausible conclusions when studying each individual case, for which treatment protocol and line of action from that point on are crucial for an adequate prognosis; it is of the outmost importance to keep in mind the diagnostic tools available to reach this goal without undermining the physical and history when in contact with patients for the first time.

References

[1]   Bageacu, S; Prades, JM; Kaczmarek, D; Porcheron, J. Images in cardiothoracic surgery. Spontaneous rupture of the inferior thyroid artery leading to life-threatening mediastinal hematoma. *Ann Thorac Surg*, 2005, 80, e20-e21.

[2]   Hoetzenecker, K; Töpker, M; Klepetko, W; Ankersmith, H. Spontaneous rupture of the inferior thyroid artery resulting in mediastinal hematoma. *Interact Cardiovas Thorac Surg*, 2010, 11, 209-210.

[3]   Stenner, M; Helmstaedter, V; Spuentrup, E; Quante, G; Huettenbrink, KB. Cervical hemorrhage due to spontaneous rupture of the superior thyroid artery: case report and review of the literature. *Head Neck*, 2010, 32(9),1277-1281.

[4]   Pickard, LR; Mattox, KL. Thoracic trauma and indications for thoracotomy. In: Mattox KL, Moore EF, Feliciano DV, editors. Trauma. Norwalk: *Appleton and Lange*, 1980, 315-320.

[5]   Rashid, MA; Wikstrom, T; Ortenwall, P. Nomenclature, classification, and significance of traumatic extrapleural hematoma. *J Trauma*, 2000, 49(2), 286-290.

[6]   Nan, YY; Chang, JP; Lu, MS; Kao, CL. Mediastinal hematoma and left main dissection following blunt chest trauma. *Eur J Cardiothorac Surg*, 2007, 31, 320-321.

[7]   Attar, S; Ayella, RJ; McLaughlin, JS. The widened mediastinum in trauma. *Ann Thorac Surg*, 1972, 13, 435-449.

[8]   Suh, JH; Kim, YH. Extra-thoracic hematoma after minor blunt chest injury. *Eur J Cardiothorac Surg*, 2008, 33, 1140.

[9]   Tsai, YF; Lu, SS. Huge extrapleural hematoma initially diagnosed as massive hemothorax. *J Med Cases*, 2013, 4(4), 247-249.

[10]   Goh, BK; Koong, HN. Massive traumatic extrapleural hematoma mimicking hemothorax: a potential pitfall of penetrating chest trauma. *J Trauma*, 2006, 61(4), 995-997.

[11]   Poyraz, AS; Kilic, D; Gultekin, B; Ozulku, M; Hatipoglu, A. Extrapleural hematoma: when is surgery indicated? *Monaldi Arch Chest Dis*, 2005, 63(3), 166-169.

[12]   Rashid, MA. Value of video-assisted thoracic surgery in traumatic extrapleural hematoma. *Thorac Cardiovasc Surg*, 1999, 47(4), 225-257.

[13] Takahashi, Y; Toyoda, Y; Okada, Y. *Thymic intracapsular hematoma caused by blunt chest trauma*, 2003, 76, 2107.

[14] Kim, KH; Choi, JB; Kim, MH. Internal thoracic vein injury presenting as extrapericardial tamponade after blunt chest trauma. *J Thorac Cardiovasc Surg*, 2013, 145, 1130.

[15] Neurofibromatosis. Conference statement. National Institutes of Health Consensus Development Conference. *Arch Neurol*, 1988, 45, 575-578.

[16] Conlon, NP; Redmond, KC; Celi, LA. Spontaneous hemothorax in a patient with neurofibromatosis type 1 and undiagnosed pheochromocytoma. *Ann Thorac Surg*, 2007, 84, 1021-1023.

[17] Zhang, K; Song, J; Xiong, W; Li, Z; Cao, D; Jiang, T; Liu, W. Massive spontaneous hemorrhage in giant type 1 neurofibromatosis in soft tissue of chest wall. *J Thorac Cardiovasc Surg*, 2012, 144, e92-e93.

[18] Lessard, L; Izadpanah, A; Williams, HB. Giant thoracic neurofibromatosis type 1 with massive intratumoral hemorrage: a case report. *J Plast Reconstructr Aesthet Surg*, 2009, 62, e325-e329.

[19] Rao, V; Afifi, RA; Ghazarian, D. Massive subcutaneous hemorrage in a chest-wall neurofibroma. *Can J Surg*, 2000, 43, 459-460.

[20] Nanjaiah, P; Agrawal, D; Prasad, SU. Pectoral hematoma mimicking a hemothorax in an octagenarian following aortic valve replacement – a near miss. *Interact Cardiovasc Thorac Surg*, 2009, 9, 847-848.

[21] Doherty, TJ. The influence of aging and sex on skeletal muscle mass and strength. *Curr Opin Clin Nutr Metabolic Care*, 2001, 4, 503-508.

[22] Agrifoglio, M; Zoli, S; Gennari, M; Annoni, A; Polvani, G. Expanding extrapleural hematoma from rib fractures after cardiac surgery. *Asian Cardiovasc Thorac Ann*, 2012, 21(3), 366-368.

[23] Pohjola-Sintonen, S; Muller, JE; Stone, PH; Willich, SN; Antman, EM; Davis, VG; Parker, CB; Braunwald, E. Ventricular septal and free wall rupture complicating acute myocardial infarction: experience in the Multicenter Investigation of Limitation of Infarct Size. *Am Heart J*, 1989, 117, 809-818.

[24] Svedjeholm, R; Håkanson, E; Lindström, M; Hjort, P. Post-infarct left ventricular free wall rupture and ventricular septal defect managed by pericardial aspiration during transport to referral hospital. *Interact Cardiovasc Thorac Surg*, 2003, 2, 193-195.

[25] Komeda, M; David, TE. Surgical treatment of postinfarction false aneurysm of the left ventricle. *J Thorac Cardiovasc Surg*, 1993, 106, 1189-1191.

[26] Pifarre, R; Sullivan, HJ; Grieco, J; Montoya, A; Bakhos, M; Scanlon, PJ; Gunnar, RM. Management of left ventricular rupture complicating myocardial infarction. *J Thorac Cardiovasc Surg*, 1983, 86, 441-443.

[27] Aslam, MS; Messersmith, RN; Gilbert, J; Lakier, JB. Successful management of coronary artery perforation with helical platinum microcoil embolization. *Catheter Cardiovasc Diagn*, 2000, 51, 320-322.

[28] Ellis, SG; Ajluni, S; Arnold, AZ; Popma, JJ; Bittl, JA; Eigler, NL; Cowley, M; Raymond, RE; Safian, RD; Whidow, PL. Increased coronary perforation in the new device era. Incidence, classification, management and outcome. *Circulation*, 1994, 90, 2725-2730.

[29] Shekar, PS; Stone, JR; Couper, GS. Dissecting sub-epicardial hematoma-challenges to surgical management. *Eur J Cardiothorac Surg*, 2004, 26, 850-853.

[30] Harpaz, D; Kriwisky, M; Cohen, AJ; Medalion, B; Rozenman, Y. Unusual form of cardiac rupture: sealed sub acute left ventricular free wall rupture, evolving to intramyocardial dissecting hematoma and to pseudoaneurysm formation-a case report and review of the literature. *J Am Soc Echocardiogr*, 2001, 14, 219-227.

[31] Prachanth, P; Mukhaini, M; Maddali, MM. Intramyocardial dissecting hematoma causing cardiac tamponade: an unusual complication after mitral valve replacement surgery. *Ann Card Anaesth*, 2009, 12, 79-80.

[32] Cheng, HW; Hung, KC; Lin, FC; Wu, D. Spontaneous intramyocardial hematoma mimicking a cardiac tumor of the right ventricle. *J Am Soc Ecocardiogr*, 2004, 17, 394-396.

[33] Panduranga, P; Valliatsu, J; Al-Mukhaini, M. Right ventricular free Wall intramyocardial hematoma after coronary bypass. *Asian Cardiovasc Thorac Ann*, 2012, 21(3), 355-357.

[34] Vargas-Barrón, J; Roldán, FJ; Romero-Cárdenas, A; Molina-Carrión, M; Vázquez-Antona, CA; Zabalgoitia, M; Martínez, Ríos MA; Pérez, JE. Dissecting intramyocardial hematoma: clinical presentation, pathophysiology, outcomes and delineation by echocardiography. *Echocardiography*, 2009, 26, 254-261.

[35] Del Nido, P; Goldman, BS. Temporary epicardial pacing after open heart surgery: complications and prevention. *J Card Surg*, 1989, 4, 99-103.

[36] Gal, ThJ; Chaet, MS; Novitzky, D. Laceration of a saphenous vein graft by an epicardial pacemaker wire. *J Cardiovasc Surg (Torino)*, 1998, 39, 221-222.

[37] Bolton, JWR; Mayer, JE. Unusual complication of temporary pacing wires in children. *Ann Thorac Surg*, 1992, 54, 769-770.

[38] Kapoor, A; Syal, S; Gupta, N; Gupta, A. Right paracardiac mass due to organized pericardial hematoma around retained epicardial pacing wires following aortic valve replacement. *Interact Cardiovasc Thorac Surg*, 2011, 13, 104-106.

[39] Chao, CP; Walker, TG; Kalva, SP. Natural history and CT appearances or aortic intramural hematoma. *Radiographics*, 2009, 29, 791-804.

[40] Sawhney, NS; DeMaría, AN; Blanchard, DG. Aortic intramural hematoma: an increasingly recognized and potentially fatal entity. *Chest*, 2001, 120, 1340-1346.

[41] Siriapisith, T; Wasinrat, J; Slisatkorn. Computed tomography and aortic intramural hematoma and thrombosed dissection. *Asian Cardiovasc Thorac Ann*, 2010, 18(5), 456-563.

[42] Robbins, RC; McManus, RP; Mitchell, RS; Latter, DR. Moon MR, Olinger GN, Miller DC. Management of patients with intramural hematoma of the thoracic aorta. *Circulation*, 1993, 88, 1-10.

[43] Nienaber, CA; von Kodolitsch, Y; Petersen, B; Loose, R; Helmchen, U; Haverich, A; Spielmann, RP. Intramural hemorrhage of the thoracic aorta, diagnostic and therapeutic implications. *Circulation*, 1995, 92, 1465-1472.

[44] Muluk, SC; Kaufman, JA; Torchiana, DF; Gertler, JP; Cambria, RP. Diagnosis and treatment of thoracic aortic intramural hematoma. *J Vasc Surg*, 1996, 24, 1022-1029.

[45] Harris, KM; Braverman, AC; Gutierrez, FR; Barzilai, B; Davila-Roman, VG. Transesophageal echocardiographic and clinical features of aortic intramural hematoma. *J Thorac Cardiovasc Surg*, 1997, 114, 619-629.

[46] Moriyama, Y; Yotsumoto, G; Kuriwaki, K; Watanabe, S; Hisatomi, K; Shimokawa, S; Toyohira, H; Taira, A. Intramural hematoma of the thoracic aorta. *Eur J Cardiothorac Surg*, 1998, 13, 230-239.

[47] Von Oppell, U; Dunne, TT; De Groot, MK; Zilla, P. Traumatic rupture: twenty-year metaanalysis of mortality and risk of paraplegia. *Ann Thorac Surg*, 1994, 58(2), 585-593.

[48] Inoue, Y; Takahashi, R; Kashima, I; Tsutsumi, K. Mediastinal hematoma: another lethal sign of aortic dissection. *Interact Cardiovasc Thorac Surg*, 2009, 8, 275-276.

[49] Bapat, VN; Brown, K; Nakas, A; Shabbo, F. Retropharyngeal hematoma--a rare complication of anticoagulant therapy. *Eur J Cardiothorac Surg*, 2002, 21(1), 117-118.

[50] Sesar, IS; Ismaeil, MF; Abdel Mageed, NA; Elsaeid, MM. Rapidly accumulating spontaneous pulmonary hematoma complicating a small parenchymal aneurysm. *Interactive Cardiovasc Thorac Surg*, 2004, 3, 243-244.

[51] Sameh, IS; Elshabrawii, M; Elsaeid, AS; Farag, YA; Abulela, S; El Salid, MM. Rapidly accumulating spontaneous pulmonary hematoma. *J Thoracic Cardiovasc Surg*, 2005, 129(1), 233.234.

[52] Okubo, K; Okamoto, T; Isobe, J; Ueno, Y. Rupture of a chronic expanding hematoma of the thorax into lung parenchyma. *J Thorac Cardiovasc Surg*, 2004, 127, 1838-1840.

In: Advances in Medicine and Biology. Volume 77
Editor: Leon V. Berhardt

ISBN: 978-1-63117-444-5
© 2014 Nova Science Publishers, Inc.

Chapter 11

Peritonitis Related to Peritoneal Dialysis (PD/Peritonitis)

Alejandro Treviño-Becerra
Clinica de Uremia y Dialisis, Mexico, D.F. Mexico

Abstract

The worldwide increases of programs to treat chronic uremia with peritoneal dialysis does not ignore that the main complication still is peritonitis and has taken special interest in the field. This type of peritonitis is different to other processes, it involves the peritoneum, as happens in abdominal trauma, perforations and surgical process.

At the earliness time (1960, the PD procedure was done with rigid catheter, fluid in glass container, added with heparin, xylocaine, and tetracycline for treating acute kidney failure, drugs intoxication and severe complications of chronic renal failure.

In June 1978, the initial group of continuous ambulatory peritoneal dialysis, results of 27 patients were shown during the First International Symposium of PD held in Chapala, Jalisco, México the incidence of episode of PD/P peritonitis was around 6 to 8 months, later the benefits of use plastic bags and soft catheter make an enormous difference. It was considered that adequate training, and treatment with new contactology and prophylaxis was the way to diminish those figures and it happens, the use of titanium connector and double bag system as the use of cyclers or automated machines the incidence of PD/P episode diminish to one episode every 18-24 months even less in the best centers. But PD/ still is the "Achilles' heel" that cause technical and patients failure, relapse episodes of peritonitis most of them severe or chronically that require prolonged hospitalizations, expenses antibiotics and surgical reinsertion of catheters. All of these troubles have dropped the figures of patients in selected countries (Canada, UK, Mexico) in chronic PD from 50% to 12% or 15% or less, except Colombia, Taiwan and Hong Kong that maintain figures 40 to 70 %.

In fact there are different types of PD-peritonitis depending of the cause, bacterial, fungi, aseptic, relapse and the worse form is sclerosing peritonitis.

But it has been demonstrated that PD fluids with glucose damage the peritoneum membrane physiological and morphology so in the last decade had been developed new more physiology PD solutions changing the osmolality substance, pH, and added some other compounds. So there are some lines of investigation inhibitors of rennin angiotensin aldosterone system, the endothelial factor, peritoneal resting, application of statins, acetylcysteine and gene therapy on stem cells. So we need to look to the future to expect a better results of PD and to avoid or disappears all the complications including severe peritonitis that even could be fatal. Keeping in mind that PD is a very good treatment for selected patients a lower cost the hemodialysis.

Introduction

The worldwide increase of programs to treat chronic uremia with peritoneal dialysis (Pd) does not ignore that the main complication still is peritonitis (P) and has taken a special interest in the field. This type of PD/P peritonitis is different to other processes, it involves the peritoneum, as happens in abdominal trauma, perforations and surgical process.

Peritonitis, a common complication of peritoneal dialysis, contributes to treatment failure, hospitalization, and death. It is important to diagnose PD/P and to initiate empiric antibiotic therapy as early as possible to prevent those serious consequences. PD/P is defined based on the presentation of symptoms, peritoneal effluent cell count, and culture of micro-organisms [1]. Patients have to recognize their symptoms-including cloudy effluent, fever and abdominal pain early in the onset of peritonitis [2]. Despite regularly update guidelines from the International Society for Peritoneal Dialysis (ISPD) related and their prevention and treatment PD/P, peritonitis continues to be a worrisome problem throughout the world.

At the earliness time (1960, the PD procedure was done with rigid catheter, fluid in glass container, added with heparin, xylocaine, and tetracycline for treating acute kidney failure, drugs intoxication and severe complications of chronic renal failure [3].

In June 1978, the initial group of continuous ambulatory peritoneal dialysis, results of 27 patients were shown during the First International Symposium of PD held in Chapala, Jalisco, México [4] the incidence of episode of PD/P peritonitis was around 6 to 8 months, later the benefits of use plastic bags and soft catheter make an enormous difference [3]. It was considerer that adequate training, and treatment with new contactology and prophylaxis was the way to diminish those figures and it happens, the use of titanium connector and double bag system as the use of cyclers or automated machines the incidence of PD/P episode diminish to one episode every 18-24 months even less in the best centers. But PD/ still is the "Achilles' heel" that cause technical and patients failure, relapse episodes of peritonitis most of them severe or chronically that require prolonged hospitalizations, expenses antibiotics and surgical reinsertion of catheters. All of these troubles have dropped the figures of patients in selected countries (Canada, UK, Mexico) in chronic PD from 50% to 12% or 15% or less, except Colombia, Taiwan and Hong Kong that maintain figures 40 to 70 %. Since the late 1990s, a significant reduction in the risk for death of patients undergoing peritoneal dialysis (PD) has occurred in many parts of the world. Studies from the United States, Canada, France, Australia, and New Zealand indicate that the reduction in death risk for patients undergoing PD in those countries has been of a significantly greater magnitude than the reduction observed for patients undergoing in-center hemodialysis [5].

In fact there are different types of PD/P depending of the cause, bacterial, fungi, aseptic, relapse and the worse form is sclerosing peritonitis [6]. But is has been demonstrated that PD fluids with glucose damage the peritoneum membrane physiological and morphology so in the last decade has been developed new more physiology PD solutions changing the osmolality substances, pH, and added some other osmotic agents [7]. So there are some lines of investigation to improve the PD/P use of some substances and procedures inhibitors of renin angiotensin aldosterone system, the endothelial factor, application of stains, acetylcysteine, gene therapy or stem cells peritoneal resting [1].

So we need to look to the future to expect better results and to avoid or reduce all the complications including severe PD/Peritonitis that even could be fatal. Keeping in mind that PD is a very good treatment for selected patients, at a lower cost than hemodialysis. In this comment paper, I stress the importance of training, educational patients on PD treatment, the more risk patients are older people and the variations of incidence of peritonitis in different parts of the world affecting by local factors and some lines about the transfer from PD to Hd.

Since first being describe by Twardowski in 1989, the PET has proved to be an essential tool to facilitate prescription management and diagnosis- and explore the factors that affect outcome-in patients on PD. The attraction of the PET has been its simplicity [8]. Fluid removal is a key component of any dialysis modality. In PD, the osmotic force exerted by osmotic agents added to dialysis fluid achieves fluid removal. Glucose is the prototypical osmotic agent in PD, although other agents such as polyglucose (icodextrin) and amino acids are also used along side. Fluid removal in PD depends on the characteristics of the dialysis fluid, especially the type and concentration of the osmotic agent, the temporal distribution of dialysis fluid exchanges, the characteristics of the peritoneal membrane, and the status of the patient. Assessment of the efficiency of fluid removal by osmosis in patients on PD is in itself a multifactor task, and several different parameters must be applied for its holistic description.

It is generally agreed that, in continuous ambulatory PD (CAPD) patients, sufficient daily UF should be achieved with absorption of glucose, both because a high concentration of glucose in the tissues induces neoangiogenesis and fibrosis and may result in a loss of UF capacity, and also glucose absorption contributes to various nutritional and metabolic disturbances [9].

A multidisciplinary approach with a precise schedule-"therapeutic education" has become an important therapeutic tool. The ISPD guidelines assert that a PD education program may be evaluated by observing changes in peritonitis rates, but the value of individual evaluation at the end of a training period is still controversial [10, 11].

The training of PD patients is extremely important and may affect technique success and clinical outcomes. Nurse training experience must also be taken into account to emphasize the importance of personalized training that considers individual circumstances and that supports self-efficacy (helping to increase the patients´ perception of their capability to cope with difficulties and to succeed). In an international survey on training, Bernardini did not find any correlation between length of training and outcome [12 – 14].

For years, the PD community has championed patient education, and it is noteworthy that the importance of greater patient involvement in long-term disease management is being increasingly recognized by many sources predicts a worse outcome in elderly individuals comparisons of the clinical characteristics and outcomes in silent and non-silent peritonitis [15, 16].

The demonstration of a higher risk of PD technique failure in individuals who are retired or disabled (or both), raises the question of whether enhancing social supports will reduce the probability of transfer to in-center hemodialysis. Indeed, to date, studies of PD patients suggest that greater social support is associated with fewer symptoms of depression and anxiety, greater satisfaction with care, better health-related quality of life, fewer hospitalizations, and higher PD technique survival patients presenting with silent peritonitis tended to be older than those presenting with non-silent peritonitis [17-19].

Although silent peritonitis is more likely to be culture-negative and less often caused by gram-negative organisms, it was not associated with a better prognosis. [8] However, the rates of treatment failure, hospitalization, and relapse were not different between the culture-positive and culture-negative episodes. Accordingly, the association between silent peritonitis and outcomes might be not influenced by that difference [14]. These issues are particularly relevant to patients with kidney diseases, because in most societies, chronic kidney disease and end-stage renal disease disproportionately affect people who are poor, less educated, and members of racial or ethnic minorities. Compared with individuals choosing in-center hemodialysis, those choosing PD therapy are required to assume a substantially greater responsibility for their own care [19, 20]. For example, it remains unclear whether the association of race with lower PD technique survival reflects unmeasured confounding with socio economical status [5, 6]. Tropical regions were associated with a higher overall peritonitis rate (including fungal peritonitis) and a shorter time to a first peritonitis episode. Augmented peritonitis prophylactic measures such as antifungal therapy and exit-site care should be considered in PD patients residing in Tropical climates [9].

Technique failure in PD is a complex problem, with causes that vary from those that can potentially be influenced by quality improvement initiatives such as lowering PD/P rates or managing ultra filtration, to those that have their roots in the patient's environment. The latter include sociologic and economic factors whose solutions lay in the domain of public health [21-24].

To attempt to prevent unplanned HD initiation, patients who are likely to fail PD should be prepared for HD. Although clinical advice and guidelines about transfer from PD to HD have been issued, predicting PD failure is still a matter of concern for clinicians [12, 25].

The literature also contains descriptions of successful programs of assisted PD in which the therapy is performed at home with the assistance of a family member or paid helper, generally a nurse [26].

References

[1]   Krishnam, M, Thodis, E, Ikonomopoulos, D., Vidgen, E, Chu, M, Bargman, J. M. et.al. Predictor outcome following bacterial peritonitis in peritoneal dialysis. *Perit. Dial. Int.* 2002.; 22: 573-81.

[2]   Chowk.M. Szeto, C.C. Cheung, K.K. Leung, C.B. Wong, S. S. Law M.C. et. Al. Predictive value of dialysate cell counts in peritonitis complicating peritoneal dialysis. *Clin. J. Am. Soc. Nephrol.* 2006; 1, 768-3.

[3]   Don S, J. Chen, Y. Impact of bag exchange procedure on risk peritonitis. *Perit. Dial. Int.* 2010; 30: 440-7.

[4]   Treviño. B. A. Boen. S. T. F. "Today's" Art of Peritoneal Dialysis, *Contribution to Nephrology* Vol. 17. Ed. Skanger A.G. Basel, 1979.

[5]   Mehrotra, R.: Translating an understanding of the determinants of technique failure to maximize patient time on Peritoneal Dialysis. *Perit. Dial. Int.* 2013. 33: 2, 112-115.

[6]   Mehrotra, R. Kerman, D, Fried, L, Kalantar Zadek, K., Khawar, O, Morris, K, et. al. Chronic peritoneal Dialysis in the United States: declining utilization despite improving outcomes *J. Am. Soc. Nephrol.* 2007, 18:2781-8.

[7]   Waniewski, J, Paniagua, R: Stachwska-Pietka, J. Ventura, M.J. Avila Diaz, M: Prado-Uribe C. Mora C. Garcia-López, E. Lindholm, B. Threefold peritoneal test of osmotic conductance, ultrafiltration efficiency, and fluid absorption. *Perit. Dial. Int.* 33.4 419-26.

[8]   Wilkie, M: Editors Introduction: Exploring unplanned transfer, Innovation in catheter placement, and more on biocompatible solutions *Perit. Dialysis Int.* 33, 4, 347-348.

[9]   Cho, Y: Badue, U.S. Hawley M.C. McDonald, P,S: Brown, G.F. Boudville, N: Wiggins, J.K., et al. Effects of climate region on peritonitis risk, microbiology, treatment and outcomes a multicenter study, *Perit. Dial. Int.* 33-1, 75-85.

[10]   Szeto, C.C. Chow, K. M. Wong, T, Y, Leung, C.B. Wang, A.Y. Lui, S. F. et. Al. Feasibility of resuming peritoneal dialysis after severe peritonitis and Tenckhoff catheter removal. *J. Am. Soc. Nephrol.* 2002, 13-1040-5.

[11]   Bunke, M; Brief, M.E. Golpert A. Culture-negative capd. Peritonitis, the network 9 study *Adv. Perit. Dial.* 1994; 10; 174-8.

[12]   Bernardini, J., Price, V, Figueiredo. A, On behalf of the International Society of Pereitoneal Dyalisis (I.S.P.D) Nursing Laison Committee Peritoneal dialysis patient training 2006. *Perit. Dial. Int.* 2006. 26: 625-32.

[13]   Neville. A, Jenkings, J, William J. D., Craig, K. J: Peritoneal dialysis training. a multisensory approach. *Perit. Dial. Int.* 2005 (Suppl 3) 5-149-51.

[14]   Dong, J, Luo, S, XU, R; Chew, Y, XU, Y: Clinical characteristics and outcomes of "silent" and "non silent" peritonitis in patients on peritoneal dialysis *Peri. Dial. Int.* 33.1 2-37.

[15]   Jassal, S.V. Tripeski, l, Zhu, N, Fenton S, Hemmelgarn, B.: Changes in survival among elderly patients initiating dialysis from 1990-1999. *C.M.A.J.* 2007: 177-1033.8.

[16]   Gadola, L. Poggi, C, Poggi, M. Saez, L., Ferrari, A. Romero V. et al. Using a multidisciplinary training program to reduce peritonitis in peritoneal dialysis patients: *Perit. Dial. Int.* 33- 1:38-45.

[17]   Russo R, Manili, L, Tiraboschi, G, Amanr, K, Deluca, M. Alberghins, E, et. al. Patients-retraining in peritoneal dialysis why and when it is needed *Kidney International suppl.* 2006: (103) S-127-32.

[18]   Plantinga LC, Fink NE, Harrington-Levey, R. Finkeistein, F. Hebathym. Powe, N. R. et. al. Association of Social support with outcomes in incident dialysis patients. *Clin J. Am Soc. Nephrol* 2010. 5. 1480-8.

[19]   Chent. W, Li.Sy, Chen, J.Y Yang W.C. Training of peritoneal dialysis patient-Taiwans experience *Perit. Dial. Int.* 2008 ; 28 (Suppl 3) 5-72-5.

[20]   Boissnot, L, Landruv, I, Cardineav, E; Zagdoun E Ryckelgenk, J.P. Lobbedez, T. Is transition between Peritoneal Dialysis and Hemodialysis really a gradual process *Perit. Dial. Int.,* 33,4, 391-97.

[21]   Plantinga LC, Fink N.E, Finkelstein F.O, Powe N.R, Jaar B.G. Association of peritoneal dialysis clinic size with clinical outcomes. *Perit. Dial. Int.* 2009; 29:285-91.

[22]   Low. W.F Peritoneal Dialysis in the Far-East and astonishing situation in 2008 *Perit. Dial. Int.* 2009. 29 (Suppl 12) S 227-9.

[23] Korbet, S.M. Vonesh, E.F, Aranek, C. A. Peritonitis in an urban peritoneal dialysis program: an analysis of infecting pathogens *Am. K. Kidney, Dis.* 1995 26: 47-53.

[24] Chern, Y. B: Ho, P.S. Kuo, L.Ch, Chen, J: B, Lower Education level is a mayor risk factor for peritonitis incidence in chronic dialysis patients a retrospective cohort study with 12-year follow-up. *Perit. Dial. Int.*: 2013, 33, 522-528.

[25] Ros, S, Remon, C; Rashid-O.A.; Ouirus, P; Lindholm, B: Carrero, J.J. Increased risk of fatal infections in women starting peritoneal dialysis. *Perit. Dial. Int.* 2013, 33, 487-494.

[26] Wilkie. M. The Complicated question of Peritoneal Dialysis Technique Survival, *Perit. Dial. Int.* 2013 33: 2, 11.

In: Advances in Medicine and Biology. Volume 77   ISBN: 978-1-63117-444-5
Editor: Leon V. Berhardt   © 2014 Nova Science Publishers, Inc.

Chapter 12

Molecular Mechanisms of Renal Tubular Acidosis

Shoko Horita[1], Osamu Yamazaki[1], Motonobu Nakamura[1], Hideomi Yamada[1], Masashi Suzuki[1] and George Seki[1,*]

[1] Department of Internal Medicine, The University of Tokyo Hospital, Hongo, Bunkyoku, Tokyo, Japan

Abstract

Acid/base balance is tightly regulated by kidney and lung. In kidney, proximal tubules and collecting ducts are the main sites of acid/base regulation. Proximal tubules reabsorb most of the bicarbonate filtered from glomeruli. On the other hand, α intercalated cells in collecting ducts secrete proton and reabsorb the regenerated bicarbonate. Carbonic anhydrase II (CAII) is located in the cytoplasm of both tubular cells, catalyzing the transformation between CO_2 and HCO_3^-. The main acid/base transporters in proximal tubules are the sodium-bicarbonate cotransporter (NBCe1) in the basolateral side and sodium-proton exchanger type 3 (NHE3) in the luminal side. Mutations in NBCe1 cause proximal renal tubular acidosis (pRTA) with ocular abnormalities and other extrarenal manifestations. In α intercalated cells, anion exchanger 1 (AE1) in the basolateral side and vacuolar type proton ATPase (V-ATPase) in the luminal side are the main transporters. Mutations in AE1 cause autosomal recessive distal renal tubular acidosis (dRTA) and/or autosomal dominant red blood cell dysmorphologies. Among multiple subunits of V-ATPase, mutations in a4 and B1 subunits cause autosomal recessive dRTA with or without impaired hearing. Mutations in CAII cause a mixed type RTA with osteopetrosis. Recent studies using genetically modified mice have significantly clarified the pathogenesis of RTA and associated extrarenal manifestations. Clinically, cases of secondary RTA due to systemic diseases such as multiple myeloma and Sjögren syndrome, or side effects of drugs are much more common than cases of hereditary RTA. In this chapter we will focus on the molecular mechanisms of RTA.

* Correspondence: George Seki, georgeseki-tky@umin.ac.jp.

Introduction

Renal tubular acidosis (RTA) represents the clinical condition that renal tubule does not reabsorb enough bicarbonate (HCO_3^-) and/or excrete enough proton (H^+) to keep acid-base homeostasis. RTA is diagnosed by acidosis with normal anion gap (i.e. hyperchloridemia). Urine acidification is impaired (urine pH > 5.5) in distal RTA (dRTA) but not in proximal RTA (pRTA). Clinically, secondary RTAs caused by systemic diseases such as Sjögren syndrome, multiple myeloma, or side effects of drugs are much more common. However, hereditary RTA is important for clarifying the mechanisms of acid-base regulation by kidney.

In a healthy individual, kidneys filtrate 180 L of the plasma each day. Among 4,000 mmol of bicarbonate (HCO_3^-) filtered from the glomeruli, approximately 80 percent is reabsorbed in the proximal tubule [1, 2]. The remaining 20 percent is reabsorbed afterwards, mainly in the loop of Henle and the connecting tubule.

In the proximal tubule, the Na^+-HCO_3^- cotransporter NBCe1 and the Na^+-H^+ exchanger NHE3 contribute to bicarbonate reabsorption. NBCe1 is located in the basolateral side of the proximal tubule, mainly in the S1 and S2 segments [3, 4]. NBCe1 transports bicarbonate coupled with Na^+ with the stoichiometric ratio of 3:1 [5]. In the luminal side, NHE3 drives H^+ out of the proximal tubule cell, in exchange for Na^+. As a result Na^+ comes into the proximal tubule cell. In the cytosole of proximal tubular cells carbonic anhydrase II (CAII) catalyzes the formation of H^+ and HCO_3^- from H_2O and CO_2.

In the collecting tubule, α intercalated cells secrete H^+ into the luminal side by V-ATPase and reabsorb HCO_3^- by the Cl^-/HCO_3^- exchanger AE1. H^+ is excreted in the form of titratable acid or NH_4^+. CAII here also catalyzes the formation of H^+ and HCO_3^-. V-ATPase is a huge complex consisted of 13 subunits, largely separated into cytosolic V0 and membrane-bound V1 domains. AE1 is encoded by *slc4a1*, which belongs to SLC4 bicarbonate transport family [6]. NBCe1, encoded by *slc4a4*, also belongs to this family. The overall structures of AE1 and NBCe1 are thought to be similar, having 33% amino acid homology [6].

Secondary RTA is caused by drugs such as valpronic acid and aminoglycosides, and diseases like diabetes mellitus, multiple myeloma, and Sjögren syndrome. Fanconi syndrome represents global dysfunction of proximal tubular functions resulting in excessive urinary excretion of amino acids, glucose, phosphate, bicarbonate, and other solutes handled by proximal tubule. Fanconi syndrome is caused by hereditary diseases like Dent disease, Lowe syndrome, and Wilson disease. However, cases of secondary Fanconi syndrome due to toxicity of heavy metals, i.e. lead and cadmium, systemic diseases such as multiple myeloma, or side effects of drugs including ifosfamide, antivirals and gentamicin are more common [7].

pRTA

pRTA is also called as RTA type 2. In this type of RTA, bicarbonate reabsorption is impaired in the proximal tubule. Normal proximal tubule reabsorbs about 80 % of the filtered bicarbonate, so this type of pRTA may occasionally lead to severe acidosis. NBCe1, CAII, and Fanconi syndrome are known as the cause of human hereditary pRTA. So far mutations of NHE3 have not been found in human hereditary pRTA.

pRTA Caused by NBCe1 Mutations

Sodium-bicarbonate cotransporter NBCe1 encoded by *slc4a4* is identified as the cause of autosomal recessive inherited pRTA. Before the first cloning of NBCe1 by Romero and colleagues [8], Igarashi and colleagues had reported a case of severe pRTA with ocular abnormalities and cerebral calcification [9]. Later they identified that the gene responsible for this acidosis is *slc4a4* [10]. So far 12 mutations of NBCe1 have been found in pRTA patients [10-19].

There are five isoforms of NBCe1, among them NBCe1A, B, and C are major variants in human. NBCe1A is expressed mainly in kidney but also detected in eye. NBCe1B is widely expressed, including pancreas, gastrointestinal ducts, eye and brain. NBCe1C is predominantly expressed in brain. The structure of NBCe1A is different from that of NBCe1B/C in the N-terminus. NBCe1C has the C-terminus different from that of NBCe1A/B. The N-terminal region of NBCe1B/C has a binding site for inositol 1,4,5-trisphosphate receptor-binding protein (IRBIT) [20]. Figure 1 shows the simplified scheme of main NBCe1 isoforms. The binding of IRBIT can activate NBCe1B/C activities.

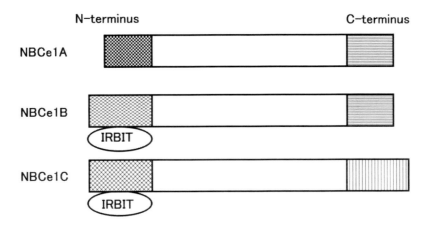

Figure 1. The simplified scheme of main NBCe1 isoforms.

Typical pRTA patients due to NBCe1 mutations present with extrarenal manifestations, especially ocular abnormalities such as glaucoma, cataract, and band keratopathy, sometimes resulting in blindness. Low stature and cerebral calcification are usually accompanied as well.

Table 1 summarizes the reported NBCe1 mutations and their manifestations. As shown, there is no tight relationship between the severity of acidosis and the magnitude of in vitro NBCe1 inactivation.

The treatment of pRTA due to NBCe1 mutations is difficult. In most of the cases the oral administration of bicarbonate cannot normalize the serum HCO_3^-. Moreover, alkali treatment often exaggerates hypokalemia. However, the developmental delay can be ameliorated to some extent if the patient is treated with alkali from infantile period [21].

Table 1. The properties and manifestations of NBCe1 mutations

	Q29X	R298S	S427L	T485S	G486R	R510H	W516X	L522P	N721TfsX29	A799V	R881C	S982NfsX4
consanguinity	+	+	-	+	+	-	-	N/A	+	+	+	-
serum HCO_3^- (mEq/L)	9.4	8.0	11	13	3	5.5	10	N/A	13.2	6.3	10.6	14.8/17.3
band keratopathy	-	+	+	+	+	+	+	+	+	+	+	+
glaucoma	+	+	+	-	-	+	+	+	+	+	+	+
migraine	-	-	N/A	-	-	+	-	+	+	-	+	+
activity in *Xenopus* oocyte (% of WT)	N/A	41%	10%	0%	4%	4%	N/A	0%	0%	14%	39%	100%
activity in HEK293 cells (% of WT)	N/A	39%	N/A	30%	42%	6%	N/A	0%	N/A	32%	4%	3%
citations	[16]	[10, 11]	[14]	[11,13]	[11, 12]	[10, 11]	[18]	[17, 19]	[15]	[11, 13]	[11, 13]	[11]

N/A: data not available.

Migraine and NBCe1

Recently we have identified two sisters presenting with relatively mild pRTA, severe ocular abnormalities, and hemiplegic migraine. A mutation in the C-terminal of NBCe1 has been identified. This mutation, S982NfsX4, shows almost normal transport function in *Xenopus* oocytes, but presents cytosolic retention in mammalian cells [11]. Re-investigation of other pRTA pedigrees revealed that homozygous NBCe1 mutations lacking plasma membrane expression in astrocytes are associated with migraine with or without hemiplegia. We think that migraine associated with NBCe1 mutations represents a primary headache most likely caused by dysfunctional local pH regulation in the brain. Interestingly, several heterozygous family members with the S982NfsX4 mutation also showed normal-tension glaucoma and migraine with or without aura. We speculated that the hetero-oligomer formation between wild-type and the mutant NBCe1 [22] might be responsible for these symptoms in the heterozygous members. Indeed, co-expression analysis identified a dominant-negative effect of S982NfsX4 mutant that prevents the plasma membrane expression of wild-type NBCe1 [11].

NHE3 in the Proximal Tubule

Na^+-H^+ exchanger (NHE) is widely distributed in many organs and tissues. There are ten isoforms in human, including NHE1 to NHE9 and sperm-specific NHE [23-27]. In the luminal side of proximal tubule NHE3 and NHE8 are known to exist. In mammals NHE3 is detected also in the luminal side of the thick ascending limb, gastrointestinal tract, gall bladder, epididymis, and brain [24].

NHE3 in the proximal tubule secrets H^+ into the lumen in exchange for Na^+. The H^+ is produced by CAII, which catalyzes the formation of H^+ and HCO_3^- from H_2O and CO_2. The counterpart HCO_3^- is reabsorbed via NBCe1.

Hereditary diseases due to NHE3 deficiency have not been discovered in human. Mice lacking NHE3 show mild to moderate acidemia [28-32].

Hereditary Fanconi Syndrome

Fanconi syndrome is a group of diseases with generalized proximal tubule dysfunction, accompanied with acidosis, aminoaciduria, glycosuria, hypophosphataemia, rickets and growth retardation. Several distinct disorders such as Lowe syndrome, Wilson disease, and nephropathic cystinosis cause Fanconi syndrome.

Cystinosis is characterized by the accumulation of cystine in all organs and tissues [33, 34]. There are three types of cystinosis, among them the nephropathic type is the severest one. The patients with this type present with Fanconi syndrome from infantile period. They will develop renal failure, if they are not appropriately treated in early time [33]. The responsible gene is *CTNS* in 17p13.3. Its product is called cystinosin, a protein of 367-amino acid. Defective cystinosin accumulates in lysosome and induces systemic manifestations such as corneal erosion, keratopathy, iris crystal formation, retinal degeneration, and endocrine disorders such as type I diabetes mellitus, hypothyroidism, and hypogonadism [35]. Cysteamine is used to prevent cystine accumulation.

Lowe syndrome is known as an X-linked oculocerebrorenal disease with renal proximal tubule dysfunction, developmental delay, blindness, and progressive renal failure [36]. The responsible gene, *OCRL1* [37], is an enzyme that regulates the metabolism of phosphoinositides. The molecular mechanism by which the dysfunction of ocrl1 leads to Lowe syndrome remains speculative.

Wilson disease is an autosomal recessive disorder, accompanied with copper accumulation in liver. This disease is also associated with aminoaciduria, nephrolithiasis, and Fanconi syndrome [38]. Mutations in copper-dependent ATPase (ATP7B) are responsible for this disease.

Recently another autosomal recessive hereditary Fanconi syndrome has been identified [39]. The affected patients, two siblings from consanguineous parents, showed pRTA, renal failure, hypophosphataemic rickets with hypercalciuria (HHRH), renal phosphate wasting and high level of serum $1,25(OH)_2D_3$ (1,25-dihydroxyvitamin D_3). The homozygous in-frame duplication of 21 bp in sodium-phosphate cotransporter IIc (NaPi-IIc), encoded by gene *SLC34A3*, was found to be responsible for this type of Fanconi syndrome. When expressed in opossum kidney cells, wild-type NaPi-IIc was colocalized with actin in the plasma membrane. However, the mutant NaPi-IIc remained in the cytoplasm [39], suggesting that the accumulation of abnormal proteins and resulting cell stress might be involved in the pathogenesis.

dRTA

In the distal tubule, acid is secreted into urine via α-intercalated cells in the collecting tubule. In the apical side of α-intercalated cells V-ATPase secrets H^+, whereas in the basolateral side anion exchanger 1 (AE1) reabsorbs HCO_3^-. CAII exists in the cytosol of collecting tubule cells and catalyzes the formation of H^+ and HCO_3^- from H_2O and CO_2. Mutations in both V-ATPase and AE1 genes result in dRTA.

Classical dRTA is also called RTA type 1. K^+ secretion is not impaired in this type of dRTA, and the patients usually show hypokalemia. These dRTA patients also have manifestations such as growth retardation, polyuria, hypercalciuria, nephrolithiasis, and sometimes osteomalacia. The magnitude of acidemia is variable, from severe to mild. The case of incomplete dRTA can be diagnosed only after acid load test.

Oral supplementation of alkali, normally taken in the form of citrate sodium/potassium, is quite effective for dRTA [40]. Usually the patients require less amount of alkali than pRTA patients. If the diagnosis of hereditary dRTA is made early in the childhood and the appropriate alkali therapy is done, the patients can avoid the occurrence of symptoms of hereditary dRTA, with normal growth. However, if the patients have hearing disorder due to hereditary dRTA, this cannot be cured [41, 42].

AE1 in Distal Tubule

Anion exchanger 1 (AE1) is expressed in the distal tubule and also in the membrane of erythrocyte. In the distal tubule AE1 is located in the basolateral side of type A (α-) intercalated cells in the connecting tubule, the cortical collecting duct and also medullary collecting duct. dRTA due to AE1 mutations occur in both autosomal dominant and recessive manners. AE1 is encoded by *SLC4A1*, a member of bicarbonate transport family, on chromosome 17q21-22 [43, 44].

AE1 has two main variants, erythrocyte AE1 (eAE1) and kidney AE1 (kAE1). Both variants differ only in the N-terminal region. AE1 is thought to have twelve transmembrane domains, a long N-terminal cytoplasmic domain, and a short C-terminal cytoplasmic domain [45]. In human, eAE1 has a longer N-terminal cytoplasmic domain than kAE1 by 66 amino acids. Figure 2 shows the simplified scheme of eAE1 and kAE1 [43, 44].

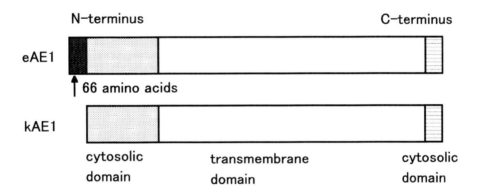

Figure 2. The simplified scheme of eAE1 and kAE1.

The Pathophysiology of AE1-related dRTA

Mutations in AE1 are known to cause dRTA of dominant inheritance. Because AE1 mutants associated with dominant dRTA retain almost normal transport function, two mechanisms have been proposed to explain the apparently dominant-negative effect of AE1 mutations [2, 46].

The first is intracellular retention of the hetero-oligomer AE1 complexes. When expressed in *Xenopus* oocytes, the kAE1 dominant-mutant R589H reached the plasma membrane and showed a moderate activity [47]. In the polarized MDCK cells, however, R589H and another dominant-mutant S613F were retained in the hetero-oligomer complexes with wild-type, preventing the plasma membrane expression of wild-type kAE1 [48]. Consistent with these data obtained from MDCK cells, the renal biopsy samples from the patient carrying the S613F mutation showed a cytoplasmic retention of kAE1 without expression in the basolateral membrane [49].

The second mechanism is mistargeting of the mutant kAE1. Devonald et al. proved that the kAE1 mutant R901X was expressed in the apical membrane in the polarized MDCK cells [50]. Toye et al. also confirmed this finding [51]. The mistargeted AE1 mutant may secrete bicarbonate into urine. The targeting of kAE1 seems to be regulated by the phosphorylation of Y904 in the C-terminal and Y359 in the N-terminal [52].

Recently several mutations of AE1 were found to cause dRTA in an autosomal recessive manner. These mutations are homozygous [53-56] or compound heterozygous [57-64]. The underlying mechanism remains speculative, but the destabilization or lack of plasma membrane expression of kAE1 may be involved.

V-ATPase

The vacuolar-type ATPase (V-ATPase) is a huge multisubunit complex involved in ATP-driven H^+ transport across the plasma membrane, the endoplasmic reticulum, lysosome, endsome, secretary vesicles, and the Golgi apparatus. V-ATPase is ubiquitously expressed in various eukaryotic cells [65, 66]. As these intracellular organelles need to keep pH in optimal range to perform the proper functions, the acidification process by V-ATPase is crucial.

The structure of V-ATPase is complicated, with two large domains, V0 and V1. V0 is located in the cell membrane, while V1 is in the cytoplasm. These domains are connected by "stalk". V0 is consisted of a, c, d, e subunits, whereas V1 is consisted of A to H subunits. There are organ specific subunits. For example, a3 in osteoclasts and a4 in the kidney, B1 in renal intercalated cells, inner ear and epididymis [67-75].

dRTA due to Mutations in Renal Specific v-ATPase Subunits

Karet et al. found that mutations in a renal specific subunit, B1, encoded by *ATP6V1B1*, cause autosomal recessive dRTA with hearing loss [71]. Subsequently, Smith et al. found that mutations in another renal specific a4 subunit, encoded by *ATP6V0A4*, cause autosomal recessive dRTA with preserved hearing [76]. At first mutations in a4 subunit were thought to be unassociated with hearing loss. However, the distinct recessive a4 mutations were later found to cause both dRTA and hearing loss [77]. The reason that why only a subset of a4 mutations causes hearing loss is not clarified.

V-ATPase in Proximal Tubule: Studies in Genetically Modified Mice

A recent study suggested that the loss of V-ATPase function might cause not only dRTA but also proximal tubule dysfunction. a4 deficient mice produced by Hennings et al. showed dRTA as well as proximal tubule dysfunction as evidenced by proteinuria, phosphaturia and lysosomal accumulation of a3 subunit, an original bone-specific isoform of V-ATPase [78]. These mice also showed accumulation of lysosomal materials in the proximal tubule. They re-analyzed the patients with V-ATPase mutations and found that patients with a4 mutations have severer acidosis than those with B1 mutations. However, whether a4 mutations indeed affect proximal tubule functions in human remains unknown.

CAII and RTA

CA catalyzes the formation of H^+ and HCO_3^- from H_2O and CO_2. Fifteen isoforms of CA have been identified up to now. In the kidney CAII, IV, and XII are expressed, among them CAII constitutes about 95% of total kidney CA activities [79, 80]. In the kidney CAII is widely expressed in proximal tubule, thin descending limb, thick ascending limb, intercalated cells of the cortical collecting duct, and inner and outer medullary collecting duct. In the cytoplasm of proximal tubule and intercalated cells it is most abundantly expressed.

Casey and colleagues have proposed that CAII, by forming physical and functional complexes known as transport metabolon, can activate both NBCe1 and AE1 [81, 82]. However, the detailed analyses by Boron and colleagues have not supported the physical and functional interaction between CAII and NBCe1 [83, 84]. We also found that co-expression of CAII does not enhance NBCe1 activity in *Xenopus* oocytes. Furthermore, acetazolamide, a CA inhibitor, failed to inhibit both wild-type and S982NfsX4 NBCe1 in the presence of CAII, speaking against the operation of transport metabolon between CAII and NBCe1 [85].

Mutations of CAII cause a mixed-type RTA (proximal and distal RTA), also called as type 3 RTA. Consanguinity is thought to be the main cause of CAII related RTA, as most of the parents of patients are cousins [86, 87]. The patients usually show the mixed type RTA with insufficient urine acidification, cerebral calcification, osteopetrosis, developmental delay, and sometimes nephrocalcinosis and nephrolithiasis [88-92].

Secondary RTA

In usual clinical practice RTA cases due to secondary factors are much more common. Diabetes mellitus causes RTA type 4 with hyperkalemia. Autoimmune diseases such as Sjögren syndrome, lupus nephritis, rheumatoid arthritis, and primary biliary cirrhosis are associated with RTA. Other diseases, such as multiple myeloma and HIV/AIDS [93] may also cause RTA. Drugs such as analgetics, amiloride, cyclosporine, lithium, pentamidine, antivirals, and trimethoprim may cause RTA.

Sjögren syndrome is frequently associated with dRTA [94], however, only a few cases of pRTA have been reported [95]. Tubulointerstitial nephropathy seems to be the cause of RTA.

Multiple myeloma is known to cause Fanconi syndrome. The association of dRTA is rare but cannot be completely excluded [96].

In diabetes mellitus, aldosterone resistance or deficiency could develop, causing hyperkalemic dRTA. Hypoaldosteronism is thought to induce hyperkalemia and impaired H^+ secretion, resulting in acidosis [97].

Conclusion

We have overviewed on the hereditary and secondary types of RTA. Generally speaking, the RTA cases due to secondary causes are much more common. However, the detailed analyses of the hereditary RTA cases have clarified the mechanisms of acid/base regulation by renal tubules.

The cases of hereditary RTA are frequently associated with multiple extrarenal symptoms, for which the effective treatments are currently not available. Therefore, future studies are still required to develop more effective therapeutic strategies for these complicated diseases.

References

[1]   Haque SK, Ariceta G, Batlle D. Proximal renal tubular acidosis: a not so rare disorder of multiple etiologies. *Nephrol Dial Transplant.* 2012;27(12):4273-87.
[2]   Alper SL. Familial renal tubular acidosis. *J Nephrol.* 2010;23 Suppl 16:S57-76.
[3]   Kondo Y, Fromter E. Axial heterogeneity of sodium-bicarbonate cotransport in proximal straight tubule of rabbit kidney. *Pflugers Arch.* 1987;410(4-5):481-6.
[4]   Boron WF, Boulpaep EL. Intracellular pH regulation in the renal proximal tubule of the salamander. Basolateral HCO_3^- transport. *J Gen Physiol.* 1983;81(1):53-94.
[5]   Yoshitomi K, Burckhardt BC, Fromter E. Rheogenic sodium-bicarbonate cotransport in the peritubular cell membrane of rat renal proximal tubule. *Pflugers Arch.* 1985;405(4):360-6.
[6]   Romero MF, Chen AP, Parker MD, Boron WF. The SLC4 family of bicarbonate (HCO_3^-) transporters. *Mol Aspects Med.* 2013;34(2-3):159-82.
[7]   Monnens L, Levtchenko E. Evaluation of the proximal tubular function in hereditary renal Fanconi syndrome. *Nephrol Dial Transplant.* 2008;23(9):2719-22.
[8]   Romero MF, Hediger MA, Boulpaep EL, Boron WF. Expression cloning and characterization of a renal electrogenic Na^+/HCO_3^- cotransporter. *Nature.* 1997;387(6631):409-13.
[9]   Igarashi T, Ishii T, Watanabe K, Hayakawa H, Horio K, Sone Y, et al. Persistent isolated proximal renal tubular acidosis--a systemic disease with a distinct clinical entity. *Pediatr Nephrol.* 1994;8(1):70-1.
[10]   Igarashi T, Inatomi J, Sekine T, Cha SH, Kanai Y, Kunimi M, et al. Mutations in SLC4A4 cause permanent isolated proximal renal tubular acidosis with ocular abnormalities. *Nat Genet.* 1999;23(3):264-6.
[11]   Suzuki M, Van Paesschen W, Stalmans I, Horita S, Yamada H, Bergmans BA, et al. Defective membrane expression of the $Na^+-HCO_3^-$ cotransporter NBCe1 is associated with familial migraine. *Proc Natl Acad Sci U S A.* 2010;107(36):15963-8.
[12]   Suzuki M, Vaisbich MH, Yamada H, Horita S, Li Y, Sekine T, et al. Functional analysis of a novel missense NBC1 mutation and of other mutations causing proximal renal tubular acidosis. *Pflugers Arch.* 2008;455(4):583-93.
[13]   Horita S, Yamada H, Inatomi J, Moriyama N, Sekine T, Igarashi T, et al. Functional analysis of NBC1 mutants associated with proximal renal tubular acidosis and ocular abnormalities. *J Am Soc Nephrol.* 2005;16(8):2270-8.
[14]   Dinour D, Chang MH, Satoh J, Smith BL, Angle N, Knecht A, et al. A novel missense mutation in the sodium bicarbonate cotransporter (NBCe1/SLC4A4) causes proximal tubular acidosis and glaucoma through ion transport defects. *J Biol Chem.* 2004;279(50):52238-46.

[15] Inatomi J, Horita S, Braverman N, Sekine T, Yamada H, Suzuki Y, et al. Mutational and functional analysis of SLC4A4 in a patient with proximal renal tubular acidosis. *Pflugers Arch.* 2004;448(4):438-44.

[16] Igarashi T, Inatomi J, Sekine T, Seki G, Shimadzu M, Tozawa F, et al. Novel nonsense mutation in the Na^+/HCO_3^- cotransporter gene (SLC4A4) in a patient with permanent isolated proximal renal tubular acidosis and bilateral glaucoma. *J Am Soc Nephrol.* 2001;12(4):713-8.

[17] Yamazaki O, Yamada H, Suzuki M, Horita S, Shirai A, Nakamura M, et al. Identification of dominant negative effect of L522P mutation in the electrogenic Na^+-HCO_3^- cotransporter NBCe1. *Pflugers Arch.* 2013;465(9):1281-91.

[18] Lo YF, Yang SS, Seki G, Yamada H, Horita S, Yamazaki O, et al. Severe metabolic acidosis causes early lethality in NBC1 W516X knock-in mice as a model of human isolated proximal renal tubular acidosis. *Kidney Int.* 2011;79(7):730-41.

[19] Demirci FY, Chang MH, Mah TS, Romero MF, Gorin MB. Proximal renal tubular acidosis and ocular pathology: a novel missense mutation in the gene (SLC4A4) for sodium bicarbonate cotransporter protein (NBCe1). *Mol Vis.* 2006;12:324-30.

[20] Shirakabe K, Priori G, Yamada H, Ando H, Horita S, Fujita T, et al. IRBIT, an inositol 1,4,5-trisphosphate receptor-binding protein, specifically binds to and activates pancreas-type Na^+/HCO_3^- cotransporter 1 (pNBC1). *Proc Natl Acad Sci U S A.* 2006; 103 (25): 9542-7.

[21] Shiohara M, Igarashi T, Mori T, Komiyama A. Genetic and long-term data on a patient with permanent isolated proximal renal tubular acidosis. *Eur J Pediatr.* 2000;159(12):892-4.

[22] Kao L, Sassani P, Azimov R, Pushkin A, Abuladze N, Peti-Peterdi J, et al. Oligomeric structure and minimal functional unit of the electrogenic sodium bicarbonate cotransporter NBCe1-A. *J Biol Chem.* 2008;283(39):26782-94.

[23] Bobulescu IA, Di Sole F, Moe OW. Na^+/H^+ exchangers: physiology and link to hypertension and organ ischemia. *Curr Opin Nephrol Hypertens.* 2005;14(5):485-94.

[24] Bobulescu IA, Moe OW. Luminal Na^+/H^+ exchange in the proximal tubule. *Pflugers Arch.* 2009;458(1):5-21.

[25] Orlowski J, Grinstein S. Emerging roles of alkali cation/proton exchangers in organellar homeostasis. *Curr Opin Cell Biol.* 2007;19(4):483-92.

[26] Slepkov ER, Rainey JK, Sykes BD, Fliegel L. Structural and functional analysis of the Na^+/H^+ exchanger. *Biochem J.* 2007;401(3):623-33.

[27] Wang D, King SM, Quill TA, Doolittle LK, Garbers DL. A new sperm-specific Na^+/H^+ exchanger required for sperm motility and fertility. *Nat Cell Biol.* 2003;5(12):1117-22.

[28] Schultheis PJ, Clarke LL, Meneton P, Miller ML, Soleimani M, Gawenis LR, et al. Renal and intestinal absorptive defects in mice lacking the NHE3 Na^+/H^+ exchanger. *Nat Genet.* 1998;19(3):282-5.

[29] Wang T, Yang CL, Abbiati T, Schultheis PJ, Shull GE, Giebisch G, et al. Mechanism of proximal tubule bicarbonate absorption in NHE3 null mice. *Am J Physiol.* 1999;277(2 Pt 2):F298-302.

[30] Choi JY, Shah M, Lee MG, Schultheis PJ, Shull GE, Muallem S, et al. Novel amiloride-sensitive sodium-dependent proton secretion in the mouse proximal convoluted tubule. *J Clin Invest.* 2000;105(8):1141-6.

[31]   Schultheis PJ, Clarke LL, Meneton P, Harline M, Boivin GP, Stemmermann G, et al. Targeted disruption of the murine Na$^+$/H$^+$ exchanger isoform 2 gene causes reduced viability of gastric parietal cells and loss of net acid secretion. *J Clin Invest.* 1998;101(6):1243-53.

[32]   Baum M, Twombley K, Gattineni J, Joseph C, Wang L, Zhang Q, et al. Proximal tubule Na$^+$/H$^+$ exchanger activity in adult NHE8$^{-/-}$, NHE3$^{-/-}$, and NHE3$^{-/-}$/NHE8$^{-/-}$ mice. *Am J Physiol Renal Physiol.* 2012;303(11):F1495-502.

[33]   Gahl WA, Thoene JG, Schneider JA. Cystinosis. *N Engl J Med.* 2002;347(2):111-21.

[34]   Nesterova G, Gahl WA. Cystinosis: the evolution of a treatable disease. *Pediatr Nephrol.* 2013;28(1):51-9.

[35]   Al-Haggar M. Cystinosis as a lysosomal storage disease with multiple mutant alleles: Phenotypic-genotypic correlations. *World J Nephrol.* 2013;2(4):94-102.

[36]   Schurman SJ, Scheinman SJ. Inherited cerebrorenal syndromes. *Nat Rev Nephrol.* 2009;5(9):529-38.

[37]   Lowe M. Structure and function of the Lowe syndrome protein OCRL1. *Traffic.* 2005;6(9):711-9.

[38]   Ala A, Walker AP, Ashkan K, Dooley JS, Schilsky ML. Wilson's disease. *Lancet.* 2007;369(9559):397-408.

[39]   Magen D, Berger L, Coady MJ, Ilivitzki A, Militianu D, Tieder M, et al. A loss-of-function mutation in NaPi-IIa and renal Fanconi's syndrome. *N Engl J Med.* 2010;362(12):1102-9.

[40]   Domrongkitchaiporn S, Khositseth S, Stitchantrakul W, Tapaneya-olarn W, Radinahamed P. Dosage of potassium citrate in the correction of urinary abnormalities in pediatric distal renal tubular acidosis patients. *Am J Kidney Dis.* 2002;39(2):383-91.

[41]   Fry AC, Karet FE. Inherited renal acidoses. *Physiology (Bethesda).* 2007;22:202-11.

[42]   Bajaj G, Quan A. Renal tubular acidosis and deafness: report of a large family. *Am J Kidney Dis.* 1996;27(6):880-2.

[43]   Alper SL, Darman RB, Chernova MN, Dahl NK. The AE gene family of Cl$^-$/HCO$_3^-$ exchangers. *J Nephrol.* 2002;15 Suppl 5:S41-53.

[44]   Alper SL. Molecular physiology and genetics of Na$^+$-independent SLC4 anion exchangers. *J Exp Biol.* 2009;212(Pt 11):1672-83.

[45]   Zhu Q, Lee DW, Casey JR. Novel topology in C-terminal region of the human plasma membrane anion exchanger, AE1. *J Biol Chem.* 2003;278(5):3112-20.

[46]   Batlle D, Haque SK. Genetic causes and mechanisms of distal renal tubular acidosis. *Nephrol Dial Transplant.* 2012;27(10):3691-704.

[47]   Jarolim P, Shayakul C, Prabakaran D, Jiang L, Stuart-Tilley A, Rubin HL, et al. Autosomal dominant distal renal tubular acidosis is associated in three families with heterozygosity for the R589H mutation in the AE1 (band 3) Cl$^-$/HCO$_3^-$ exchanger. *J Biol Chem.* 1998;273(11):6380-8.

[48]   Cordat E, Kittanakom S, Yenchitsomanus PT, Li J, Du K, Lukacs GL, et al. Dominant and recessive distal renal tubular acidosis mutations of kidney anion exchanger 1 induce distinct trafficking defects in MDCK cells. *Traffic.* 2006;7(2):117-28.

[49]   Walsh S, Turner CM, Toye A, Wagner C, Jaeger P, Laing C, et al. Immunohistochemical comparison of a case of inherited distal renal tubular acidosis (with a unique AE1 mutation) with an acquired case secondary to autoimmune disease. *Nephrol Dial Transplant.* 2007;22(3):807-12.

[50]   Devonald MA, Smith AN, Poon JP, Ihrke G, Karet FE. Non-polarized targeting of AE1 causes autosomal dominant distal renal tubular acidosis. *Nat Genet.* 2003;33(2):125-7.

[51]   Toye AM, Banting G, Tanner MJ. Regions of human kidney anion exchanger 1 (kAE1) required for basolateral targeting of kAE1 in polarised kidney cells: mis-targeting explains dominant renal tubular acidosis (dRTA). *J Cell Sci.* 2004;117(Pt 8):1399-410.

[52]   Williamson RC, Brown AC, Mawby WJ, Toye AM. Human kidney anion exchanger 1 localisation in MDCK cells is controlled by the phosphorylation status of two critical tyrosines. *J Cell Sci.* 2008;121(Pt 20):3422-32.

[53]   Ribeiro ML, Alloisio N, Almeida H, Gomes C, Texier P, Lemos C, et al. Severe hereditary spherocytosis and distal renal tubular acidosis associated with the total absence of band 3. *Blood.* 2000;96(4):1602-4.

[54]   Bruce LJ, Wrong O, Toye AM, Young MT, Ogle G, Ismail Z, et al. Band 3 mutations, renal tubular acidosis and South-East Asian ovalocytosis in Malaysia and Papua New Guinea: loss of up to 95% band 3 transport in red cells. *Biochem J.* 2000;350 Pt 1:41-51.

[55]   Tanphaichitr VS, Sumboonnanonda A, Ideguchi H, Shayakul C, Brugnara C, Takao M, et al. Novel AE1 mutations in recessive distal renal tubular acidosis. Loss-of-function is rescued by glycophorin A. *J Clin Invest.* 1998;102(12):2173-9.

[56]   Yenchitsomanus PT, Sawasdee N, Paemanee A, Keskanokwong T, Vasuvattakul S, Bejrachandra S, et al. Anion exchanger 1 mutations associated with distal renal tubular acidosis in the Thai population. *J Hum Genet.* 2003;48(9):451-6.

[57]   Jamard B, Allard J, Caron P, Corberand JX, Blanchard A, Vargas-Poussou R, et al. Distal renal tubular acidosis and ovalocytosis: a case report. *Osteoporos Int.* 2008;19(1):119-22.

[58]   Wrong O, Bruce LJ, Unwin RJ, Toye AM, Tanner MJ. Band 3 mutations, distal renal tubular acidosis, and Southeast Asian ovalocytosis. *Kidney Int.* 2002;62(1):10-9.

[59]   Chu C, Woods N, Sawasdee N, Guizouarn H, Pellissier B, Borgese F, et al. Band 3 Edmonton I, a novel mutant of the anion exchanger 1 causing spherocytosis and distal renal tubular acidosis. *Biochem J.* 2010;426(3):379-88.

[60]   Chang YH, Shaw CF, Jian SH, Hsieh KH, Chiou YH, Lu PJ. Compound mutations in human anion exchanger 1 are associated with complete distal renal tubular acidosis and hereditary spherocytosis. *Kidney Int.* 2009;76(7):774-83.

[61]   Sritippayawan S, Sumboonnanonda A, Vasuvattakul S, Keskanokwong T, Sawasdee N, Paemanee A, et al. Novel compound heterozygous SLC4A1 mutations in Thai patients with autosomal recessive distal renal tubular acidosis. *Am J Kidney Dis.* 2004;44(1):64-70.

[62]   Toye AM, Williamson RC, Khanfar M, Bader-Meunier B, Cynober T, Thibault M, et al. Band 3 Courcouronnes (Ser667Phe): a trafficking mutant differentially rescued by wild-type band 3 and glycophorin A. *Blood.* 2008;111(11):5380-9.

[63]   Choo KE, Nicoli TK, Bruce LJ, Tanner MJ, Ruiz-Linares A, Wrong OM. Recessive distal renal tubular acidosis in Sarawak caused by AE1 mutations. *Pediatr Nephrol.* 2006;21(2):212-7.

[64]   Kittanakom S, Cordat E, Akkarapatumwong V, Yenchitsomanus PT, Reithmeier RA. Trafficking defects of a novel autosomal recessive distal renal tubular acidosis mutant (S773P) of the human kidney anion exchanger (kAE1). *J Biol Chem.* 2004;279(39):40960-71.

[65]   Wagner CA, Finberg KE, Breton S, Marshansky V, Brown D, Geibel JP. Renal vacuolar H$^+$-ATPase. *Physiol Rev.* 2004;84(4):1263-314.

[66]   Nishi T, Forgac M. The vacuolar H$^+$-ATPases--nature's most versatile proton pumps. *Nat Rev Mol Cell Biol.* 2002;3(2):94-103.

[67]   Peng SB, Crider BP, Xie XS, Stone DK. Alternative mRNA splicing generates tissue-specific isoforms of 116-kDa polypeptide of vacuolar proton pump. *J Biol Chem.* 1994;269(25):17262-6.

[68]   Peng SB, Li X, Crider BP, Zhou Z, Andersen P, Tsai SJ, et al. Identification and reconstitution of an isoform of the 116-kDa subunit of the vacuolar proton translocating ATPase. *J Biol Chem.* 1999;274(4):2549-55.

[69]   Frattini A, Orchard PJ, Sobacchi C, Giliani S, Abinun M, Mattsson JP, et al. Defects in TCIRG1 subunit of the vacuolar proton pump are responsible for a subset of human autosomal recessive osteopetrosis. *Nat Genet.* 2000;25(3):343-6.

[70]   Smith AN, Borthwick KJ, Karet FE. Molecular cloning and characterization of novel tissue-specific isoforms of the human vacuolar H$^+$-ATPase C, G and d subunits, and their evaluation in autosomal recessive distal renal tubular acidosis. *Gene.* 2002;297(1-2):169-77.

[71]   Karet FE, Finberg KE, Nelson RD, Nayir A, Mocan H, Sanjad SA, et al. Mutations in the gene encoding B1 subunit of H$^+$-ATPase cause renal tubular acidosis with sensorineural deafness. *Nat Genet.* 1999;21(1):84-90.

[72]   Nelson RD, Guo XL, Masood K, Brown D, Kalkbrenner M, Gluck S. Selectively amplified expression of an isoform of the vacuolar H$^+$-ATPase 56-kilodalton subunit in renal intercalated cells. *Proc Natl Acad Sci U S A.* 1992;89(8):3541-5.

[73]   van Hille B, Richener H, Schmid P, Puettner I, Green JR, Bilbe G. Heterogeneity of vacuolar H$^+$-ATPase: differential expression of two human subunit B isoforms. *Biochem J.* 1994;303 (Pt 1):191-8.

[74]   Bernasconi P, Rausch T, Struve I, Morgan L, Taiz L. An mRNA from human brain encodes an isoform of the B subunit of the vacuolar H$^+$-ATPase. *J Biol Chem.* 1990;265(29):17428-31.

[75]   Smith AN, Finberg KE, Wagner CA, Lifton RP, Devonald MA, Su Y, et al. Molecular cloning and characterization of Atp6n1b: a novel fourth murine vacuolar H$^+$-ATPase a-subunit gene. *J Biol Chem.* 2001;276(45):42382-8.

[76]   Smith AN, Skaug J, Choate KA, Nayir A, Bakkaloglu A, Ozen S, et al. Mutations in ATP6N1B, encoding a new kidney vacuolar proton pump 116-kD subunit, cause recessive distal renal tubular acidosis with preserved hearing. *Nat Genet.* 2000;26(1):71-5.

[77]   Stover EH, Borthwick KJ, Bavalia C, Eady N, Fritz DM, Rungroj N, et al. Novel ATP6V1B1 and ATP6V0A4 mutations in autosomal recessive distal renal tubular acidosis with new evidence for hearing loss. *J Med Genet.* 2002;39(11):796-803.

[78]   Hennings JC, Picard N, Huebner AK, Stauber T, Maier H, Brown D, et al. A mouse model for distal renal tubular acidosis reveals a previously unrecognized role of the V-ATPase a4 subunit in the proximal tubule. *EMBO Mol Med.* 2012;4(10):1057-71.

[79]   Saari S, Hilvo M, Pan P, Gros G, Hanke N, Waheed A, et al. The most recently discovered carbonic anhydrase, CA XV, is expressed in the thick ascending limb of Henle and in the collecting ducts of mouse kidney. *PLoS One.* 2010;5(3):e9624.

[80] Purkerson JM, Schwartz GJ. The role of carbonic anhydrases in renal physiology. *Kidney Int.* 2007;71(2):103-15.

[81] Cordat E, Casey JR. Bicarbonate transport in cell physiology and disease. *Biochem J.* 2009;417(2):423-39.

[82] McMurtrie HL, Cleary HJ, Alvarez BV, Loiselle FB, Sterling D, Morgan PE, et al. The bicarbonate transport metabolon. *J Enzyme Inhib Med Chem.* 2004;19(3):231-6.

[83] Lu J, Daly CM, Parker MD, Gill HS, Piermarini PM, Pelletier MF, et al. Effect of human carbonic anhydrase II on the activity of the human electrogenic Na/HCO$_3$ cotransporter NBCe1-A in Xenopus oocytes. *J Biol Chem.* 2006;281(28):19241-50.

[84] Piermarini PM, Kim EY, Boron WF. Evidence against a direct interaction between intracellular carbonic anhydrase II and pure C-terminal domains of SLC4 bicarbonate transporters. *J Biol Chem.* 2007;282(2):1409-21.

[85] Yamada H, Horita S, Suzuki M, Fujita T, Seki G. Functional role of a putative carbonic anhydrase II-binding domain in the electrogenic Na$^+$-HCO$_3^-$ cotransporter NBCe1 expressed in Xenopus oocytes. *Channels (Austin).* 2011;5(2):106-9.

[86] Shah GN, Bonapace G, Hu PY, Strisciuglio P, Sly WS. Carbonic anhydrase II deficiency syndrome (osteopetrosis with renal tubular acidosis and brain calcification): novel mutations in CA2 identified by direct sequencing expand the opportunity for genotype-phenotype correlation. *Hum Mutat.* 2004;24(3):272.

[87] Batlle D, Ghanekar H, Jain S, Mitra A. Hereditary distal renal tubular acidosis: new understandings. *Annu Rev Med.* 2001;52:471-84.

[88] Sly WS, Hewett-Emmett D, Whyte MP, Yu YS, Tashian RE. Carbonic anhydrase II deficiency identified as the primary defect in the autosomal recessive syndrome of osteopetrosis with renal tubular acidosis and cerebral calcification. *Proc Natl Acad Sci U S A.* 1983;80(9):2752-6.

[89] Whyte MP, Murphy WA, Fallon MD, Sly WS, Teitelbaum SL, McAlister WH, et al. Osteopetrosis, renal tubular acidosis and basal ganglia calcification in three sisters. *Am J Med.* 1980;69(1):64-74.

[90] Guibaud P, Larbre F, Freycon MT, Genoud J. [Osteopetrosis and renal tubular acidosis. 2 cases of this association in a sibship]. *Arch Fr Pediatr.* 1972;29(3):269-86.

[91] Vainsel M, Fondu P, Cadranel S, Rocmans C, Gepts W. Osteopetrosis associated with proximal and distal tubular acidosis. *Acta Paediatr Scand.* 1972;61(4):429-34.

[92] Ismail EA, Abul Saad S, Sabry MA. Nephrocalcinosis and urolithiasis in carbonic anhydrase II deficiency syndrome. *Eur J Pediatr.* 1997;156(12):957-62.

[93] Isa WY, Daud KM. Distal renal tubular acidosis in HIV/AIDS patient. *Intern Med.* 2011;50(16):1765-8.

[94] Maripuri S, Grande JP, Osborn TG, Fervenza FC, Matteson EL, Donadio JV, et al. Renal involvement in primary Sjögren's syndrome: a clinicopathologic study. *Clin J Am Soc Nephrol.* 2009;4(9):1423-31.

[95] Bridoux F, Kyndt X, Abou-Ayache R, Mougenot B, Baillet S, Bauwens M, et al. Proximal tubular dysfunction in primary Sjögren's syndrome: a clinicopathological study of 2 cases. *Clin Nephrol.* 2004;61(6):434-9.

[96] Hoorn EJ, Zietse R. Combined renal tubular acidosis and diabetes insipidus in hematological disease. *Nat Clin Pract Nephrol.* 2007;3(3):171-5.

[97]   Karet FE. Mechanisms in hyperkalemic renal tubular acidosis. *J Am Soc Nephrol.* 2009;20(2):251-4.

In: Advances in Medicine and Biology. Volume 77
Editor: Leon V. Berhardt

ISBN: 978-1-63117-444-5
© 2014 Nova Science Publishers, Inc.

Chapter 13

The Importance of Regulation of Body Fluid pH in the Development and Progression of Metabolic Diseases

Wataru Aoi[1] and Yoshinori Marunaka[2]

[1]Laboratory of Health Science, Graduate School of Life and Environmental Sciences, Kyoto Prefectural University, Kyoto, Japan
[2]Departments of Molecular Cell Physiology and Bio-Ionomics, Graduate School of Medical Science, Kyoto Prefectural University of Medicine, Kyoto, Japan

Abstract

The pH of body fluids is maintained constant by various internal buffering systems and acid excretion. However, in pathological metabolic conditions such as diabetes, the body fluid pH becomes acidic, mainly due to the elevated levels of production of organic acids, which further advances the disease severity. In addition, drastic changes in the interstitial fluid of the local metabolic tissues are observed even before the clinical onset of disease. It has been suggested that a reduction in the interstitial fluid pH during the early developmental stage of insulin resistance mediates the onset of insulin resistance. On the other hand, intake of several nutrients and exercise therapy can improve lipid metabolism, buffering capacity, and proton clearance in muscle, which may partly explain their preventive and therapeutic effects in metabolic diseases.

Introduction

Regulation of body fluid pH is one of the most important systems for maintenance of physiological functions homeostasis, because activity of most enzymes is dependent on the fluid pH. To avoid disturbance of homeostasis of body fluid pH, it is kept in a fixed state by various buffering systems and acid excretion. However, in metabolically pathological conditions, it changes to acidic mainly due to elevation of organic acids production. A typical example is diabetic ketoacidosis which leads to further advancing in severity of the disease [1, 2]. In the physiological condition, an elevation of lactic acid production in metabolic tissues is also involved in the body fluid acidosis. Physical exercise generates lactic acid in skeletal muscle depending on its intensity; therefore, strenuous exercise accumulates lactic acid in muscle tissues and leads to preventing muscle contraction by transient acidosis [3]. In addition, recent findings suggest that pH would be drastically changed in interstitial fluid of local metabolic tissues even if in pre-disease state [4, 5], which would be closely associated with development of diseases. We here reviewed the involvement of body fluid pH reduction in development and progression of common diseases, and importance of the pH regulation.

The regulation of body fluid pH is one of the most important systems that maintain the physiological homeostasis, considering that an optimal body fluid pH is essential for all enzymatic activity in the living systems. To avoid fluctuations in the body fluid pH, it is maintained constant by various buffering systems and acid excretion mechanisms. However, in metabolically pathological conditions, an increase in the organic acid production leads to a more acidic pH. A typical example is diabetic ketoacidosis, in which, acidic pH leads to the advancement and severity of the disease [1, 2]. Under physiological conditions, elevated lactic acid production in the metabolic tissues leads to body fluid acidosis. Physical exercise, depending on its intensity is known to generate lactic acid in skeletal muscle. Strenuous exercise accumulates lactic acid in the muscle inhibiting its contractility through transient acidosis [3]. In addition, recent findings suggest that drastic changes in pH in the interstitial fluid of local metabolic tissues is observed even before the manifestation of clinical symptoms [4, 5], which is often associated with the development of diseases. Here, we review the involvement of body fluid pH reduction and the importance of pH regulation in the development and progression of common diseases.

The Regulation and Abnormalities in Body Fluid pH

The normal physiological pH of mammalian body fluids (arterial blood) is accurately maintained at 7.40. Abnormal conditions such as acidosis or alkalosis are associated with a change of more than 0.05 units from the normal pH of 7.40. The pH of the body fluids is determined by the content of protons (H^+) generated from the organic acids produced within the living cells. Lactic acid (Lactate$^-$/H^+) is a typical source of proton and is involved in the regulation of physiological pH. In metabolic tissues such as skeletal muscle and adipose tissue, the glycolytic anaerobic metabolism mediates the conversion of glucose and glycogen into lactic acid. Because the pKa of lactic acid is 3.86, it is immediately dissociated into lactate (Lactate$^-$) and protons under physiological conditions, resulting in reduced intracellular pH. In addition, pyruvic acid (Pyruvate$^-$/H^+) converted to lactic acid under anaerobic conditions is also a source of protons but as an intermediate metabolite, although it generates much less protons compared to lactic acid. In addition, materials such as the ketone bodies also behave as sources of protons. Beta-hydroxybutyric acid (beta-hydroxybutyrate$^-$ /H^+), a typical ketone body, is generated as a result of fatty acid metabolism in liver and is also dissociated into beta-hydroxybutyrate anions and protons, leading to the reduction of intracellular pH.

Metabolic acidosis is caused by an imbalance in the rate of proton release and the rate of proton buffering and removal. Several intracellular buffering systems exist to prevent from abnormal pH resulting from excess proton production [6]. One such effective buffering system is the bicarbonate-carbonate system. The bicarbonate system includes two major ionic forms: HCO_3^- and CO_3^{2-}. The HCO_3^- is of primary importance in buffering body fluids because it may be protonated to H_2CO_3 and establishes equilibrium with the dissolved CO_2 and H_2O. The acid/base metabolism in the body is thus regulated by the following equation: $CO_2 + H_2O \leftrightarrows H_2CO_3 \leftrightarrows H^+ + HCO_3^-$. Finally, the CO_2 is exhaled or removed via urine or breathing gas, thus accounting for the removal of a proton equivalent. Another system that mediates pH buffering is the protein-proton bindings. Proteins are composed of amino acids and their functional groups act as weak acids and bases to stabilize the pH within the living bodies. In addition, phosphoric acid acts as a buffering factor by the following equation: $H_2PO_4^- \leftrightarrows H^+ + HPO_4^{2-}$. These intracellular buffering systems maintain the physiological pH (7.40) and protect cellular events.

Protons are also removed from the cytosol via the plasma membrane or mitochondrial membrane transporters. It is known that most of the cellular lactate is consumed through oxidation as a respiratory fuel, while the remainder is converted into glucose and glycogen [7]. Thus, the cytosolic lactate produced in the contracting muscle is transported into the blood and mainly delivered to oxidative tissues through extracellular lactate shuttle [8]. It has been hypothesized that lactate is readily oxidized in the mitochondria, accounting for most of the intracellular lactate shuttles [9]. The lactate transport across the membrane occurs primarily via the H^+-monocarboxylate cotransporters (MCTs) [10, 11]. In most mammalian cells, MCTs participate in the transport of lactate and other monocarboxylic acids such pyruvate, beta-hydroxybutyrate, and acetoacetate across the cellular membrane is responsible for MCTs [12-14]. The MCT carrier system thus functions as a proton symport, facilitating the electroneutral cotransport of protons and monocarboxylate anions. Other transporters such as the Na^+/H^+ exchanger and the bicarbonate-dependent exchanger also contribute to the proton output from the cytosol to the extracellular space [15-17]. These buffering mechanisms thus contribute to the intracellular pH homeostasis.

Abnormal Body Fluid pH in the Development and Progression of Metabolic Diseases

It is well known that the body fluids of diabetes patients is acidic and exhibit characteristic ketoacidosis caused by an increased level of ketone bodies in the blood [1, 2]. Ineffectiveness of insulin action due to insulin resistance in these metabolic tissues accelerates the utilization of lipids as an energy substrate instead of glucose, which in turn accumulates in these conditions, leading to hyperglycemia. Lipolysis leads to increased circulating free fatty acids, the oxidation of which facilitates gluconeogenesis, causing large quantities of ketone bodies (i.e. acetoacetic and β-hydroxybutyric acids), often due to their increased synthesis in liver. This further overloads the normal buffering mechanisms, resulting in metabolic ketoacidosis (pH < 7.35). Thus, metabolic acidosis prevents metabolic enzyme activity such as phosphofructokinase and further accelerates the progression of pathological conditions, accompanied by physical fatigue in these patients [18-20].

The acidosis induced by organic acids could also contribute to the early stages in the development of insulin resistance. Several studies [5, 21, 22] have suggested a close correlation between organic acid production and insulin sensitivity not only in type 2 diabetes patients, but also in healthy subjects. Otsuki et al. [5] have investigated over 1,000 subjects who are not treated for any common diseases, and demonstrated that body weight and waist circumference showed a negative correlation with both insulin sensitivity and urine pH. Maalouf et al. [21] have also reported that subjects with the metabolic syndrome had a significantly lower value of 24-h urine pH compared with the normal subjects and that the mean 24-h urine pH decreased with the increasing number of metabolic syndrome abnormalities. It has been suggested that the presence of lower levels of serum bicarbonate and the higher levels of anion gap resulting from metabolic acidosis are associated with lower insulin sensitivity [23]. Recently, we reported that the interstitial fluid pH in ascites and metabolic tissues in Otsuka Long-Evans Tokushima Fatty (OLETF) rats prior to the development of diabetic symptoms was lower than the normal pH (7.40) [4]. In general, the buffering capacity is relatively high in the cytosol and in the blood, but rather low in the interstitial fluid, owing to the limited availability of the buffering factors such as proteins. Therefore, interstitial fluid pH in metabolic tissues is vulnerable, and undergoes drastically changes defining the onset of insulin resistance development. In this regard, we examined the effects of the extracellular pH on the insulin signaling pathway in the L6 rat skeletal muscle-derived cell line. The phosphorylation status of the insulin receptor and the binding affinity of insulin with insulin receptors were significantly diminished in media with low pH conditions [24]. In addition, the levels of phosphorylated Akt, which is a downstream target of the insulin signaling pathway, was also decreased in low pH media, further reducing the glucose uptake in lower pH conditions. These *in vitro* results support that lower extracellular pH conditions may cause insulin resistance in skeletal muscle cells.

Metabolic syndromes refer to several common metabolic disorders that occur worldwide and include visceral obesity, high blood glucose levels, dyslipidemia, and hypertension. In particular, metabolic syndrome primarily manifests as insulin resistance, which is the causative of type 2 diabetes. In addition, it is well known that insulin resistance plays a critical role in the development of cardiovascular disease and cancer. Therefore, pH abnormalities cause abnormal metabolic regulation in a pre-disease state. We recently found that the interstitial pH around the hippocampus, an important region for memory [25] was lower in diabetic OLETF rats (26 week age) than in normal Wistar rats [26]. It has been reported that diabetic patients have a high risk of developing dementia and alzheimer's disease [27], and may experience defective memory functions. The action of insulin is necessary for neuronal survival within the central nervous system [28, 29]. It has been suggested that fluctuating glucose levels resulting from defective insulin leads to apoptosis and formation of neuritic plaques and neurofibillary tangles, hallmark lesions of Alzheimer's disease, energy starvation, and altered acetylcholine levels in the hippocampus [30, 31]. Therefore, we suggest that maintenance of the interstitial fluid pH at the normal level or the recovery of the interstitial pH to normal levels would be a key factor in developing molecular and cellular therapies for metabolic brain disorders.

Nutritional and Exercise Approaches on Insulin Resistance and pH Regulation

Regulating the pH or the buffering capacity through diet could be a major approach in the prevention and treatment of metabolic diseases. It is well known that adequate diet is important to control pathological conditions in diabetes patients. In addition, intervention studies in humans have reported that several bioactive factors included in foods such as polyphenols [32-34], n-3 unsaturated fatty acids [35, 36], and vitamins [37, 38] improve insulin sensitivity. Additional factors such as carotenoids, alpha lipoic acids, amino acids/peptides, and minerals may also offer preventive or therapeutic effects to combat hyperglycemia and several animal and culture studies have demonstrated their efficacy in improving insulin sensitivity [39-43]. However, the effects of these nutrients, when administered in combination, are beneficial rather than the administration of a particular nutrient alone. Indeed, in contrast to the successful application of combined nutrients or dietary approaches [44-46], several intervention studies using single nutrients have failed to confirm their beneficial effects on insulin resistance and cardiovascular risk [47, 48]. Therefore, it is considered that multiple nutrients are more effective compared with bioactive factors administered alone.

Propolis is a natural product derived from the plant resins collected by honeybees and contains many compounds such as polyphenols, phenolic aldehydes, sequiterpene quinines, coumarins, amino acids, steroids, and inorganic compounds [49]. It is known that propolis possesses anti-microbial, anti-oxidant, anti-inflammation, and anti-tumor properties [50-53]. In addition, some compounds present in propolis might potentially improve insulin sensitivity. Previously, propolis extracts have been reported to attenuate diabetic nephropathy and β-cell damage in animal model experiments [54, 55]. Recently, we reported that propolis improves metabolic defects caused by abnormal blood glucose and insulin in the younger (18 week age) OLETF rats [5]. The rats were characterized by hyperphagia, obesity, decreased glucose infusion rate in a euglycemic clamp at 16-18 weeks of age, and hyperinsulinemia around 25 weeks of age in response to an intravenous glucose infusion and later development of type 2 diabetes [56, 57]. Thus, our observations suggest a beneficial and preventive effect of propolis on diabetes mellitus for use during the early stages of development of insulin resistance. In addition, we found that intake of propolis increased the pH of ascites and metabolic tissues compared with normal diet, suggesting that dietary propolis suppressed the production of organic acids or elevated buffering capacity in those tissues. Therefore, propolis may improve insulin sensitivity by preventing metabolic acidosis.

Habitual exercise regimen is another major life-style option for reducing the risk of metabolic disease. Many large cohort studies have found that higher level of physical activity is associated with reduced risk of developing diabetes and cardiovascular disease (CVD) [58–60]. Accumulating evidence obtained from *in vitro* and *in vivo* studies has demonstrated that a single bout of exercise generally improves glucose uptake in skeletal muscles through insulin-dependent and insulin-independent signal transduction mechanisms [61, 62]. Insulin sensitivity in skeletal muscle in resting state is adaptively improved by habitual exercise, which facilitates the translocation of the glucose transporter 4 (GLUT4) to the plasma membrane, thereby elevating glucose uptake. In addition to several mechanical and chemical stimulations induced by exercise, it may mediate the maintenance of body fluid pH and offer preventive and therapeutic effects in the management of metabolic diseases.

The maintenance of pH through exercise is achieved partly through the acceleration of lipid utilization with improved aerobic metabolism. Habitual exercise adaptively accelerates the entry of fatty acids from the plasma into the muscle cell, from the cytosol into the mitochondria, and enhances the Krebs cycle function in the resting state, all of which is caused by elevating the expression and activity of related enzymes in the skeletal muscle [63-66]. In particular, regular exercise accelerates lipid utilization and increases the peroxisome proliferator-activated receptor gamma coactivator-1 alpha, which plays an important role in the improvement of the metabolic rate through mitochondrial biogenesis and elevation of aerobic enzyme expression [67, 68]. Since the energy consumed in muscle during exercise is mainly supplied by carbohydrates and lipids, the exercise-induced lipid utilization may decrease the energy obtained from carbohydrates, further decreasing the lactate/proton production, referred to as lactic acidosis. In addition, intramuscular and circulating buffering capacities are improved by habitual exercise due to an increase in the buffering factors such as proteins, amino acids, and phosphate [69-71]. As a physiological adaptation to exercise, peripheral circulation is improved through vasodilation [72], which further facilitates the proton wash-out. Further evidence suggests that excretion of protons from the cytosol to extracellular space or circulation via transporters located on plasma membrane contributes to the prevention of intracellular acidosis. It has been shown that the expression of two MCT isoforms (MCT1 and MCT4) is associated with the lactate disposal in muscle [10]. High levels of MCT1 are located in both the sarcolemmal and the mitochondrial membranes of the oxidative muscle [9, 11, 73]; on the other hand MCT4 is predominantly located on the plasma membranes of the glycolytic muscle and is assumed to contribute to the lactate efflux [73]. It has reported that exercise training increases the MCT levels in the skeletal muscle and the heart of humans and rats [74-76]. Although the regulation of MCT levels is not clearly understood, these findings indicate that exercise mediated increase in lactate movement across the membrane may induce the upregulation of MCT protein synthesis as an adaptation mechanism. Lactic acid must be transported into or out of skeletal muscle to maintain pH homeostasis and the lactate concentration gradient. In addition, we reported that MCT1 content in the erythrocyte membranes is increased by exercise training in rats [77, 78]. A proportion of the lactate released from the skeletal muscle into the plasma is taken up by the erythrocytes. The mature erythrocytes generate ATP only through the glycolytic pathway because they lack the mitochondrial machinery. Therefore, erythrocytes cannot metabolize lactate produced as a respiratory fuel and this necessitates the release of lactate into the plasma via MCT1 [79]. However, one of the most important role for erythrocytes is to take up and distribute the monocarboxylates released from other tissues, since the erythrocytes produce much less lactate than the other tissues. Indeed, the skeletal muscle may be entirely dependent on the MCT1-mediated lactate-uptake by the erythrocytes, to regulate pH homeostasis, on the basis of our *in vitro* study [78]. Also, there is a high correlation between the athletic performance in horse and the erythrocyte lactate concentration after the trotters race [80]. Therefore, efficient proton transport via MCTs induced by habitual exercise may contribute to the improvement of insulin sensitivity and muscle fatigue caused by pH reduction.

Conclusion

The interstitial fluid pH could be easily reduced by acid stress even when the intracellular and blood pH remain normal (Figure 1). Such an acidic environment disturbs homeostasis of the intracellular circumstance, leading to the onset and development of metabolic diseases. Thus, it is important to maintain the interstitial fluid pH for prevention of metabolic disease. In addition, the pH value of interstitial fluid may be used as a biomarker to reflect the developmental state of the metabolic disease. However, detailed mechanisms responsible for the reduction of interstitial fluid pH are unknown, although the roles of several possible factors including the excessive production of acids, reduction of buffering factors and transmembrane output, and respiratory and urinary excretion have been speculated. Therefore, further studies are required to examine both the detailed mechanisms and the physiological relevance of altered body fluid pH, along with possibility of usage of interstitial pH as a biomarker for disease diagnosis.

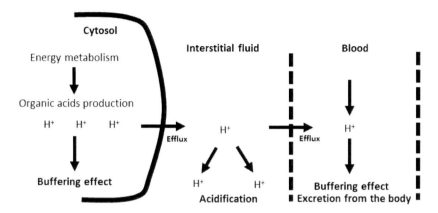

Figure 1. Regulation of pH in intracellular and extracellular body fluid. Body fluid pH is kept in a fixed state by various buffering systems and acid excretion. The buffering capacity is relatively high in the cytosol and in the blood, but rather low in the interstitial fluid, owing to the limited availability of the buffering factors such as proteins. Consequently, the interstitial fluid pH could be easily reduced by acid stress.

Acknowledgments

This work was supported by Grants-in-Aid from Japan Society of the Promotion of Science (25282199, 25670111), Salt Science Foundation (1235) and Cell Research Conference.

References

[1]   Felig, P. (1974). Diabetic ketoacidosis. *N. Engl. J. Med.*, 290, 1360-1363.
[2]   Reaven, G. M. and Olefsky, J. M. (1978). The role of insulin resistance in the pathogenesis of diabetes mellitus. *Adv. Metab. Disord.*, 9, 313-331.

[3]   McKenna, M. J. (1992). The roles of ionic processes in muscular fatigue during intense exercise. *Sports Med.*, 13, 134-145.

[4]   Aoi, W., Hosogi, S., Niisato, N., Yokoyama, N., Hayata, H., Miyazaki, H., Kusuzaki, K., Fukuda, T., Fukui, M., Nakamura, N., and Marunaka, Y. (2013). Improvement of insulin resistance, blood pressure and interstitial pH in early developmental stage of insulin resistance in OLETF rats by intake of propolis extracts. *Biochem. Biophys. Res. Commun.*, 432, 650-653.

[5]   Otsuki, M., Kitamura, T., Goya, K., Saito, H., Mukai, M., Kasayama, S., Shimomura, I., and Koga, M. (2011). Association of urine acidification with visceral obesity and the metabolic syndrome. *Endocr. J.*, 58, 363-367.

[6]   Heinemann, H. O. and Goldring, R. M. (1974). Bicarbonate and the regulation of ventilation. *Am. J. Med.*, 57, 361-370.

[7]   Brooks, G. A. (1986). The lactate shuttle during exercise and recovery. *Med. Sci. Sports Exerc.*, 18: 360-368.

[8]   Brooks, G. A. (1991). Current concepts in lactate exchange. *Med. Sci. Sports Exerc.*, 23, 895-906.

[9]   Brooks, G. A., Dubouchaud, H., Brown, M., Sicurello, J. P., and Butz, C. E. (1999). Role of mitochondrial lactate dehydrogenase and lactate oxidation in the intracellular lactate shuttle. *Proc. Natl. Acad. Sci. USA*, 96, 1129-1134.

[10] Bonen, A. (2000) Lactate transporters (MCT proteins) in heart and skeletal muscles. *Med. Sci. Sports Exerc.*, 32, 778-789.

[11] Juel, C. (1997). Lactate-Proton cotransport in skeletal muscle. *Physiol. Rev.*, 77, 321-358.

[12] Garcia, C. K., Goldstein, J. L., Pathak, R. K., Anderson, R. G., and Brown, M. S. (1994). Molecular characterization of a membrane transporter for lactate, pyruvate, and other monocarboxylates: implications for the Cori cycle. *Cell*, 76, 865-873.

[13] Xu, A. S. and Kuchel, P. W. (1993). Characterisation of erythrocyte transmembrane exchange of trifluoroacetate using 19F-NMR: evidence for transport via the monocarboxylate transporter. *Biochim. Biophys. Acta.*, 1150, 35-44.

[14] Robert, C. P. and Andrew, P. H. (1993). Transport of lactate and other monocarboxylates across mammalian plasma membranes. *Am. J. Physiol.*, 264, C761-C782.

[15] Ward, C. A. and Moffat, M. P. (1995). Modulation of sodium-hydrogen exchange activity in cardiac myocytes during acidosis and realkalinisation: effects on calcium, pHi, and cell shortening. *Cardiovasc. Res.*, 29, 247-253.

[16] Park, C. O., Xiao, X. H., and Allen, D.G. (1999). Changes in intracellular Na^+ and pH in rat heart during ischemia: role of Na^+/H^+ exchanger. *Am. J. Physiol.*, 276, H15-H90.

[17] Loh, S. H., Chen, W. H., Chiang, C. H., Tsai, C. S., Lee, G. C., Jin, J. S., Cheng, T. H., and Chen, J. J. (2002). Intracellular pH regulatory mechanism in human atrial myocardium: functional evidence for Na(+)/H(+) exchanger and Na(+)/HCO(3)(-) symporter. *J. Biomed. Sci.*, 9, 198-205.

[18] Sumi, S., Mineo, I., Kono, N., Shimizu, T., Nonaka, K., and Tarui, S. (1984). Decreases in hepatic fructose-2,6-bisphosphate level and fructose-6-phosphate, 2-kinase activity in diabetic mice: a close relationship to the development of ketosis. *Biochem. Biophys. Res. Commun.*, 120, 103-108.

[19] Lemieux, G., Aranda, M. R., Fournel, P., and Lemieux, C. (1984). Renal enzymes during experimental diabetes mellitus in the rat. Role of insulin, carbohydrate metabolism, and ketoacidosis. *Can. J. Physiol. Pharmacol.*, 62, 70-75.

[20] Gil, J., Carreras, J., and Bartrons, R. (1986). Effects of diabetes on fructose 2, 6-P2, glucose 1, 6-P2 and 6-phosphofructo 2-kinase in rat liver. *Biochem. Biophys. Res. Commun.*, 136, 498-503.

[21] Maalouf, N. M., Cameron, M. A., Moe, O. W., Adams-Huet, B., and Sakhaee, K. (2007). Low urine pH: a novel feature of the metabolic syndrome. *Clin. J. Am. Soc. Nephrol.*, 2, 883-888.

[22] Maalouf, N. M., Cameron, M. A., Moe, O. W., and Sakhaee, K. (2010). Metabolic basis for low urine pH in type 2 diabetes. *Clin. J. Am. Soc. Nephrol.*, 5, 1277-1281.

[23] Farwell, W. R. and Taylor E. N. (2008). Serum bicarbonate, anion gap and insulin resistance in the National Health and Nutrition Examination Survey. *Diabet. Med.*, 25, 798-804.

[24] Hayata, H., Miyazaki, H., Niisato, N., Yokoyama, N., and Marunaka, Y. (2013). Involvement of the extracellular pH in skeletal muscle insulin resistance. *J. Physiol. Sci.*, 63, S199.

[25] Packard, M. G. and Goodman, J. (2013). Factors that influence the relative use of multiple memory systems. *Hippocampus,* in press.

[26] Marunaka, Y., Yoshimoto, K., Aoi, W., Hosogi, S., and Ikegawa, Y. (2013). Low pH of interstitial fluid around hippocampus of the brain in diabetic OLETF rats. *Mol. Cell. Therap.* in press.

[27] Mirza, Z., Kamal, M. A., Abuzenadah, A. M., Al-Qahtani, M. H., and Karim, S. (2013). Establishing Genomic/Transcriptomic Links between Alzheimer's Disease and Type II Diabetes Mellitus by Meta-Analysis Approach. *CNS Neurol. Disord. Drug Targets,* in press.

[28] Dudek, H., Datta, S. R., Franke, T. F., Birnbaum, M. J., Yao, R., Cooper, G. M., Segal, R. A., Kaplan, D. R, and Greenberg, M. E. (1997) Regulation of neuronal survival by the serine-threonine protein kinase Akt. *Science*, 275, 661-665.

[29] Recio-Pinto, E., Rechler, M. M., and Ishii, D. N. (1986). Effects of insulin, insulin-like growth factor-II, and nerve growth factor on neurite formation and survival in cultured sympathetic and sensory neurons. *J. Neurosci.*, 6, 1211-1219.

[30] Rasgon, N. and Jarvik, L. (2004). Insulin resistance, affective disorders, and Alzheimer's disease: review and hypothesis. *J. Gerontol. A Biol. Sci. Med. Sci.*, 59, 178-183.

[31] Steen, E., Terry, B. M., Rivera, E. J., Cannon, J. L., Neely, T. R., Tavares, R., Xu, X. J., Wands, J. R., and de la Monte, S. M. (2005). Impaired insulin and insulin-like growth factor expression and signaling mechanisms in Alzheimer's disease--is this type 3 diabetes? *J. Alzheimers Dis.*, 7, 63-80.

[32] Nagao, T., Meguro, S., Hase, T., Otsuka, K., Komikado, M., Tokimitsu, I., Yamamoto, T., and Yamamoto, K. (2009). A catechin-rich beverage improves obesity and blood glucose control in patients with type 2 diabetes. *Obesity (Silver Spring)*, 17, 310-317.

[33] Llaneza, P., González, C., Fernández-Iñarrea, J., Alonso, A., Díaz, F., and Pérez-López, F. R. (2012) Soy isoflavones improve insulin sensitivity without changing serum leptin among postmenopausal women. *Climacteric.*, 15, 611-620.

[34] Squadrito, F., Marini, H., Bitto, A., Altavilla, D., Polito, F., Adamo, E. B., D'Anna, R., Arcoraci, V., Burnett, B. P., Minutoli, L., Di Benedetto, A., Di Vieste, G., Cucinotta, D., de Gregorio, C., Russo, S., Corrado, F., Saitta, A., Irace, C., Corrao, S., and Licata, G. (2013). Genistein in the metabolic syndrome: results of a randomized clinical trial. *J. Clin. Endocrinol. Metab.*, 98, 3366-3374.

[35] Ramel, A., Martinéz, A., Kiely, M., Morais, G., Bandarra, N. M., and Thorsdottir, I. (2008). Beneficial effects of long-chain n-3 fatty acids included in an energy-restricted diet on insulin resistance in overweight and obese European young adults. *Diabetologia*, 51, 1261-1268.

[36] Vessby, B., Uusitupa, M., Hermansen, K., Riccardi, G., Rivellese, A. A., Tapsell, L. C., Nälsén, C., Berglund, L., Louheranta, A., Rasmussen, B. M., Calvert, G. D., Maffetone, A., Pedersen, E., Gustafsson, I. B., Storlien, L. H.; KANWU Study. (2001). Substituting dietary saturated for monounsaturated fat impairs insulin sensitivity in healthy men and women: The KANWU Study. *Diabetologia*, 44, 312-319.

[37] Yoshida, M., Jacques, P. F., Meigs, J. B., Saltzman, E., Shea, M. K., Gundberg, C., Dawson-Hughes, B., Dallal, G., and Booth, S. L. (2008). Effect of vitamin K supplementation on insulin resistance in older men and women. *Diabetes Care*, 31, 2092-2096.

[38] Asemi, Z., Samimi, M., Tabassi, Z., Shakeri, H., and Esmaillzadeh, A. (2013). Vitamin D supplementation affects serum high-sensitivity C-reactive protein, insulin resistance, and biomarkers of oxidative stress in pregnant women. *J. Nutr.*, 143, 1432-1438.

[39] Bhuvaneswari, S. and Anuradha, C. V. (2012). Astaxanthin prevents loss of insulin signaling and improves glucose metabolism in liver of insulin resistant mice. *Can. J. Physiol. Pharmacol.*, 90, 1544-1552.

[40] Takikawa, M., Inoue, S., Horio, F., and Tsuda, T. (2010). Dietary anthocyanin-rich bilberry extract ameliorates hyperglycemia and insulin sensitivity via activation of AMP-activated protein kinase in diabetic mice. *J. Nutr.*, 140, 527-533.

[41] Greene, E. L., Nelson, B. A., Robinson, K. A., and Buse, M. G. (2001). alpha-Lipoic acid prevents the development of glucose-induced insulin resistance in 3T3-L1 adipocytes and accelerates the decline in immunoreactive insulin during cell incubation. *Metabolism*, 50, 1063-1069.

[42] Lee, H. S., Lee, H. J., and Suh, H. J. (2011). Silk protein hydrolysate increases glucose uptake through up-regulation of GLUT 4 and reduces the expression of leptin in 3T3-L1 fibroblast. *Nutr. Res.*, 31, 937-943.

[43] Wang, Y. Q. and Yao, M. H. (2009). Effects of chromium picolinate on glucose uptake in insulin-resistant 3T3-L1 adipocytes involve activation of p38 MAPK. *J. Nutr. Biochem.*, 20, 982-991.

[44] Lindström, J., Ilanne-Parikka, P., Peltonen, M., Aunola, S., Eriksson, J. G., Hemiö, K., Hämäläinen, H., Härkönen, P., Keinänen-Kiukaanniemi, S., Laakso, M., Louheranta, A., Mannelin, M., Paturi, M., Sundvall, J., Valle, T. T., Uusitupa, M., Tuomilehto, J.; Finnish Diabetes Prevention Study Group. (2006). Sustained reduction in the incidence of type 2 diabetes by lifestyle intervention: follow-up of the Finnish Diabetes Prevention Study. *Lancet*, 368, 1673-1679.

[45] Plantinga, Y., Ghiadoni, L., Magagna, A., Giannarelli, C., Franzoni, F., Taddei, S., and Salvetti, A. (2007). Supplementation with vitamins C and E improves arterial stiffness

and endothelial function in essential hypertensive patients. *Am. J. Hypertens.*, 20, 392-397.

[46] Zureik, M., Galan, P., Bertrais, S., Mennen, L., Czernichow, S., Blacher, J., Ducimetiere, P., and Hercberg, S. (2004). Effects of long-term daily low-dose supplementation with antioxidant vitamins and minerals on structure and function of large arteries. *Arterioscler. Thromb. Vasc. Biol.*, 24, 1485-1491.

[47] Eskurza, I., Monahan, K. D., Robinson, J. A., and Seals, D. R. (2004). Ascorbic acid does not affect large elastic artery compliance or central blood pressure in young and older men. *Am. J. Physiol. Heart Circ. Physiol.*, 286, H1528-H1534.

[48] Woods, M. N., Wanke, C. A., Ling, P. R., Hendricks, K. M., Tang, A. M., Knox, T. A., Andersson, C. E., Dong, K. R., Skinner, S. C., and Bistrian, B. R. (2009). Effect of a dietary intervention and n-3 fatty acid supplementation on measures of serum lipid and insulin sensitivity in persons with HIV. *Am. J. Clin. Nutr.*, 90, 1566-1578.

[49] Khalil, M. L. (2006). Biological activity of bee propolis in health and disease. *Asian Pac. J. Cancer Prev.*, 7, 22-31.

[50] Aga, H., Shibuya, T., Sugimoto, T., Kurimoto, M., and Nakajima, S. (1994). Isolation and identification of antimicrobial compounds in Brazilian Propolis. *Biosci. Biotech. Biochem.*, 58, 945-946.

[51] Krol, W., Czuba, Z., Scheller, S., Gabrys, J., Grabiec, S., and Shani, J. (1990). Antioxidant property of ethanolic extract of propolis (EEP) as evaluated by inhibiting the chemiluminescence oxidation of luminol. *Biochem. Int.*, 21, 593-597.

[52] Song, Y. S., Park, E. H., Jung, K.J., and Jin, C. (2002). Inhibition of angiogenesis by propolis. *Arch. Pharm. Res.*, 25, 500-504.

[53] Kimoto, T., Arai, S., Kohguchi, M., Aga, M., Nomura, Y., Micallef, M. J., Kurimoto, M., and Mito, K. (1998). Apoptosis and suppression of tumor growth by artepillin C extracted from Brazilian propolis. *Cancer Detect. Prev.*, 22, 506-515.

[54] Abo-Salem, O. M., El-Edel, R. H., Harisa, G. E., El-Halawany, N., and Ghonaim, M. M. (2009). Experimental diabetic nephropathy can be prevented by propolis: Effect on metabolic disturbances and renal oxidative parameters. *Pak. J. Pharm. Sci.*, 22, 205-210.

[55] Matsushige K., Basnet P., Hase K., Kadota S., Tanaka K., Namba T. (1996). Propolis protects pancreatic β-cells against the toxicity of streptozotocin (STZ). *Phytomedicine*, 3, 203-209.

[56] Yagi, K., Kim, S., Wanibuchi, H., Yamashita, T., Yamamura, Y., and Iwao, H. (1997). Characteristics of diabetes, blood pressure, and cardiac and renal complications in Otsuka Long-Evans Tokushima Fatty rats. *Hypertension*, 29, 728-735.

[57] Kawano K., Hirashima T., Mori S., and Natori T. (1994). OLETF (Otsuka Long-Evans Tokushima Fatty) rat: a new NIDDM rat strain. *Diabetes Res. Clin. Pract.*, 24, S317-S320.

[58] Hu, F.B., Leitzmann, M.F., Stampfer, M.J., Colditz, G.A., Willett, W.C., and Rimm, E. B. (2001). Physical activity and television watching in relation to risk for type 2 diabetes mellitus in men. *Arch. Intern. Med.*, 161, 1542-1548.

[59] Hu, F. B., Manson, J. E., Stampfer, M. J., Colditz, G., Liu, S., Solomon, C. G., Willett, W. C. (2001). Diet, lifestyle, and the risk of type 2 diabetes mellitus in women. *N. Engl. J. Med.*, 345, 790-797.

[60] Hu, F. B., Sigal, R. J., Rich-Edwards, J. W., Colditz, G. A., Solomon, C. G., Willett, W. C., Speizer, F. E., and Manson, J. E. (1999). Walking compared with vigorous physical activity and risk of type 2 diabetes in women: a prospective study. *JAMA*, 282, 1433-1439.

[61] Aoi, W., Naito, Y., and Yoshikawa, T. (2011). Dietary exercise as a novel strategy for the prevention and treatment of metabolic syndrome: effects on skeletal muscle function. *J. Nutr. Metab.*, 2011:676208.

[62] Röckl, K. S., Witczak, C. A., and Goodyear, L. J. (2008). Signaling mechanisms in skeletal muscle: acute responses and chronic adaptations to exercise. *IUBMB Life*, 60, 145-153.

[63] Holloway, G. P., Bezaire, V., Heigenhauser, G. J., Tandon, N. N., Glatz, J. F., Luiken, J. J., Bonen, A., and Spriet, L. L. (2006). Mitochondrial long chain fatty acid oxidation, fatty acid translocase/CD36 content and carnitine palmitoyltransferase I activity in human skeletal muscle during aerobic exercise. *J. Physiol.*, 571, 201-210.

[64] Wibom, R., Hultman, E., Johansson, M., Matherei, K., Constantin-Teodosiu, D., and Schantz, P. G. (1992). Adaptation of mitochondrial ATP production in human skeletal muscle to endurance training and detraining. *J. Appl. Physiol. (1985).*, 73, 2004-2010.

[65] Bradley, N. S., Snook, L. A., Jain, S. S., Heigenhauser, G. J., Bonen, A., and Spriet, L. L. (2012). Acute endurance exercise increases plasma membrane fatty acid transport proteins in rat and human skeletal muscle. *Am. J. Physiol. Endocrinol. Metab.*, 302, E183-E189.

[66] Greiwe, J. S., Holloszy, J. O., and Semenkovich, C. F. (2000). Exercise induces lipoprotein lipase and GLUT-4 protein in muscle independent of adrenergic-receptor signaling. *J. Appl. Physiol.(1985)*, 89, 176-181.

[67] Russell, A.P., Feilchenfeldt, J., Schreiber, S., Praz, M., Crettenand, A., Gobelet, C., Meier, C.A., Bell, D.R., Kralli, A., Giacobino, J.P., and Dériaz, O. (2003). Endurance training in humans leads to fiber type-specific increases in levels of peroxisome proliferator-activated receptor-α coactivator-1 and peroxisome proliferator-activated receptor- α in skeletal muscle. *Diabetes,* 52, 2874-2881.

[68] Baar, K. (2004). Involvement of PPAR gamma co-activator-1, nuclear respiratory factors 1 and 2, and PPAR alpha in the adaptive response to endurance exercise. *Proc. Nutr. Soc.*, 63, 269-273.

[69] Susuki, Y., Ito, O., Takahashi, H., and Takamatsu, K. (2004). The effect of sprint training on skeletal muscle carnosine in humans. Int. J. Sport. Health. Sci. 2, 105-110.

[70] Parkhouse, W. S., McKenzie, D. C., Hochachka, P. W., and Ovalle, W. K. (1985). Buffering capacity of deproteinized human vastus lateralis muscle. *J. Appl. Physiol. (1985)*, 58, 14-17.

[71] Arthur, P. G., Hogan, M. C., Bebout, D. E., Wagner, P. D., and Hochachka, P. W. (1992). Modeling the effects of hypoxia on ATP turnover in exercising muscle. *J. Appl. Physiol. (1985)*, 73, 737-742.

[72] DeSouza, C. A., Shapiro, L. F, Clevenger, C. M., Dinenno, F. A., Monahan, K. D., Tanaka, H., and Seals, D. R. (2000). Regular aerobic exercise prevents and restores age-related declines in endothelium-dependent vasodilation in healthy men. *Circulation*, 102, 1351-1357.

[73] Bonen, A. (2001). The expression of lactate transporters (MCT1 and MCT4) in heart and muscle. *Eur. J. Appl. Physiol.*, 86, 6-11.

[74] Dubouchaud, H., Butterfield, G. E., Wolfel, E. E., Bergman, B. C., and Brooks, G. A. (2000). Endurance training, expression, and physiology of LDH, MCT1, and MCT4 in human skeletal muscle. *Am. J. Physiol. Endocrinol. Metab.*, 278, E571-E579.

[75] Baker, S. K., McCullagh, K. J. A., and Bonen, A. (1998). Training intensity-independent and tissue-specific increases in lactate uptake and MCT-1 in heart and muscle. *J. Appl. Physiol.*, 84, 987-994.

[76] Bonen, A., McCullagh, K. J. A., Putman, C. T., Hultman, E., Jones, N. L., and Heingenhauser, G. J. F. (1998). Short-term training increases human muscle MCT1 and femoral venous lactate in relation to muscle lactate. *Am. J. Physiol.*, 274, E102-E107.

[77] Aoi, W., Tsuzuki, M., Fujie, M., Iwashita, S., and Suzuki, M. (2002). Sustained voluntary climbing exercise increases erythrocytes MCT1 in rats. *J. Clin. Biochem. Nutr.*, 32, 23-29.

[78] Aoi, W., Iwashita, S., Fujie, M., and Suzuki, M. (2004). Sustained swimming increases erythrocyte MCT1 during erythropoiesis and ability to regulate pH homeostasis in rat. *Int. J. Sports Med.*, 25, 339-344.

[79] Skeleton, M. S., Kremer, D. E., Smith, E. W., and Gladden, L. B. (1998). Lactate influx into red blood cells from trained and untrained human subjects. *Med. Sci. Sports Exerc.*, 30, 536-342.

[80] Rassanan, L. A., Lampinen, K. J., and Poso, A. R. (1995). Responses of blood and plasma lactate and purine concentrations to maximal exercise and their relation to performance in Standardbred trotters. *Am. J. Vet. Res.*, 56, 1651-1656.

In: Advances in Medicine and Biology. Volume 77
Editor: Leon V. Berhardt

ISBN: 978-1-63117-444-5
© 2014 Nova Science Publishers, Inc.

Chapter 14

Lactic Acidosis in HIV-Infected Patients: Causes, Treatment and Prevention

Gordana Dragovic, M.D., PhD[1],*, Jovana Kusic, M.D.[1],
Danijela Sekulic, M.D.[2] and Djordje Jevtovic, M.D., PhD[2]

[1]Department of Pharmacology, Clinical Pharmacology and Toxicology, School of
Medicine, University of Belgrade, Belgrade, Serbia
[2]HIV Center of Infectious and Tropical Diseases Hospital, School of Medicine,
University of Belgrade, Belgrade, Serbia

Abstract

Lactic acidosis is the most serious, sometimes life-threatening, adverse effect of nucleoside reverse transcriptase inhibitor (NRTI) usage in HIV infected patients. The reported incidence rate of lactic acidosis due to an NRTI based regimen is low, but the fatality rate is estimated at around 60 - 80% in those HIV-infected patients who develop lactic acidosis during NRTI usage. The mechanism of NRTI induced lactic acidosis is based on inhibition of mitochondrial DNA polymerase - γ and consequent mitochondrial depletion and deficit in the respiratory chain function.

All NRTIs may interact with polymerase – γ, but dideoxynucleosides, such as stavudine (d4T), zalcitabine (ddC) and didanosine (ddI), also known as d-drugs, are the most potent. In resource limited settings, where d-drugs still remain the first line treatment option, the highest incidence of NRTI-induced lactic acidosis is due to stavudine (d4T), followed by didanosine (ddI) usage. Lactic acidosis developed even more frequently when stavudine and didanosine were prescribed together.

Zidovudine (AZT) could potentially induce lactic acidosis, while significant events are not reported with other NRTI drugs, such as lamivudine, abacavir and tenofovir. Risk factors associated with lactic acidosis are female sex, advanced HIV-1 induced

---

* Correspondence: Department of Pharmacology, Clinical Pharmacology and Toxicology, School of Medicine, University of Belgrade, Dr Subotica 1, 11129 Belgrade, Serbia; phone: + 381 65 27 21 180; fax: +381 11 36 43 397; e-mail: gozza@beotel.net.

immunodeficiency, obesity and prolonged duration of NRTI-based antiretroviral treatment. Renal and liver abnormalities, especially hepatitis B and hepatitis C virus co-infection, are associated with a higher incidence of lactic acidosis. Lactic acidosis induced with NRTI usage is treated by NRTI withdrawal, especially in life-threatening clinical conditions with serum lactate level of 5 mmol/L and higher. Within several days the outcome is favourable in most cases. Recovery is complete, especially when no other d-drug is re-administered.

Even though current HIV/AIDS treatment guidelines discourage the usage of d-drugs, national HIV treatment guidelines from low-middle income countries are still unable to abandon these drugs. Thus, NRTI-associated lactic acidosis is still issue of concern in the resource limited settings.

Keywords: Lactic acidosis, nucleoside reverse transciptase inhibitors, antiretroviral therapy, risk factors

1. Introduction

As we step into the third decade of antiretroviral therapy usage, the survival rate of patients with human immunodeficiency virus (HIV) infection and acquired immune deficiency syndrome (AIDS) has been improved increasingly [1]. However, adverse effects of a combination antiretroviral therapy (cART) are becoming more often recognized as a reason for treatment discontinuation [2, 3].

Thus, numerous efforts have been made in order to anticipate, treat or prevent drug related adverse effects and therefore improve expectancy and quality of life in HIV infected patients while on cART. It still remains essential to prevent life-threatening adverse effect [2, 4, 5].

European AIDS Clinical Society (EACS), as well as International AIDS Society-USA panel and the British HIV Association guidelines for HIV together with World Health Organisation (WHO) guidelines have been suggesting the usage of nucleoside reverse transcriptase inhibitors (NRTIs) as a backbone within the first-line antiretroviral therapy [6 – 9]. Despite the initial positive impact of NRTI-based regimen, severe adverse effects have been associated with their use. Lactic acidosis is rare, but most severe and sometimes fatal adverse effect that may occur during the NRTI usage [10, 11]. In this chapter we will focus exclusively on lactic acidosis in HIV-infected patients, its causes, treatment and prevention.

2. Aetiology of Lactic Acidosis

Lactic acidosis is defined as a physiological condition characterized by low pH values (pH < 7.35) in body tissues and blood accompanied by the buildup of lactate (above the upper limit of the reference range) and/or low serum bicarbonate level (< 20 mmol/L) [12]. Potential causes of development of lactic acidosis include genetic background, sepsis, shock, muscular exercise, diabetic ketoacidosis, hepatic or renal disease, medication (e.g. NRTIs, acetaminophen, ethanol, methanol, propylene glycol, beta-adrenergic agents such as epinephrine, ritodrine, terbutaline, biguanides such as phenformin, metformin, cocaine, 5-Fluorouracil, halothane, isoniazid, propofol, salicylates, sulfasalazine, valproic acid, etc) [10,

12]. On the other hand, hyperlactatemia is defined as a physiological condition with mildly to moderately elevated lactate levels, but still normal CO_2 levels, normal pH values and normal serum bicarbonate levels [13]. It may occur in both physiological circumstances, e.g. exercise and hyper-metabolic status, or within pathological conditions, including drug related toxicity [10].

By Cohen-Woods classification, aetiology of lactic acidosis is categorized into two types. Type A is overproduction of lactate due to tissue hypo-perfusion and hypo-oxygenation, thus stimulating the anaerobic metabolism (e.g. liver disease, sepsis, hypovolaemic shock, haemorrhage, pulmonary or circulatory problems, etc). Type B lactic acidosis develops in circumstances with no evident tissue hypo-perfusion or ischemia. It may be present due to drug use, toxins, diseases that do not alter tissue oxygenation, or within congenital abnormalities [10, 12, 14].

3. Clinical Symptoms of Lactic Acidosis

Symptoms associated with lactic acidosis range from dyspnea, nausea, vomiting, hyperventilation, abdominal pain, tachycardia, lethargy, body weakness, all the way to severe life threatening complications such as liver and/or renal failure, clotting abnormalities, seizures, cardiac arrhythmia [10, 15]. Although these symptoms are non-specific and may not seem serious, they can potentially be a predicting sign of a severe life-threatening condition. Thus, HIV-infected patients should be encouraged to inform their doctors when these symptoms occur [16, 17].

4. Incidence of Lactic Acidosis in HIV-Infected Patients

A number of studies have proved almost all of the NRTI drugs to be associated with lactic acidosis, as their most serious adverse effect [1, 10, 11, 14-19]. Initial cases of lactic acidosis due to NRTI use were reported in the early 1990s, at the very beginning of cART use [18, 19].

The reported incidence rate of lactic acidosis due to NRTI based regimen is low, and varies from 1.3 - 10 per 1.000 person years on cART. However, the fatality rate is estimated at around 60 - 80% in those HIV patients who develop lactic acidosis during NRTI usage [20, 21]. On the other hand, asymptomatic hyperlactataemia in patients on cART is reported in around 9 – 16 % of patients on NRTI, but only 1% of them would have lactate levels above 5 mmol/L. Actually, hyperlactataemia without acidosis remains a common feature of NRTI use and often a transient event when cART is initiated [4, 5]. Finally, the incidence rate of symptomatic patients with moderately raised lactate level (2.5 – 5 mmol/L) is estimated at between 8 - 20.9 cases per 1.000 person years at risk [17].

5. Risk Factors for Lactic Acidosis Development

Systematic review of lactic acidosis due to cART presented in medical literature reveals risk factors associated with development of lactic acidosis. The list of main risk factors for lactic acidosis development in HIV-infected patients on NRTI based cART regimens includes: antiretroviral drugs usage, especially duration of NRTI usage; patients' age; gender; advanced immunosuppression; various metabolic conditions; liver and renal abnormalities; co-administered drugs together with NIRT drugs [1, 5, 13, 14, 16, 17, 20-22].

5.1. NRTI Use and Lactic Acidosis

A number of studies have shown that NRTIs increase the risk of lactic acidosis development [1 - 3, 11, 13, 16-20, 22]. NRTIs could potentially induce the side effect by inducing mitochondrial toxicity. In fact, all NRTIs inhibit mitochondrial DNA polymerase – γ action. Thus, all NRTIs may interact with polymerase – γ, but it has been shown that dideoxynucleosides, such as stavudine (d4T), zalcitabine (ddC) and didanosine (ddI) - also known as d-drugs, are the most potent in this respect [11, 22, 23]. The usage of other NRTIs such as abacavir and lamivudine did not appear to increase the risk for developing lactic acidosis [3, 16, 24, 25]. Thus, WHO suggests switching the treatment towards abacavir and tenofovir–based first line regimens due to better toxicity profiles in comparison with d-drugs and low risk of lactic acidosis development [9].

In the resource limited settings, where d-drugs still remain the first line option, the highest incidence of NRTI-induced lactic acidosis is due to stavudine (d4T), followed by didanosine (ddI) usage [1, 3, 17]. Furthermore, the lactic acidosis developed even more frequently when stavudine and didanosine were prescribed together [25]. Zidovudine (AZT) is also known to be able to induce lactic acidosis, while other NRTI drugs, such as lamivudine, abacavir and tenofovir, are not associated with significant events [10, 16, 24, 26].

As mentioned before, d-drugs are nowadays mostly used in resource limited setting, which explains the high incidence of lactic acidosis due to HAART in these countries. Additionally, fatal events due to lactic acidosis were increasingly connected to treatment regimens containing d-drugs [1, 11, 13].

Concomitant use of other antiretroviral drugs, such as PIs or non-NRTI drugs are not associated with a risk for the development of lactic acidosis [25, 27, 28].

Recent studies of drugs from the class of both integrase inhibitors and fusion inhibitors showed safer adverse effect profiles. Lactic acidosis is not even mentioned as a potential adverse effect due to integrase and/or fusion inhibitors usage [2, 29].

5.2. Duration of NRTI Usage

In most studies the estimated time spent on NRTI until lactic acidosis developed was approximately 8 months [5, 30]. Some studies have reported even shorter period of time for lactic acidosis development, in which lactic acidosis appeared after only 4 weeks of NRTI treatment [16, 24]. Anyhow, there is no doubt that the cumulative NRTI treatment was a definite risk factor for lactic acidosis development. Long-term therapy was recognized to lead to mitochondrial depletion and onset of toxicity despite relatively low NRTI dosage. Also, prolonged usage of NRTI regimen was associated with more severe lactic acidosis events [14, 17, 24, 30]. The Swiss cohort study showed that the risk of hyperlactataemia increases 4 times in patients receiving d-drugs for 6 - 24 months, compared to patients receiving a d-drug for less than 6 months. Nevertheless, if exposure to d-drugs extends beyond 24 months there is no additional increase of the risk [25]. Usually, asymptomatic hyperlactatemia followed by cART initiation is a transient rather than persisting phenomenon [1, 4, 5].

5.3. Patients' Age

Regarding demographic data, median age of HIV - infected patients with lactic acidosis was 37 - 40 years [3, 10, 16]. The Swiss cohort study found that the risk of development of lactic acidosis due to NRTI usage was independent of age [25]. Similar observation was reported by Bonnet et al. [24]. Age-adjusted data show no significant difference in outcome prognosis by age groups (30).

5.4. Gender

In most studies, the incidence of lactic acidosis in HIV infected patients treated with NRTIs varied significantly between males and females. Women are known for a higher incidence of adverse effects when treated with NRTI drugs [1, 16, 22, 24, 25, 31]. For example, a research group from Botswana reported a 3-year follow-up of patients receiving cART where lactic acidosis and symptomatic hyperlactataemia developed in 20 patients who were all female (p < 0.01) [13]. Geddes et al. reported a significantly higher risk of NRTI-related toxic events in terms of lactic acidosis in females compared to males [32]. Similar observations were reported by Boulassel et al. [33]. Arenas-Pinto et al. also estimated the risk of lactic acidosis to be 2.5 times higher in women than in men [16]. Conversely, in a Swiss cohort study examining hyperlactataemia, the males were predominant; actually 74% of them had increased lactate levels. The possible reason for the discordant data among these studies is that the Swiss cohort study evaluated mainly hyperlactataemia, with only one patient, out of 54 with hyperlactataemia, with a condition that evolved into acidosis [25]. Furthermore, pharmacokinetic studies show that women, contrary to men, present with 2-fold higher NRTI triphosphate concentrations, thus increasing the risk of drug related toxicity [17, 34].

Decreased likelihood for initiation of HAART, together with poor adherence, among women has been reported in a number of studies [31, 32]. Consequently, women tend to develop more advanced disease when cART is eventually initiated, which potentially leads to development of adverse effects, including lactic acidosis [17]. Supporting this, patients starting NRTI based regimen with lower CD4+ T-cells count and more advanced disease present with higher rates of intracellular NRTI phosphorylation [35 – 37].

5.5. Level of Immunosuppression

Advanced immunosuppression itself is described as a risk factor for the development of lactic acidosis [17, 22]. Higher baseline CD4+ T cells counts are found to protect from development of hyperlactatemia and/or lactic acidosis [35]. Patients with baseline CD4+ T cells count of less than 100 cells/mm^3 had 2.5 times higher levels of NRTI intracellular triphosphate levels shortly after initiation of cART, thus a higher risk of development of adverse effects, than patients with better immunological status at the cART initiation. During the follow-up triphospate levels decreased despite continuation of antiretroviral treatment; however patients with low baseline CD4+ T cells counts were significantly more vulnerable to NRTI-associated toxicities [35, 38]. Additionally, report from Lactic Acidosis Group suggested a strong association between both development of lactic acidosis and fatality rate with low CD4+ T cells count at the time of event [11, 17].

5.6. Metabolic Conditions

Higher baseline weight has been addressed as an additional predisposing factor for the development of lactic acidosis. Significantly higher risk was observed in female patients who were overweight [13, 39]. Data from Botswana suggest that HIV-infected females with body mass index above 25 experience an increased risk of life-threatening NRTI-induced toxicities, especially symptomatic hyperlactatemia and lactic acidosis [13]. Conversely, Lo et al. demonstrated a low rate of lactic acidosis among obese women. Actually, their results suggest only NRTI duration to be connected to the high lactate levels, but this correlation has also been decreased by adjustment for insulin resistance [30].

Both hyperlipidemia and insulin resistance may lead to increased lactate levels, through decreased liver function and consequently reduced lactate clearance [40]. It has been shown that hyperglycaemia and hyperinsulinaemia may increase cellular lactate release, thus the higher incidence of hyperlactataemia reported in patients with diabetes [41, 42]. Furthermore, increased fatality in patients with NRTI-induced lactic acidosis was seen when diabetes is a co-morbidity (P=0.04), whereas hypertension, tuberculosis, prior stroke and coronary artery disease were found irrelevant in this respect [1].

5.7. Liver Abnormalities

Liver diseases, especially hepatitis B virus (HBV) and hepatitis C virus (HCV) co-infection, were a common finding in observed patients with lactic acidosis [5, 24]. Mild to severe liver abnormalities, with elevation of transaminase levels above the upper limit of normal, were connected to higher incidence rates of lactic acidosis. Hepatic steatosis was a frequently observed pathological finding [16].

5.8. Renal Abnormalities

Bonnet et al. have been the first to investigate renal function and its association to lactic acidosis. According to their results, impaired renal function leads to reduced drug clearance. Consequentially, drug accumulation promotes toxic effects. Potential contributors may be a concomitant use of nephrotoxic drugs or previous renal disease [25]. Leung et al. presented increased risk of NRTI-associated death due to lactic acidosis in people with elevated serum creatinine [1].

5.9. Co-Administered Drugs

Usage of cART improved and increased life expectancy. Accordingly, many drugs are used simultaneously with cART in order to prevent and cure non-AIDS illnesses. Some may interact with cART, thus potentiating the toxicity and should be used with caution [44]. Synergistic toxicity with NRTI has been shown for valproate. Drug-drug interactions studies confirmed that didanosine interacts with allopurinol and hydroxyurea [45]. Moreno et al. reported a high incidence of ddI-related adverse effects when used concomitantly with ribavirin in HIV-infected patients co-infected with HCV. Their results confirmed the significant difference; more than 50% of patients developed toxicity when both drugs were administered versus just 11% of patients using only ddI [44].

6. Mechanism of NRTI Induced Lactic Acidosis

Nucleoside reverse transcriptase inhibitors are zidovudine (AZT), didanosine (ddI), stavudine (d4T), zalcitabine (ddC), lamivudine (3TC), abacavir (ABC), emtricitabine (FTC) and tenofovir (TDF). As NRTIs have been frequently used in the last couple of decades as a backbone of cART, their toxic profiles have been increasingly recognized and investigated [2].

In order to exercise their mechanism of action, they must undergo the intracellular phosphorylation process first [34 – 38].

The mechanism of NRTI induced lactic acidosis is based on inhibition of mitochondrial DNA polymerase - γ and consequently mitochondrial depletion and deficit in the respiratory chain function [28, 34]. Thus, aerobic respiration is inhibited, which leads to oxidative stress and mutation in mtDNA. As a result, mitochondrial and/or tissue failure increases. Contrary to other NRTIs, zidovudine is proven to act through some other mechanisms, as well, not only by inhibition of polymerase – γ [35, 46]. The best known include inhibition of adenylate kinase, impairment of the mitochondrial adenosine diphosphate adenosine triphosphate (ADP-ATP) translocator, and uncoupling of the electron transport chain [46]. Pharmacokinetic studies focused at intracellular NRTI triphosphate concentrations, related to both NRTI pharmacodinamic effects and long-term toxicity, reviled that the lactic acidosis is caused by the over activation of intracellular hyperphosphorylation process [34, 36].

7. Screening for Lactic Acidosis

Lactic acidosis is still a rare condition, thus screening is not recommended [5]. However, as the risk factors predisposing to lactic acidosis while on NRTI treatment are well known, monitoring of patients at risk may be helpful in reducing the incidence of lactic acidosis [1, 10, 11, 13].

Elevated serum lactate level, low blood pH or/and low bicarbonate level are required for establishing the diagnosis of lactic acidosis [10]. Patients must be well hydrated and abstain from any vigorous physical activity and alcohol use for at least 10 hours before the blood is sampled. Clenching the fist while blood sampling should be limited to the shortest time possible in order to prevent prolonged ischemia and therefore artificially increased blood lactate levels. Blood should be processed to the laboratory within 4 hours after collection [30, 43]. Though hepatic steatosis was a frequently observed pathological finding when lactic acidosis developed, liver biopsy should not be included in the regular testing algorithm [18].

Other causes of lactic acidosis, such as sepsis, renal or liver failure, exercise, alcohol intoxication, regional hypoperfusion, should be ruled out before the diagnosis of NRTI induced lactic acidosis is established [43].

8. Treatment of Lactic Acidosis Induced with NRTIs

Lactic acidosis induced with NRTI use is treated by NRTI withdrawal, especially in life-threatening clinical conditions with serum lactate level of 5 mmol/L and above. Usually discontinuation of all antiretrovirals, not only NRTIs, is recommended [13]. If patient's immunological status requires immediate withdrawal of antiretrovirals, switching to a treatment regimen with different toxicity profile is an alternative [45].

Substitution of riboflavin, thiamine (vitamin B1), coenzyme Q, L-carnitine, or vitamins C, E, and K in patients with lactic acidosis did not produce desirable benefit, but may safely be used [26, 43]. Substitution therapy with fluids is usually required.

9. Outcome

When lactic acidosis is diagnosed, immediate discontinuation of treatment is advised. Within several days the outcome is favourable in most cases. Especially when no other d-drug is re-administered, immunological recovery is complete [13]. In some cases, when NRTI was re-administered after some time, another episode of lactic acidosis occurred. In some other cases, however, no further lactic acidosis event recurred although NRTI was re-administered [16].

10. Prevention

NRTIs associated with lactic acidosis are currently mostly used in resource limited settings, because of their affordability and effectiveness [1, 3, 13]. Though the European AIDS Clinical Society (EACS), International AIDS Society, British HIV Association and World Health Organization (WHO) HIV/AIDS treatment guidelines discourage the use of d-drugs, national HIV management guidelines from low-middle income countries are still unable to withdraw these drugs from the first-line regimens [6 – 9].

Conclusion

NRTI based cART regimens are still the first-line antiretroviral treatment proposed by HIV/AIDS guidelines. In resource limited settings, because of beneficial effect and low treatment costs, availability of NRTIs is mainly reduced to dideoxynucleosides. Exposure to these drugs, stavudine and didanosine in particular, is strongly associated with the likelihood of developing lactic acidosis. In rare occasions lactic acidosis leads to a life-threatening condition.

Risk factors associated with lactic acidosis are female sex, advanced HIV-1-induced immunodeficiency, obesity and prolonged duration of NRTI-based antiretroviral treatment. Renal and liver abnormalities, especially hepatitis B and hepatitis C virus co-infection, are associated with a higher incidence of lactic acidosis. Treatment of NRTI-induced lactic acidosis implies discontinuation of NRTI, and pertinent switch to cART regimens with better toxicity profiles.

References

[1]   Leung L, Wilson D, Manini AF. Fatal toxicity from symptomatic hyperlactatemia. *Drug saf.* 2011; 34:521-527.

[2]   Reust CE. Common Adverse Effects of Antiretroviral Therapy for HIV Disease. *Am. Fam. Physician.* 2011; 83:1443-1451.

[3]   Dragovic G, Smiths C, Jevtovic D, Johnson MA, Ranin J, Salemovic D, et al. Comparison of nucleoside reverse transcriptase inhibitor use as part of first-line therapy in a Serbi and a UK HIV clinic. *HIV Clin. trials.* 2009; 10:306-313.

[4]   Brinkman K. Management of hyperlactatemia: no need for routine lactate measurements. *AIDS.* 2001; 13:795-7.

[5]   Houcqueloux L, Alberti C, Feugeas JP, Lafaurie M, Lukasiewicz E, Bagnard G, et al. Prevalence, risk factors and outcome of hyperlactatemia in HIV-infected patients. *HIV Medicine.* 2003; 4:18-23.

[6]   European AIDS Clinical Society (EACS) Guidelines, Version 7.0. 2013. http://www.eacsociety.org/Portals/0/*Guidelines_Online_*131014.pdf [viewed at 13th December 2013].

[7]	Thompson MA, Aberg JA, Hoy JF, Telenti A, Benson C, Cahn P, et al. Antiretroviral Treatment of Adult HIV Infection: 2012 Recommendations of the International Antiviral Society–USA Panel. *JAMA.* 2012; 308:387-402.

[8]	Williams I, Churchill D, Anderson J, Boffito M, Bower M, Cairns G, et al. British HIV Association guidelines for the treatment of HIV-1 -positive adults with antiretroviral therapy. *HIV Medicine.* 2012; 13:1-85.

[9]	Doherty M, Ford N, Vitoria M, Weiler G, Hirnschall G. The 2013 WHO guidelines for antiretroviral therapy: evidence-based recommendations to face new epidemic realities. *Curr. Opin. HIV AIDS.* 2013; 8:528-534.

[10]	Moyle G. Hyperlactatemia and Lactic Acidosis: Should Routine Screening Be Considered, *AIDS Read.* 2002; 12:344-348.

[11]	Arenas-Pinto A, Grant A, Bhaskaran K, Copas A, Carr A, Worm SW, et al. Risk factors for fatality in HIV-infected patients with dideoxynucleoside-induced severe hyperlactataemia or lactic acidosis. *Antivir. Ther.* 2011; 16:219-26.

[12]	Luft, FC. Lactic acidosis. *Journal of the American Society of Nephrology (American Society of Nephrology).* 2001; 12:15–19.

[13]	Wester CW, Eden SK, Shepherd BE, Bussmann H, Novitsky V, Samuels DC, et al. Risk factors for symptomatic hyperlactatemia and lactic acidosis among combination antiretroviral therapy-treated adults in Botswana: results from a clinical trial. *AIDS Res. Hum. Retroviruses.* 2012; 28:759-65.

[14]	Moyle GJ, Datta D, Mandalia S, Morlese J, Asboe D, Gazzard BG. Hyperlactataemia and lactic acidosis during antiretroviral therapy: relevance, reproducibility and possible risk factors. *AIDS.* 2002; 16:1341-1349.

[15]	John M, Moore CB, James IR, Nolan D, Upton RP, McKinnon EJ, et al. Chronic hyperlactatemia in HIV-infected patients taking antiretroviral therapy. *AIDS.* 2001; 15:717-23.

[16]	Arenas-Pinto A, Grant AD, Edwards S, Weller IV. Lactic acidosis in HIV infected patients: a systematic review of published cases. *Sex Transm. Infect.* 2003; 79:340-3.

[17]	Lactic Acidosis International Study Group. Risk factors for lactic acidosis and severe hyperlactataemia in HIV-1-infected adults exposed to antiretroviral therapy. *AIDS.* 2007; 21:2455-2464.

[18]	Lai KK, Gang DL, Zawacki JK, Cooley TP. Fulminant hepatic failure associated with 2,3-dideoxyinosine (ddI). *Ann. Intern. Med.* 1991; 115: 283–4.

[19]	Bissuel F, Bruneel F, Habersetzer F, Chassard D, Cotte L, Chevallier M, et al. Fulminant hepatitis with severe lactate acidosis in HIV-infected patients on didanosine therapy. *J. Intern. Med.* 1994; 235:367–72.

[20]	Falco V, Rodriguez D, Ribera E, Martínez E, Miró JM, Domingo P, et al. Severe nucleoside associated lactic acidosis in human immunodeficiency virus infected patients: Report of 21 cases and review of the literature. *Clin. Infect. Dis.* 2002; 34:838–846.

[21]	Stenzel MS, Carpenter CCJ. The management of the clinical complications of antiretroviral therapy. *Infect. Dis. Clinics North Am.* 2000; 14:851–878.

[22]	Dragovic G, Jevtovic D. The role of nucleoside reverse transcriptase inhibitors usage in the incidence of hyperlactatemia and lactic acidosis in HIV/AIDS patients. *Biomedicine&Pharmacotherapy.* 2012; 66:308-311.

[23] Walker UA, Bäuerle J, Laguno M, Murillas J, Mauss S, Schmutz G, et al. Depletion of mitochondrial DNA in liver under antiretroviral therapy with didanosine, stavudine, or zalcitabine. *Hepatology.* 2004; 39:311-7.

[24] Bonnet F, Bonarek M, Morlat P, Mercie P, Dupon M, Gemain MC. Risk factors for lactic acidosis in HIV-infected patients treated with nucleoside reverse-transciptase inhibitors: a case-control study. *CID.* 2003; 36:1324-1328.

[25] Boubaker K, Flepp M, Furrer H, Haenesl A, Hirschel B, Boggian K Hyperlactatemia and antiretroviral therapy: the Swiss HIV cohort study. *Clinical infectious diseases.* 2001; 33:1931-1937.

[26] Margolis AM, Heverling H, Pham PA, Stolbach A. A Review of the Toxicity of HIV Medications. *J. Med. Toxicol.* 2013. DOI 10.1007/ s13181-013-0325-8.

[27] Tymchuk CN, Currier JS. The safety of antiretroviral drugs. *Expert Opin. Drug Saf.* 2008; 7:1-4.

[28] Fichtenbaum CJ. Metabolic abnormalities associated with HIV infection and antiretroviral therapy. *Curr. Infect. Dis. Rep.* 2009; 11:84-92.

[29] Lennox JL, DeJesus E, Lazzarin A, Pollard RB, Madruga JV, Berger DS, et al. Safety and efficacy of raltegravir-based versus efavirenz-based combination therapy in treatment-naive patients with HIV-1 infection: a multicentre, double-blind randomised controlled trial. *Lancet.* 2009; 374:796-806.

[30] Lo JC, Kazemi a MR, Hsue PY, Martin JN, Deeks SG, Schambelan M. The relationship between nucleoside analogue treatment duration, insulin resistance, and fasting arterialized lactate level in patients with HIV infection. *Clinical Infectious diseases.* 2005; 41:1335-1340.

[31] Nicastri E, Leone S, Angeletti C, Palmisano L, Sarmati L, Chiesi A. Sex issues in HIV-1-infected persons during highly active antiretroviral therapy: a systematic review. *Journal of Antimicrobial Chemotherapy.* 2007; 60:724–732.

[32] Geddes R, Knight S, Moosa MY, Reddi A, Uebel K, Sunpath H. A high incidence of nucleoside reverse transcriptase inhibitor (NRTI)-induced lactic acidosis in HIV-infected patients in a South African context. *S. Afr. Med. J.* 2006; 96:722–724.

[33] Boulassel MR, Morales R, Murphy T, Lalonde RG, Klein MB. Gender and long-term metabolic toxicities from antiretroviral therapy in HIV-1 infected persons. *J. Med. Virol.* 2006; 78:1158–63.

[34] Lewis W, Day BJ, Copeland WC. Mitochondrial toxicity of NRTI antiviral drugs: an integrated cellular perspective. Nature Reviews Drug Discovery. 2003; 2:812-822.

[35] Anderson PL, Kakuda TN, Lichtenstein KA. The Cellular Pharmacology of Nucleoside- and Nucleotide-Analogue Reverse-Transcriptase Inhibitors and Its Relationship to Clinical Toxicities. *Clinical Infectious Diseases.* 2004; 38:743–753.

[36] Walker UA, Venhoff N. Uridine in the prevention and treatment of NRTI-related mitochondrial toxicity. *Antivir. Ther.* 2005; 10:117-23.

[37] Cressey TR, Lallemant M. Pharmacogenetics of antiretroviral drugs for the treatment of HIV-infected patients: an update. *Infect. Genet. Evol.* 2007; 7:333-342.

[38] Anderson PL, Brundage RC,Weller D, Kawle SP, Bushman L, Fletcher CV. The pharmacokinetics of zidovudine-triphosphate (ZDV-TP) in HIV-infected adults [abstract 6.3]. In: Program and abstracts of the 3rd International Workshop on Clinical Pharmacology of HIV Therapy (Washington, DC). Utrecht, The Netherlands: *Virology Education*, 2002: abstract 6.3.

[39] Osler M, Stead D, Rebe K, Meintjes G, Boulle A. Risk factors for and clinical characteristics of severe hyperlactataemia in patients receiving antiretroviral therapy: a case-control study. *HIV Med.* 2010; 11:121-129.

[40] Moyle G. Mitochondrial toxicity hypothesis for lipoatrophy: a refutation. *AIDS* 2001, 15:413–415.

[41] Henry S, Schneiter P, Jequier E, Tappy L. Effects of hyperinsulinaemia and hyperglycaemia on lactate release and local blood flow in subcutaneous adipose tissue of healthy humans. *J. Clin. Endochrinol. Metab.* 1996, 81:2891–2895.

[42] Novel-Chate V, Rey V, Chioléro R, Schneiter P, Leverve X, Jéquier E, et al. Role of Na-K–ATPase in the insulin-induced lactate release by skeletal muscle. *Am. J. Physiol. Endochrinol. Metab.* 2001, 280:E296–E300.

[43] Walker UA. Update on mitochondrial toxicity: where are we now? *J. HIV Ther.* 2003; 8:32-5.

[44] Moreno A, Quereda C, Moreno L, Perez-Elías MJ, Muriel A, Casado JL, et al. High rate of didanosine-related mitochondrial toxicity in HIV/HCV-coinfected patients receiving ribavirin. *Antiviral. Therapy.* 9:133-138.

[45] Carr A. Lactic acidemia in infection with human immunodeficiency virus. *Clin. Infect. Dis.* 2003; 36:S96-S100.

[46] Arnaudo E, Dalakas M, Shanske S, Moraes CT, DiMauro S, Schon EA. Depletion of muscle mitochondrial DNA in AIDS patients with zidovudine-induced myopathy. *Lancet.* 1991; 337:508–10.

Index

B

C

F

G

H

I

M

Q

R

S